Look who's raving about <u>The Detox Solution</u>. . .

"If you want to maintain or regain your health and your life and stay out of the doctor's office and hospital, read Dr. Patricia Fitzgerald's *The Detox Solution*. It provides you with timely authoritative, easy-to-understand, practical information. I give it my highest recommendation."
— William G. Crook, M.D.
Author of *The Yeast Connection Handbook* and
Tired – So Tired! and the "Yeast Connection"

"Dr. Patricia Fitzgerald's *The Detox Solution* is a very informative and helpful book which is a must read for anyone who desires to take responsibility for their own health. Because her approach to health is holistic, she includes the spiritual aspect of the human being which I believe is essential to healing not only the whole person, but one's life as well."
— Ron Roth, Ph.D., Author of *Holy Spirit for Healing:*
Merging Ancient Wisdom with Modern Medicine

"I highly recommend *The Detox Solution* to all of my patients. It is an excellent resource to aid in healing a main contributing factor to illness – that of toxic buildup in the body. I am very impressed with the increased health and well being resulting when patients follow Dr. Patricia Fitzgerald's plan in her outstanding book. Anyone who wants abundant health and energy must read this book!"
— Harold Ravins, D.D.S., Center for Holistic Dentistry,
Los Angeles

"Dr. Patricia Fitzgerald's *The Detox Solution* is a must read for anyone who wishes to attain optimal levels of health in the 21st Century. With the increase of toxins from the environment, as well as bacteria and parasites from increased travel, *The Detox Solution* is necessary protection from the dangers of modern living."
— Dr. Omar Amin, Professor of Parasitology and
Epidemiology; Director, Institute of Parasitic Diseases
Founder, Parasitology Center, Inc.

"A great treatise for those ready to take control!"
— Sherry A. Rog   6 *Weeks*
(prestigepublis

D1053892

The DETOX SOLUTION

The Missing Link to
Radiant Health, Abundant Energy,
Ideal Weight, and Peace of Mind

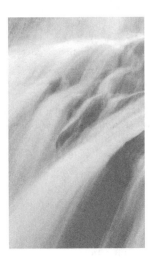

Dr. Patricia Fitzgerald

Illumination
PRESS

Illumination Press
P.O. Box 269
Santa Monica, CA 90406
www.thedetoxsolution.com

First printed July 2001

10   9   8   7   6   5   4

Manufactured in the United States of America

Fitzgerald, Patricia, 1964-
    The detox solution : the missing link to radiant
health, abundant energy, ideal weight, and peace of mind
/ Patricia Fitzgerald, -- 1st ed.
    p. cm.
    Includes bibliographical references and index.
    LCCN 2001088962
    ISBN 0-9708299-0-6

    1. Rejuvenation--Nutritional aspects. 2.
Detoxification (Health) 3. Environmental health 4.
Aging--Prevention. 5. Herbs--Therapeutic use. 6.
Alternative medicine. I. Title.

RA776.75F58 2001   613
                                QBI01-700410

Edited by Robin Quinn
Cover and interior design by Lightbourne

To the Creator of Abundant Health
Whose Healing Power and Unconditional Love
Resides Within Each and Every One of Our Hearts

ACKNOWLEDGEMENTS

I have been so blessed to know so many wonderful people who have inspired the journey that has resulted in the presentation of this book.

First of all, thanks Mom and Dad for always supporting my dreams, for your constant prayers and faith, and for being amazing demonstrations of Love. You gave me roots and wings, a foundation that I am so grateful for.

For the many teachers who have inspired me tremendously, especially Dr. Bernard Jensen, a pioneer of cleansing and detoxification, who helped thousands regain their health, and who continued to teach the truth about healing until his death at 93 years young.

To my "little" brother Ed—thanks for letting me experiment on you with health food and magic potions when we were kids; most people raised their eyebrows, but you opened your mouth with faith in your big sister's curiosity.

To the entire gang at the Institute of Applied Ontology—your invisible and visible support and encouragement is something I treasure tremendously.

To Beth and Mona, the years of encouragement regarding this project and especially your friendship are priceless to me.

To my colleagues who have provided amazing inspiration and support over the past twenty years—you are too numerous to mention, you know who you are.

Thanks to Dr. Omar Amin and Michael O'Brien for your dedication to truth and special assistance with this project.

To the staff and friends at the Santa Monica Wellness Center, especially Kathy, Tanna, Lauren, May, and Jackie. Your support and dedication is so deeply appreciated.

Lauren, Angela, Kathy, Rachel, Judy, and Barbara, your dedication to excellent proofreading and copyediting is so deeply appreciated.

Thanks to Dan Poynter for expert publishing advice.

To all of the patients who have given me the privilege to join them on their healing journeys. You teach and inspire me daily. You have no idea how much I appreciate each and every one of you. Thank you for your trust and confidence.

A special thanks to Robin Quinn, of Quinn's Word to Word—your editorial magic and writing assistance have been nothing short of miraculous. You are an angel straight from God who came at the perfect time and hung in there always with a smile, great attitude, and amazing talent.

For those who I am so grateful to but have failed to name, may God Bless You abundantly with the Spirit of Forgiveness.

A Brief History of Healing

"I don't feel well."

2000 BC – Here, drink this brew.
400 AD – That brew is of the devil.
Here, say this prayer.
1100 AD – That prayer is superstition.
Here, drink this potion.
1930 AD – That potion is snake oil.
Here, swallow this pill.
1970 AD – That pill is inferior.
Here, take this antibiotic.
2000 AD – That antibiotic has side effects
and has lost its effectiveness.

Here, drink this brew and meditate.

It is fascinating to observe how attitudes toward health and wellness have changed throughout history. It wasn't too long ago when eating organic food, drinking bottled water, participating in regular exercise, and engaging in a spiritual practice was considered weird and labeled "unproven." Fortunately, enough research has shown that those habits are now considered worthwhile and contribute to a healthier life.

It is difficult to believe that the obvious link of diet and toxicity to disease and health has only become common knowledge within the past decade. As a teenager, when I added whole foods to my diet, the neighbors thought I was on a "crazy health kick," shrugging their shoulders wondering why I would choose that weird brown (whole wheat) bread over the squeaky clean white version. They wondered why I exercised since I wasn't fat. My dear grandmother, God rest her soul, frequently expressed her concern that I wasn't getting enough sugar. As some of the relatives commented on my strange behavior, I loved my supportive father's comeback, "Leave her alone, she's not doing drugs. If her teenage rebellion consists of rebelling against junk food, I am blessed."

I have had a passion for the healing arts since I was young. In my teens, I read every nutrition book I could get my hands on. I sought out sources of herbs with which I used to experiment in our family kitchen. My parents graciously ignored the stench. When I developed the teenage maladies of pimples and PMS, I enjoyed experimenting with nutrition and herbal medicine, which I experienced as "miracle cures."

My first official introduction to natural health and detoxification is a vivid memory. In the early 80s, I dragged my little brother to a health convention in Philadelphia, where we heard the legendary Dr. Bernard Jensen speak. Dr. Jensen is *the* pioneer of natural healing. He has written over fifty books, and continued to teach until his death at the age of ninety-three. When I first heard him speak, he presented the theory shared by many medical experts throughout history—that toxicity is a major contributing factor to compromised health. His presentation had a great impact on my brother and myself. We came home, and in addition to our abandonment of white sugar and white flour, we set out on a quest for high fiber, organic foods. Twenty years later, Dr. Jensen's "controversial" ideas have been accepted by medical science, as the link of toxicity and disease continues to be validated.

Approximately ten years ago, my Dad telephoned me and said, "Well, Patricia, what you have been saying for years is finally recognized by the mainstream." On the front page of the *Los Angeles Times* that morning was the "breaking" news that a correlation between diet and cancer had been found. Now that this fact is so ingrained in our society, it is hard to believe it was only a decade ago when the seemingly obvious notion started to gain acceptance.

The acceptance of the diet-disease connection could have been helpful five years earlier, as my mother was receiving experimental chemotherapy treatments for cancer. When I presented research to a group of physicians on how vitamin E taken before a certain chemotherapy drug was administered would prevent heart damage, the chief oncologist of a major university hospital patted me on the back and said, "That's nice, dear, but nutrition has nothing to do with cancer." Almost twenty years later, I remember his words as clear as a bell. Back then, when I was sneaking vitamin E to my mother and her heart didn't show the same damage as without the supplement, the doctors scratched their heads in bewilderment, calling it a mere "coincidence."

My initial professional venture in the natural health field was in 1985, when I accepted a position as the clinical nutritionist at the first holistic health facility in Philadelphia. It was there I had my first television interview. The reporter was a spy from one of those consumer watch segments on the news. He came to our clinic and interviewed me, attempting to expose a "quack" who actually believed that healthy food could improve health. The reporter thought he had successfully created a story that would trash the clinic or force us to close our doors. Instead, our phone rang off the hook with interested people, desperately seeking nontoxic assistance in improving their health.

As a budding nutritionist at this clinic, I taught patients how to incorporate a whole foods diet—something that was considered "out there" at the time—into their lives. I still have letters from patients who claimed their conditions such as difficulty losing weight, arthritis, allergies, fatigue, etc., improved because of simple, common sense dietary changes.

At that time, herbs and nutritional supplements weren't as ubiquitous as they are today. As I observed the seemingly miraculous improvements from just simple nutritional changes, I could hardly wait to get "hard core" and learn more about herbs and other healing techniques.

On a business trip to Santa Monica, California, I had the overwhelming knowingness that I had to move there. I went home, packed my bags, and came out to explore the West, where most of the other "health nuts" lived. I also knew I had better educational opportunities there.

While enjoying the surf and sand, I continued my nutritional practice. I was able to expand the modalities offered as I completed my Master's in Traditional Chinese Medicine and my Doctorate in Homeopathy. I also gained licensure as an acupuncturist. It was then I decided to open a holistic health center, which I named the Santa Monica Wellness Center. Another sign of the times: my patients and friends adamantly begged me to reconsider the name of the clinic. They were worried that people wouldn't identify with the word "wellness," which wasn't even in Webster's dictionary at the time.

After fifteen years in the health field, I have observed that what seems to aid people most in their quest to experience the fullness of life is their ability and desire to make choices that serve them best. We make choices every moment of every day. Our choices result in patterns and outcomes. As we become more conscious of the choices we are making, and their beneficial or toxic nature, we can create a life that has meaning, purpose, and harmony. When we make choices to create health, we spend less time worrying that we will "catch" a disease (as we lessen our chances), and we can enjoy life with more enthusiasm.

Making choices for nontoxic influences used to be easy. Most food was health food until the turn of the century. It was grown organically. Water contamination and air pollution were rare. We now must assume the responsibility to learn about the effects of what is coming into our daily experience.

The effect of these toxins on our health is more than just a scientific theory; it is becoming an increasing part of the daily experience. "I know this sounds crazy, but I just feel toxic" is a common expression I hear from patients after they present their symptoms to me in the clinic. Ironically, most people expressing this concern aren't even aware that detoxification protocols are available.

It is my vision that the world will learn to embrace the blessings that are available in every moment. We don't have to hit rock bottom to realize the beauty that is ours. When I started my practice, genetically-modified foods were only something in science fiction movies, such as *Attack of the Killer Tomatoes*; pre-Nintendo kids had to be more creative in play, forced to use their imaginations more than their parents' credit cards; regular medication was something associated mostly with the elderly; the school nurse dispensed the occasional aspirin—instead of the common ADD drugs; knowing someone who had cancer was a rare experience, not the norm of today; an allergy was an occasional occurrence, not a chronic debilitating condition treated with immunosuppressive steroids; candy was an occasional treat, not disguised as a daily breakfast cereal; and kids got in trouble in school for talking in class, not for carrying guns.

In this new millennium, we have the opportunity to realize our full potential instead of accepting "just getting by" as our choice of life expression. *The Detox Solution* provides a blueprint to assist in making this dream a reality. This book is not just about avoiding illness; it's about living life to the fullest. Do we have to see how bad it can get before we decide to take responsibility for our choices? Let's be part of the solution, not add to the problem.

We also must not forget to nurture our Spirit. "God can only do for you what God can do through you." I remember as a little girl, hearing that we were temples of the Holy Spirit. I used to wonder why people would treat their own temples so poorly, dumping junk food and drugs into them, and not even feeling good from those choices. Now modern research supports this observation. If our spiritual life is seen as something to be experienced only on Sunday, no wonder why our lives aren't working. Every breath we breathe, every thought we think, every action we take, and every word we speak is an expression of Spirit. Let's cleanse our temple; let our light shine to the world.

Someone Very Famous once said, "The kingdom of heaven is within." We make choices daily to experience heaven or hell on some level. Life-supporting choices create more heaven; life-draining choices create more hell.

As a society, we have made numerous choices that have had a life-draining impact on our health. Consider these facts:

Fact: The fourth leading cause of death in the United States is from interactions from prescription drugs, commonly known for their toxicity and dangerous side effects. Most of these medications haven't been around for very long; their cumulative effects are virtually unknown.

Fact: There are very few complications from the use of herbal medicine, a therapy that is dramatically more cost effective, virtually nontoxic, and has thousands of years of safe use behind it.

Fact: Complications from the occasional misuse of herbs tend to be dramatically sensationalized in the media; the millions of problems occurring from prescription medication are mysteriously underreported.

Fact: Most synthetic medication is symptom management oriented; herbal medicine tends to focus on strengthening tissues, organs, and systems of the body, as well as identifying and removing the cause of the health concern.

Hmmm . . .

Isn't it *common sense* that we use our research money to look into nontoxic alternatives with a safe history rather than creating more synthetic medication with hazardous side effects that contribute to preventable deaths? Doesn't it make more sense to use substances that actually *build health* rather than merely cover up symptoms of an unhealthy body?

Fact: The American Cancer Society confirms that diet and exercise can help fight cancer and cancer death.

Fact: The American Cancer Society also reports that environmental factors can account for three-quarters of all cancers.

Fact: It is expected that one in three adults will develop cancer, a statistic that is the highest in human history. Pediatric cancers are also increasing at an alarming rate.

Hmmm...

Isn't is *common sense* that we should change our focus in industry to create products and services that are not toxic and support health, instead of those that drain our well-being and take our loved ones from the planet? Isn't it strange that we put profit before life? Doesn't *common sense* also tell us that as we put profit before life and create disease in the process, we will end up spending the profits treating our own preventable diseases instead of using the money for products and services that actually enhance our lives?

Fact: We are spending billions of dollars looking for the cure.

Fact: We are spending billions of dollars creating the causes.

Hmmm...

Wouldn't *common sense* tell us to use the money to eliminate the causes of disease from our environment and our bodies?

Fact: Thousands of chemicals are infiltrating our environment.

Fact: Thousands of studies show that these chemicals are toxic and endanger our health and life.

Hmmm...

Wouldn't *common sense* tell us to use our research to find nontoxic alternatives?

Why do we need expensive studies to prove poisons are not good for us?

Couldn't we find better use of our resources?

Fact: Over one trillion dollars annually is spent in the United States alone on "health" care.

Fact: America spends more money on health care than any other industrialized nation, yet we have higher disease rates.

Hmmm...

Wouldn't *common sense* tell us that if we know the majority of diseases involve lifestyle factors, then we should spend a majority of the money providing healthier food, opportunities for exercise, and wellness education? Isn't it *common sense* that the answer to the poor health of America is not more technology, but to encourage people to make healthier choices?

Fact: Medical experts agree that stress is a major contributing factor to chronic illness.

Fact: Stress management is not part of most treatment plans for chronic illness.

Hmmm . . .

Wouldn't it make sense (and save dollars) to address what is an obvious impediment to healing?

If you have a thorn in your finger, and it starts bleeding, you are not going to try to find a cure for your problem. You simply remove the thorn, and the skin will heal naturally.

Identifying causes to problems and removing them seems like *common sense.*

The Detox Solution is a humble attempt to bring common sense into the confusion. It is my privilege to present to you insights and inspirations that have been shared with many patients, colleagues, and friends throughout the years. I have learned so much from the many who have come to the Santa Monica Wellness Center. They have shared their stories, their struggles, their laughter, their pain, their love, and their willingness to create better lives for themselves.

It is my hope that you will refer to this book from time to time and incorporate some of the suggestions offered. It is not expected that all of the changes will be made overnight. The road to wellness is traveled one step at a time.

CONTENTS

CHAPTER FIFTEEN

CHAPTER SIXTEEN

ONE

The Decision to Detoxify:
Essential in the New Millennium

*If we put fresh, new wine into an old wineskin,
the new wine will turn sour and be worthless.*

The same principle is at work in matters of health.

*A healthy body begins with cleaning out the
accumulated toxins of the past and preparing
it to accept new and efficient nutrients.*

*When the body is cleared of poisons, nature
will take over and provide us the gift of health.*

— **Dr. Hazel Parcells,** legendary healer and pioneering
nutritionist who lived with boundless energy to age 106

The new millennium is an exciting and empowering time to be living. Many people are discovering that there are actions they can take to significantly improve their health. If you're thinking it's not enough to just eat more fruits and vegetables plus get regular exercise, you're right. The real truth is that *the quality of our life and health is greatly affected by the many choices we make throughout our lifetime.* We make choices about what to eat, what items to purchase, what activities to participate in, what people to spend time with, what conclusions to make, how to prioritize, how to enjoy life. We have the ability to make wonderful decisions not only about improving our state of health but also our quality of life. One great decision that can enhance the quality of our lives at every level is the decision to detoxify—that is, to remove what is in our life that does not serve our highest good.

When people think of detoxification, what tends to come to mind is

THE IMMORTAL CELL

A remarkable experiment by the perceptive Nobel-prize-winning scientist Dr. Alexis Carrell illustrates the power of detoxification and proper nourishment. In 1912, at the Rockefeller Institute, Carrell began a groundbreaking test that continued for over 34 years. The scientist took living tissue from a chicken heart and submerged it in a solution that provided optimal nourishment. Every day the used solution—which then contained toxic waste materials excreted from the cells—was replaced with a fresh nutrient solution. Carrell's goal was to show that under the best conditions, cells could live for a long period—possibly indefinitely.

Under these ideal conditions, the tissue continued to live for 34 years—more than three times a chicken's natural life expectancy of 11 years and two years beyond the life of Carrell himself! It is reported that the tissue died after a worker forgot to change the waste-polluted solution on *just one day*. For this and other scientific efforts, Carrell became associated with the notion of the possible "immortality" of the cell.

The underlying principles of *The Detox Solution* are vividly demonstrated by Carrell's novel experiment. First, every organism is as healthy as what it takes in and absorbs, because *that makes up what it becomes.* Second, if an organism holds onto things it does not need (such as toxins), this is going to have a negative effect. For humans, these two principles are played out on many levels—including the physical, emotional, and spiritual. If your body accumulates toxins that come from air pollution, it's going to detract from the quality of how you feel and may contribute to illness. If you hold onto anger, your emotional health may be compromised. If you embody beliefs that are not life-affirming, you may feel disconnected from your soul.

The concept of cellular immortality, the possibility of living cells surviving forever, is still being debated today. Scientists continue to explore the reasons why we age and methods for extending our longevity. Yet we can see from Carrell's experiment that the potential of living things can be maximized. *We **can** improve the quality of our life and even influence its length by making wise decisions every day.*

someone who is in drug rehab or going "on the wagon" from alcohol. The reality is that we are all exposed to toxins daily that affect our health and well-being. *The Detox Solution* is a plan to assist you in examining everything that you're taking into your body, mind, and spirit. You will be guided to determine what is beneficial and what is toxic. As you evaluate your influences, you will be provided with suggestions on how to choose what is best for your physical, emotional, and spiritual health. As you begin making better choices, you will notice an improvement in your vitality. This book is intended to be a guide to help you understand how you can begin to recognize and utilize the best of everything.

The Detox Solution also takes this concept a step further. Once you have improved what you are taking in, then you will be shown how to reduce the toxic residues stored in your body. Though our bodies are detoxifying every second (for instance, we breathe in cell-nourishing oxygen and exhale the toxic metabolic by-product carbon dioxide), they cannot cleanse efficiently without help. Extra detoxification assistance is needed as a result of the unprecedented load of toxins imposed on us by our modern world. This toxic overload is the price we've paid for the noteworthy progress which has been made over the past 150 years in technology and science. Among the many toxins we encounter today are pesticides, industrial wastes, synthetic medicine, food additives, car exhaust, and cigarette smoke. Most of these chemicals are foreign to our bodies.

As a health practitioner for over fifteen years, it has been my observation that many health challenges have toxins and toxic behaviors as either their main causes or as significant contributing factors. The concept of detoxification, however, is valuable to everyone regardless of his or her current health status. *Detoxification is not just a way to prevent or heal illness. It can also bring a level of vibrant, energetic health that you may never have thought possible.* Detoxification is the link to better health that is missing in our society today.

WHY STANDARD MEDICAL CARE ISN'T ENOUGH

Some people believe that if they don't have a diagnosed condition, then they are healthy. But *health is not just the absence of disease or symptoms.* We will look at the prominent traits of optimal health later in this chapter. However one realistic barometer would be whether you leap out of bed each morning with a high level of joyful energy that is sustained throughout the day. Is this true for you?

As Americans, we tend to think of ourselves as having better health than citizens of other countries around the world. Though this was the situation at one time, it no longer is. In 1900, the U.S. was rated #1 in terms of health among 100 other developed countries. Today we are near the bottom of that list!![1] And according to the National Centers for Disease Control, one-third of Americans are chronically ill—a term defined as suffering from an ailment of long duration or frequent recurrence. In 1950, it was only about 5%.[2] These sad statistics exist in spite of the fact that the United States spends more than any other country in the world on health care—over $1.3 trillion a year. *Apparently, more money and more technology are not the answer to optimal health.*

In addition to the Standard American Diet (S.A.D.), which is currently high in fat and nutrient-deficient processed foods, another contributor to this state of affairs is the way our health system is designed. It's geared toward dealing with developed diseases and crisis care. Yes, America has the technology to treat the symptoms of a health crisis. If you're leading a stressful life, eating all the wrong foods, and then have an All-American heart attack, you can go to a great hospital to have high-quality heart surgery. If you're diagnosed with a disease like diabetes, your doctor can prescribe a drug that is likely to bring some relief from symptoms. But in these situations, we must not fool ourselves. Managing the body with surgery and drugs is not healing and strengthening it. What about looking at the original causes of these problems? Why not deal with the factors contributing to the compromise in optimal health?

Many early signs of health degeneration go untreated because they are not considered serious

Author's Note to the Reader:

BACK TO BASICS

Some of the information in this book may seem to be very basic. That's the idea! Basic information which can save your life has often been overlooked in the search for more "sophisticated solutions." Reflecting on this, I sometimes comment, "It seems that common sense has gone out of style!" The ideas contained in "The Detox Solution" are intended to be a fundamental program for optimal health care, supporting the body to function as it was designed to, not for disease management care, which focuses mostly on alleviating symptoms.

enough to warrant concern. For instance, constipation (lack of one to three daily, easy-to-pass bowel movements) is often not detected as a significant cause for attention at a routine office visit. Yet constipation and slow bowel transit time have been linked to colon cancer—a disease that kills nearly 48,000 Americans a year! According to the American Cancer Society, colorectal cancers (the colon and rectal varieties combined) are the third most common cancers in men and women, causing 11% of deaths related to the "big C."

As you can see, waiting to receive an official medical diagnosis before you do something to improve your health is very dangerous. By the time a condition is identified as treatable within traditional Western medicine, years of degeneration are likely to have gone into creating it. Why not decide to start rejuvenating and purifying the body earlier so that such degeneration is avoided as much as possible? The information you'll find on these pages is about moving toward regeneration rather than degeneration.

Although there are significant limitations to the current medical system, I want to acknowledge that Western medicine has certainly saved thousands of lives. For instance, Caesarean sections have provided a viable alternative for mothers whose babies were not able to safely pass through the birth canal. Antibiotics have come to the rescue of many people with life-threatening infections. But even in these cases, there are problems because the modern medical system has come to rely too frequently on these measures. Today C-sections are vastly overused. Antibiotics are overprescribed, which has lead to a new health threat— potent antibiotic-resistant bacteria. (See "Antibiotics: The Magic Bullet Goes Off Target.") In response to the often-risky options offered by Western medicine (surgery, prescription and over-the-counter drugs, etc.), people are beginning to wonder what they can do for themselves. *The Detox Solution* sets many answers before you.

A REAL INSURANCE PLAN

The term "health insurance" seems to be a contradiction in terms. Having health insurance does not insure you of good health. Instead it could be called "sick insurance" because it only makes money available if your symptoms are severe enough to deem them worth treating. Unfortunately most health plans do not acknowledge the early signs of

ANTIBIOTICS:
The Magic Bullet Goes Off Target

How did we get to the point where the annual production of antibiotics adds up to an astounding 40 million pounds? Well, when scientists first observed antibacterial properties in various organisms during the 1920s, this gave hope for defeating a wide range of life-threatening bacterial infections. These discoveries eventually led to the development and manufacturing of penicillin, an antibiotic that did, in fact, save many lives during World War II. Antibiotics began to be viewed as a "magic bullet." Between 1940 and 1990, many of these drugs became available, and their use became routine over time for a growing number of maladies—from the minor to the more serious. Based upon the impressive track record of these medications, caution was often set aside for expediency's sake.

Unfortunately there was an unforeseen development that accompanied the naïve overuse of antibiotics. Bacteria have an extraordinary ability to become resistant to the very antibiotics designed to combat them. In fact, bacteria appear to even be able to share drug resistance information and genes with bacteria of different strains. An additional problem is that bacteria can adapt faster than we are able to develop new antibiotics to attempt to subdue them!

Another issue, which was not anticipated, is the deterioration in health, which often results from the shotgun way the most commonly used antibiotics work. Today, because of drug resistance, physicians often write prescriptions for the potent broad-spectrum antibiotics. These drugs cause the massive die-off of beneficial bacteria along with harmful ones. Since the friendly bacteria are part of the human body's immunity arsenal, the patient's defenses against infection and disease become weakened. In addition, internal imbalances occur as unfriendly organisms (yeast, fungi, "bad guy" drug-resistant bacteria, parasites) proliferate because "good guy" bacteria are no longer there to keep them in check. These changes can produce an array of health complaints—heartburn, acid reflux, diarrhea, constipation, skin eruptions, abdominal pain, food allergies, depression, yeast infections, fatigue, etc.

Sadly, many times this unhealthy state develops unnecessarily because the prescription for antibiotics was not the correct choice for the situation. Antibiotics can only affect bacteria, not viruses. The Centers for Disease Control estimates that half of all antibiotics are inappropriately prescribed for colds or other viral conditions.[3]

Fortunately the Centers for Disease Control and other medical groups began a campaign in 1995 to alert the medical community and the public of the dangers of the overuse of antibiotics in children. The response has been significant. A survey shows that the antibiotic prescription rate in the United States dropped 34% from 1989-90 to 1997-98 for children under the age of 15.[4]

While antibiotics have their place, cautious judgment needs to be part of the determination to use them and in setting the duration of the prescription. When the body's complex internal flora is upset, health becomes compromised. Any prescription for antibiotics should be followed by treatment to restore the original beneficial bacteria, necessary for healthy immunity. This is not occurring in most cases. You'll learn more about preventing the health complications that can be related to antibiotic use in Chapter 6.

toxicity. Many signs go undetected and evolve into more serious conditions. Important preventive care is regularly not being covered, although this is changing slowly among more progressive programs.

Note also that many of the medical treatments that are available under standard insurance plans do not actually *create optimal health*. They are, at best, Band-Aid solutions, suppressing the symptoms of an unhealthy body. This care can be limited because the root causes of illnesses are often not addressed.

A real insurance plan is one in which you take responsibility for your own health by educating yourself and taking action on a daily basis. I'm not suggesting that you cancel your insurance policy. Instead, it is wise to focus on becoming proactive with your own health and longevity.

There are basically two approaches to living: *proactive* and *reactive*. Most people live somewhere in between. When it comes to their health, a proactive person will tend to eat healthfully, exercise, and take other positive actions. At the other end of the spectrum, a reactive individual might sit on the couch downing chips and cola, foolishly expecting "them" to successfully treat whatever ill health is being created; i.e., a cancer cure to be discovered just in time. Wouldn't you prefer *to create* a healthier future for yourself rather than *just accepting* the next way that your body will break down? You can make the decision right now to explore detoxification and to incorporate health-promoting habits into your daily life.

You are with your body 24 hours a day. Your doctor may be with you for the average office visit of seven minutes once every few years. Where does the power of optimal health lie?

WHAT IS HEALTH?

If health is not just the absence of disease, what is it exactly? What is our goal? *Optimal health can be defined as experiencing the fullness of life physically, mentally, and spiritually.* According to the World Health Organization, "Health is more than the absence of disease. Health is a state of optimal well-being."

It seems that many people are willing to accept feeling just "okay"; they expect to be tired and to show the "normal" signs of aging. But if you have ever been in the presence of a golden senior who vibrates with health, wisdom, and joy, you know that there's another alternative available despite your age. *That is a state of exuberant health!!*

Take a moment now to look over the list on the following page. Are these characteristics currently part of your way of being? If not, are they traits that you would like to acquire?

The approach in *The Detox Solution* will address ways to create a healthy life beyond just the physical. Detoxification is really about boosting *the quality of your life.*

In addition, you will also be improving your physical well-being. You may have noticed that it is difficult to be joyful and creative when your physical energy is not at its optimum level. The good news is that the detoxification and rejuvenation plan outlined in this book can help bring back the energy you experienced as a youth. Remember how alive you felt and how exciting it was to be part of this world? You can still get back in touch with that enthusiastic and energetic you. *The authentic you.* Once you feel more alive, it will be easier to make other improvements in your overall quality of living.

TRAITS OF OPTIMAL HEALTH

- A feeling of energy is available throughout the day.

- A youthful and age-defying physical appearance is evident.

- Sleep comes easily and lasts till morning.

- There's a feeling of being refreshed upon awakening.

- Digestion is comfortable.

- Energy is present after meals.

- Bowel movements occur comfortably, one to three times a day.

- Urination takes place every few hours.

- The skin is clear and glowing.

- The hair has a glossiness and shine.

- Illness is rare and departs quickly.

- The mind is clear and alert.

- A wide range of activities can be enjoyed.

- There's a feeling of being challenged without feeling overwhelmed.

- The body is toned and flexible.

- A comfortable weight is maintained.

- The eyes are shiny and clear.

- There's a feeling of gratitude.

- Obstacles and setbacks are seen as opportunities for growth.

- Emotions are stable.

- Joy, laughter, and happiness are experienced daily.

- Sexual energy is balanced.

- Relationships are supportive, enjoyable, meaningful, and fulfilling.

- There is a sense of purpose in life.

- Inner peace is attained and enjoyed.

- A profound awareness of the Presence of Unconditional Love is realized.

ROOM FOR IMPROVEMENT: Average Life Expectancy Vs. Maximum Life Span

Though statistics show that the *"average life expectancy"* is greater today than it was at the turn of the 20th Century, merely looking at the raw numbers can be deceiving. In 1900, the life expectancy at birth in the U.S. was only 44 years. In 1999, it was 76. So the increase appears to be dramatic. However, the lower number at the turn of the 20th Century is largely due to figuring in the deaths of children caused by infections. More children survive today because of improved sanitation. When the two statistics are adjusted to take infant mortality into account, the increase over the 99-year period is only 3.7 years!

Here are some other enlightening numbers. Fewer people alive at age 70 today will survive to 90 than was seen just 40 years ago. Also, at the dawn of the 20th Century, conditions like heart disease and cancer were rare. For instance, in 1900, only one person in 33 had cancer, and heart disease was uncommon. Today, one out of three Americans die of cancer, and one in five will develop some form of a heart condition. Yet we are currently pouring billions into research into these areas and have extensive diagnostic and other medical tools. Americans are now spending one out of every 14 dollars for medical care, which translates into $800 billion a year. Looking at the results, it is clear that the time has come to rethink where we are headed with our health care. Certainly we can afford to take the time to make the type of changes that can result in a real difference in the quality of our health and the length of our lives.

When thinking of our longevity, it's important to remember that the average *life expectancy* is different from our potential *"maximum life span."* Our life expectancy, again, is only an average based on how long other human beings have lived. In contrast, the maximum life span is the genetically determined longevity that is possible for humans to achieve. This figure for our species has remained around 120 years since the time of ancient Rome—and possibly longer. As you can see, there is a lot of room for improvement in how much of this potential we realize.

PHYSICAL DETOXIFICATION

As you may have guessed, the unique, life-enhancing detoxification plan presented in this book uses cleansing of the body as a core element. (Please note that the terms "detoxification" and "cleansing" can be used interchangeably.) Some readers may be more familiar with physical detoxification than others. Some of you have undoubtedly tried the one-day, weekend, or week-at-a-time cleansing or detoxification protocols. I have found that the results you can achieve through these programs are limited. *How can we expect to rid our bodies of the toxins that have built up over a lifetime through a program that lasts only a day or two or even seven?* The plan presented here is more extensive, it is not as extreme as many others, there is no fasting, and the plan can be followed as you go about your normal life.

Those of you who have never tried cleansing or detoxifying and who may just be discovering this process need to know the basics. "Just what is physical detoxification?" you may wonder. "What parts of the body are involved?" may be another question. We'll start by looking at the fundamentals.

Our bodies detoxify naturally every single day. Besides the breath, another basic example of natural detoxification is the way the body reacts to food poisoning. Think of how quickly your body works to eliminate poisons at these times! Yet when people get food poisoning, they often reach for something to stop the diarrhea or vomiting. They don't realize these are actually signs of our body healing itself.

The major parts of our body involved in physical detoxification are the digestive tract, the liver, our lungs, the lymphatic system, our skin, and the urinary system. These systems and organs are the sites designed within the body to process toxins either by eliminating them or transforming them into less threatening substances. You'll learn more about specific detoxification processes in Parts 2 and 3.

We are currently living in a very toxic time. Our exposure to toxins has increased through pollution and other sources. The amount of toxic residues in our bodies has also increased, as they accumulate in our human fat, tissues, and organs. This build-up of toxicity results in numerous illnesses and health complications. Detoxification—using herbs, pure food, water, and other elements—helps to cleanse the body of this toxicity. An effective and innovative physical detoxification plan will be fully presented later in this book. Keep in mind that a body that is cleansed of toxins is stronger, healthier, and more vibrant.

DO YOU NEED A COMPREHENSIVE DETOXIFICATION PLAN?

Most people today will benefit from a detoxification program that addresses physical, emotional, and spiritual health. How do you know if this is something you need? Scan the list below to see if you are experiencing any of the items mentioned. (Note that a more extensive list of symptoms is presented in the following chapter.)

INDICATORS OF TOXICITY

- Frequent fatigue
- Compromised digestion
- Chronic constipation
- Unpleasant skin eruptions
- Excess weight
- Poor stress management
- Powerful food cravings
- Debilitating depression
- Frequent colds and flu
- Recurring headaches
- Insomnia or sleeping too many hours
- Pain in joints
- No sense of purpose
- Self-defeating belief systems
- Wide mood swings
- Compromised sexual function
- Limited sense of joy and inner peace

If you identified one or more of the indicators as part of your current state of being, detoxification is something to consider. Keep in mind that our bodies have an uncanny ability to rejuvenate if they are given the proper conditions. By clearing undesirable factors from your life, you will be creating an environment conducive to the natural healing process.

LOW ENERGY OR HIGH ENERGY —YOUR CHOICE!

Lack of energy and feelings of fatigue are among the most common complaints voiced by those who need a detoxification plan. Some new patients report that even a full night's sleep doesn't relieve them from feeling exhausted. Others say that meals leave them feeling even more lethargic than before they ate. Fatigue is an important symptom to recognize. Not only is it an indicator of toxicity, but fatigue is often a forerunner of numerous serious diseases. Many people who have been diagnosed with cancer and other life-threatening illnesses look back and realize that they hadn't felt "right" for years.

Let's turn again to the physical aspect of detoxification. When toxins build up in the body, one result is that they can prevent you from fully utilizing the foods you eat. Even if you are on a very healthy diet, your body may not be able to convert the food you consume into the energy you require. If your system is clogged with toxins, you may only have access to less than 50% of the nutrients that you are taking in. It is easy to understand why you might be feeling exhausted!!

The digestive tract is a major player in the body's detoxification process. It is where food is converted into energy and toxins are processed for elimination. After a cleanse of the digestive tract has been accomplished, your body once again will become an efficient food processing machine. The result will be higher energy overall and an end to lethargy after eating.

As you have learned in this chapter, the digestive tract is just part of your body's extensive detoxification system. The program in *The Detox Solution* emphasizes cleansing of the colon and liver (two vital parts of the digestive system), and also addresses the lungs, skin, kidneys, and lymph. This approach is based on the system I have used for over a decade in my practice in Santa Monica, California. Time and again, many patients have witnessed improvement of various health conditions and have soared to high levels of radiant health through detoxification.

OTHER BENEFITS OF DETOXIFICATION

High energy is just one of the many benefits that you can gain through a comprehensive effective detoxification program. Here are some of the others.

The Prevention of Illness – Have you ever noticed how some people never seem to catch colds or the flu while others are frequently sick with such common ailments? Among the people who are more susceptible to colds and flu are those whose bodies are struggling to function due in part to a buildup of toxins. These toxins challenge immune function and interfere with nutrient absorption, resulting in vulnerability to disease. I describe this to my patients by saying, "We don't catch diseases, we host them." The body needs to be a welcoming landscape in order for illness to take hold. Is your body a friendly host or aloof stranger to germs?

Some diseases in this country are the result of specific toxins that we take in as part of our American diet. Heart disease is one such example, developing in part because of the increased ingestion of junk food in this country. Two essential parts of the plan in this book are eliminating toxins from your diet and learning about proper nutrition.

An Improvement in Physical Appearance – People who cleanse tend to glow. Freed from carrying around the burden of toxicity, their body systems can work more efficiently. As a result, their complexions clear and their cheeks become rosy. When you reach your detoxification goals, you too will become healthier overall. You will begin to project a feeling of radiant well-being that is very attractive.

A Boost in Emotional Well-Being – When you feel better physically, it brings relief to you emotionally. Energy you may have had to use to compensate for ill health can now be directed towards activities you enjoy. When you take care of yourself by doing a cleanse, you give your self-esteem a lift.

In addition to physical well-being, *The Detox Solution* specifically addresses the emotional dimensions of detoxification. In Chapter 13, you will learn techniques and strategies for efficiently managing your emotions so you can experience more joy and inner peace. You can take inventory of your emotional habits, learn how to let go of self-defeating patterns and how to reinforce positive approaches to working with challenging situations. In addition, you can incorporate proactive tools into your daily life that can reduce your emotional stress.

A Sharpening of Mental Capabilities – Do you feel like there's a fog that often drifts across your mind? Or do you need a cup of coffee to push your brain to its full capabilities? Toxicity is a major cause of dull thinking. Eliminating toxins from your life and removing toxic residues from your body can result in a sharper mental focus.

An Enhancement in Digestion – When you begin to improve the quality of the foods you take in, you'll notice that your digestion will become more comfortable. Instead of intensely battling toxins taken in as part of your diet, your digestive tract will be able to concentrate on processing and assimilating the foods you eat. When you then clean out the toxic residues in your digestive tract, food absorption will be further enhanced.

The Elimination of Unhealthy Food Addictions & Allergies – When the body is coping with a toxic overload, it experiences a chemical imbalance. Unhealthy food cravings are the body's attempt to get back into equanimity. Also, foods that otherwise would not trouble you can be perceived as allergens by a body coping with toxicity. Detoxification can help you develop a healthier and safer relationship with food.

The Attainment of Ideal Weight – It's been very common for patients to lose weight with little effort during and after detoxifying. I've seen this occur even in people who have had weight challenges for a long time. The reason? Detoxification supports a healthy metabolism. By removing toxicity, you allow the cells to process nutrients in a more efficient way. This will significantly boost the rate at which you metabolize the foods you eat. When you clean up your diet at the same time you detoxify, metabolism is further enhanced.

A Minimizing of the Effects of Aging – Toxins block nutrients from adequately nourishing the cells of your body. This can lead to premature aging. In contrast, when you improve what you take into your body and clean out the toxins, your cells are revitalized. Detoxification can help you remain more youthful.

Spiritual Renewal – When the body is clear of toxins, there is a feeling of spiritual renewal. The physical cleanse can serve as a metaphor for healing on a spiritual level. Traditionally, physical detoxification has been linked with spiritual renewal.

Due to its comprehensive nature, the program in *The Detox Solution* can also assist you directly in getting in touch with your Spirit. As you examine your current belief system and elevate your use of language, thoughts, and actions, you can look forward to increased awareness. As you embrace the spiritual, you will be rewarded with a greater sense of fulfillment, purpose, and wonder.

A LONG HISTORY OF DETOXIFICATION

Though detoxification is overlooked as a key tool for health by modern medicine, it has always been a part of other healing traditions. These other traditions emphasize bringing the body back into balance, and they recognize detoxification as a natural recovery process. So while detoxification is trendy today, it's nothing new. As you have learned, this is in fact a perfectly natural process; your body is detoxifying every second of your life!

Let us look at a few of these other healing traditions.

▪ The Amazon Rain Forest Tradition

With a strong basis in Nature, this system of detoxification utilizes the abundance and diversity of medicinal herbs available within the verdant Amazon rain forest. Shamans (spiritual healers) have long been the keepers of this tradition's knowledge about cleansing herbs. For centuries, information was passed on orally through shamans to their students. Within this system of cleansing, herbs are viewed as having spiritual influences as well as physical effects on the body.

Practices were extensive within this tradition and many are still in use in the 21st Century. For instance, herbs to improve digestion are often delivered today in chewing gum. Liver cleanses utilize Brazil nut tree bark, various herbal teas, and papaya. Massage enhances the effects of the detoxifying herbs. Hot steam mixed with medicinal herbs is used in therapeutic baths to purge toxins through sweat.

▪ The Ayurvedic Tradition

This tradition from India is part of a comprehensive approach to medicine, which dates back as far as 3000 B.C. The primary goal of Ayurvedic medicine is to maintain the health, balance, and energy of the mind and body. Detoxification is strongly emphasized. Herbs, aromatherapy oils, special foods, massage, and sweat baths are utilized in cleansing. Yoga, breathing exercises, adjustments in mental perspective, and meditation are also part of this approach. Medicated enemas may be administered.

Juice fasts lasting from a few days to two weeks are part of this tradition. Sweet juices are avoided, as they are believed to foster a buildup of toxins.

The European Tradition

Cleansing traditions come from various sources in Europe. For instance, the ancient Romans are famous for their cleansing baths, which were the center of their social life. Treatments there involved exercise, oiling of the body, immersion in water of various temperatures, exposure to steam, and scraping of the skin. Also, the Finns have long turned to saunas during the winter months to sweat impurities out of their bodies. A Finnish saying describes the sauna as "a sacred place, a place of silence, a place of recreation, a place of peace, and a place of health."

Today spas for cleansing can be found throughout Europe, and some, like the German and Austrian Kur (cure) spas, emphasize detoxification of specific organs such as the liver. You'll find further information on the importance of saunas and other forms of hydrotherapy in Chapter 12, which focuses on different ways to stimulate your circulation for enhanced detoxification.

The Naturopathic Tradition

The Naturopathic tradition has developed within the past century. Naturopath doctors use cleansing techniques from various ancient traditions. The use of herbal medicine, nutritional counseling, and hydrotherapy are some of the most common therapies employed.

Naturopathic medicine has always placed a specific emphasis on detoxification. The naturopathic physician is trained to address the underlying cause of illness, which is often a toxic influence. They often provide guidance to patients on how to remove influences of disease from their lifestyle and environment.

Many herbal cleansing protocols have their origin in the naturopathic tradition. Naturopathic physicians have been extensively trained in the safe use of herbs to enhance detoxification.

The Native American Tradition

One of the best known aspects of the Native American approach to detox are sweat lodges which are used for both spiritual and physical cleansing. These domed structures are made with a wood frame, which is covered with animal hides. Hot rocks are piled in a pit at the center of the lodge and water is poured over the rocks to create steam. Herbs, such as sage, may be wrapped around body parts, spread on the floor of the sweat lodge, or burned to create medicinal smoke.

Herbal cleansing formulas are also used internally in the Native American tradition to detoxify the body in the spring as part of a celebration of new life.

▪ Traditional Chinese Medicine

Traditional Chinese Medicine (TCM) has a history of over 5,000 years. The basic premise is one of health and harmony. TCM has a sophisticated system of prevention, detecting potential disease before it would be diagnosed by traditional Western standards. Understanding patterns of balance and harmony in each organ is a developed skill in the TCM practitioner. Detoxification with herbs and/or acupuncture to improve the function of imbalanced organs is a common protocol in Traditional Chinese Medicine. Chinese medicine addresses the issues of toxicity from a physical, emotional, and spiritual perspective. Currently, acupuncture has been gaining media attention for its success with drug detoxification.

As you read through this book and work with the detox practices, you will be reminded of the processes described above. Many of the basic ideas have been tested over the centuries within these various traditions.

It's interesting to note how detoxification has been used for both prevention and healing throughout history, even without the toxic bombardment we have in the 21st Century. Efficient detoxification is needed today like never before. It is quite amazing that our present medical system addresses detoxification usually only as part of a drug or alcohol problem. In fact, Western medicine is the only medical system that doesn't emphasize detoxification as a therapy in treating and preventing disease!

WHAT'S AHEAD

When you've decided to detoxify, the chapters to come will assist you in moving forward. As you progress with the plan laid out in *The Detox Solution*, you may be surprised by how much better you feel. Allow these new feelings of clarity and well-being to confirm your decision to explore detoxification; you'll know that you're on the right path.

At this point, let's look at the steps you'll be taking as you travel through the chapters ahead. In Chapter 2, you'll assess your current level of exposure to toxicity and your motivations and goals in detoxifying. This will be followed by a chapter on external toxins, which will help you further identify exposures that you can eliminate or limit in your life. In Chapter 3, you'll also be supplied with many nontoxic alternatives to make new choices easy for you. Part I will then conclude with Chapter 4, which addresses internal toxins. Here you'll discover how internal toxins are formed, their negative impacts on health, and preventive measures.

In Part II (Chapters 5 through 8), you can explore the miraculous ways your body naturally detoxifies. You will come to understand the roles of the major detoxification organs and systems, such as the colon, liver, and digestive tract. Health challenges that commonly afflict those needing detoxification will also be described.

Part III (Chapters 9 through 16) will walk you through the core components of the plan. You will learn a way of eating that supports a continuous feeling of energy, as well as how to use supplements and "superfoods" to provide further support. You'll be presented with a proven herbal detoxification program that has worked for thousands of people. In addition, you will learn how circulation improves detoxification and the steps that you can take to optimize the way your body cleanses itself. You'll also become familiar with the emotional and spiritual dimensions of detoxification. Just in case you need it, you will learn how, and when, to seek assistance from a health professional. Finally, you will be sent on your way with ideas for continuing the benefits of detoxification and for staying committed to a lifetime of optimal physical, emotional, and spiritual well-being.

Ready for a health-enhancing adventure? Let's get started. In the next chapter, "Toxins in Your Life: An Assessment," you'll find a series of easy questionnaires that will help you see your world from a new perspective. With this new vision, you can understand more clearly why toxicity is the most important health concern facing us in modern times.

TWO

Toxins in Your Life:
An Assessment

The doctor of the future will give no medicine
but will interest his patients in the care of
the human frame, in diet, and in the
cause and prevention of disease.

—Thomas Edison

Each week, people come to the clinic for natural, nontoxic solutions for a variety of health challenges. Again and again, I hear of chronic health complaints, such as digestive disturbances, fatigue, allergies, chronic pain, hormonal imbalances, and skin disorders. Perhaps you purchased this book because you too are coping with a chronic health condition. A common and highly effective solution for bringing patients to a superior state of health has been detoxification. Time and time again, I've seen dramatic improvements from a comprehensive detoxification program—one that not only pays attention to improving your diet and gaining support from supplements and herbs, but also considers an individual's environment, level of stress, daily habits, emotional health, and spiritual outlook.

Some of you have purchased this book even though you consider your health to be relatively good. Perhaps you were drawn to the title

The Detox Solution because your goal is to reach high levels of vibrant health. Yes, you've also come to the right place! There are many ways that you too can benefit from reading and using the ideas in this book. For instance, you may want to achieve the healthy glow that comes when your body is detoxifying at an optimal level. Or you may wish to clear a persistent mental fog, which could be the result of your toxic exposures.

In this chapter, we'll start by looking at an extensive list of common symptoms of toxicity. Keep in mind that when most of these symptoms are treated within the modern medical system, the underlying issue of toxicity is often ignored. Next, we'll concentrate on identifying the types of toxins that you may be encountering in your life today. This identification process is a major focus of the chapter. It marks the beginning of your detoxification program. Later, in Chapter 3, you'll learn more about these modern-day toxins and how you can eliminate them or reduce their impact.

If you lived on a pristine island where there was an ample supply of fresh food, a supportive loving community, a relaxed lifestyle, spiritual awareness, and no pollution, you probably wouldn't have to do an assessment of the toxins in the environment. Your body could simply rely on its built-in detoxification abilities because the level of toxins would be so low. However, in the 21st Century, such ideal conditions are the rare exception, and it is becoming increasingly important to become aware of the types of toxins that could be draining your energy and eroding your health.

The bottom line is that the human body can only remove a certain amount of toxicity on its own. When overwhelmed by toxins like it is today, the body will give us warning signals in the form of symptoms. The toxicity symptoms listed on the following checklist are among those that are often experienced; yet the connection to toxicity is unnoticed by many.

TOXICITY SYMPTOM CHECKLIST

Are you experiencing any of the following symptoms of toxicity? These are all health complaints that many colleagues and myself have heard from patients who later improved through detoxification practices. As you read in Chapter 1, such early symptoms are often not treated effectively in people using the traditional medical system, and so these initial indicators of deterioration in health can develop into chronic conditions and diseases. Don't let this happen to you! Take some time now to consider which symptoms apply to you.

Digestive System

- Indigestion/heartburn
- Gas (burping or flatulence)
- Bad breath
- Coated tongue
- Body odor
- Constipation
- Diarrhea
- Bloating
- Nausea
- Abdominal pain
- Hemorrhoids
- Gallstones
- Irritable bowel syndrome
- Protruding abdomen
- Candida
- Parasites

Dermal System (Skin)

- Rashes
- Acne
- Hives
- Eczema
- Extremely dry skin
- Extremely oily skin
- Plugged pores
- Slowly healing wounds
- Dark circles under eyes
- Puffiness under eyes

Immune System

- Allergies
- Frequent colds/flu
- Fatigue
- Cancer

Musculoskeletal System

- Sore joints
- Frequent headaches
- Neck/back pain
- Aches/pain
- Fibromyalgia

Lymphatic System

- Swollen lymph nodes
- Sore lymph nodes

Endocrine System

- Hypoglycemia/diabetes
- Food cravings
- Overweight/underweight
- Cellulite
- Excess sweating/night sweats
- Infertility

Nervous System

- Insomnia
- Hyperactivity
- Mental fog
- Dizziness
- Attention Deficit Disorder (ADD)
- Attention Deficit Disorder with Hyperactivity (ADHD)

Urinary System

- Kidney stones
- Fluid retention
- Darkly colored urine

Respiratory System

- Coughing
- Wheezing
- Sinus infections
- Sneezing
- Shallow breathing
- Congestion

Cardiovascular System

- High blood pressure
- Heart disease
- High cholesterol

Reproductive System

- PMS
- Fibroid tumors
- Fibrocystic breast disease
- Yeast infections
- Irregular periods

Psychological Indications

- Depression
- Mood swings
- Anxiety
- Irritability

Did you find symptoms that are troubling you? If you have mild symptoms, you may notice improvements just by following the basics of *The Detox Solution*. If you have a chronic health challenge, you would probably benefit from the basics of the plan coupled with assistance from a health care professional who is trained in detoxification.

If you cannot identify with any of the above symptoms, congratulations, you are probably in great health. Periodic detoxification can be a wonderful addition to help you maintain excellent health as you grow older.

Most Americans would claim at least one symptom on the checklist. Many are living with numerous symptoms of toxicity, thinking that they are just the result of "bad luck" or the aging process. Though toxicity is not the sole reason such symptoms occur, it is often a major contributing factor. Remember, although your body is programmed for healing, when it is pushed to the limit, life-threatening conditions can develop.

PREPARING TO DETOX

In the first chapter, the importance of taking personal responsibility for our health was presented, noting that there is ever-increasing evidence that we can make a huge difference in our state of well-being. A major part of this self-help effort involves educating ourselves and improving our habits and outlook.

When it comes to detoxifying, personal responsibility starts with setting yourself up for success rather than failure. To begin on the right foot, take a moment to consider what's going on in your life right now. If you're going through a major transition—such as a divorce or new job—you may want to start the detoxification process slowly by making only a few minor changes. If your life is less challenging, you can do more.

Detoxification doesn't have to be an "all or nothing" matter. You can start by picking a few changes that you want to begin with. As the saying goes, "a journey of a thousand miles begins with a single step." Select your first step, and then move forward with the plan at a pace you are comfortable with. *Remember, life is a journey, not a destination—a process, not a product.*

WHAT TOXINS ARE IN YOUR LIFE?

When embarking on a detoxification program, it is advised to begin by taking stock of the toxins you are encountering. Once you've pinpointed them, you'll be in a position to eliminate or minimize those exposures.

Removing toxins from your everyday environment, diet, etc., will be a crucial step in detoxifying. In fact, it is an *essential* one. Yet this sort of effort is overlooked in many of the programs that are currently available. Too frequently, people are encouraged to jump headfirst into a one-day, one-weekend, or one-week "cleansing" regimen, without being advised to first assess the toxins they're exposed to every single day. Reducing these daily exposures has made a big difference with patients in the clinic. This important change has made it possible for many to become healthier consistently.

So, are you ready to begin? The questionnaires ahead will help you discover toxins in many areas of your life. First, we'll consider the toxins that might be in your diet and environment, but we won't stop there. In addition, we'll look at emotional and spiritual factors, as well as your stress response. In the approach in this book, all the elements that are taxing to your system are considered toxins, whether on a physical, emotional, or spiritual level.

■ Diet

The foods and liquids you consume daily can be major sources of toxins. If you piled up all the meals you ate in one year, the mound formed would be huge. Can you imagine if all the food you ate in a lifetime were heaped in one place? The average American eats 25 *tons* of food by the time they hit age 65.[1] Considering this amount, it's quite apparent that the foods you take in can either be a major contributor to your well-being or to ill health. Answering the questions below will help you detect which foods may be adding to your toxic load.

Diet Questionnaire

- When you shop for groceries, do you toss convenience/processed foods into your cart?
- Do you purchase nonorganic produce, meat, and/or dairy?
- Are you unaware that the foods you buy might be genetically engineered or irradiated?
- Is red meat on your plate more than once a week?
- Do you add commercial salt rather than sea salt to your food?
- Do you cook with aluminum pots and pans?
- Are you unsure if your plates, bowls, and cups might be tinted with lead paint?
- Do you eat fried foods regularly at home or at restaurants?
- Are fast foods part of your regular diet?
- Do you order take-out foods or eat in restaurants frequently?
- Are barbecued foods on your plate often during warm weather?
- Do you snack on junk foods?
- Do you experience food cravings?
- Do you have a sweet tooth and regularly consume candies and desserts?
- Do you buy foods or soft drinks that contain artificial sweeteners?
- Do you add artificial sweeteners to your hot beverages?
- Are sodas one of the main liquids you drink?

- Do you regularly consume caffeinated drinks, such as coffee, tea, or colas?
- Do you rely on coffee to provide extra energy to get you through the day?
- Do you drink alcohol regularly?
- Do you consume less than eight 8-10 ounce glasses of water each day?
- Is the water you drink from the tap or plastic bottles?
- Is the environment where you eat hectic and stressful rather than relaxed and nurturing?
- Do you swallow your food without chewing it thoroughly?

If you answered yes to three or more questions, then diet could be a significant part of your toxic load.

This questionnaire covers a lot of ground. For now, just give some thought to how you might start reducing some of the toxins you've identified in your diet. The next chapter provides further suggestions for lowering the toxicity associated with the foods and drinks you consume.

▪ Environment

Our increasingly toxic environment—both outside and indoors—is a major reason why detoxification is more important than ever. In January 2000, Bill Clinton proposed a 56% funding increase for research into environmental toxins that are suspected to cause cancer. Part of the goal of the research would be to investigate the relationship between rising toxicity in the environment and heightened cancer risk. *At the time, the American Cancer Society reported that environmental toxins might account for as many as three-quarters of all cancers.* The following questionnaire highlights some of the major sources of environmental toxins.

Environment Questionnaire

- Is your residence and/or job in a city?
- Is your office or house located close to a factory?

HOLD THE PESTICIDES, PLEASE!

Chemical Use in Pounds per Acre

Strawberries	148
Sweet potatoes	127
Carrots	68
Brussels sprouts	53
Potatoes	35
Watermelons	28
Oriental eggplant	27
Peppers	25
Cilantro	13
Tomatoes	12
Blueberries	11
Raspberries	11
Basil	10
Pears	10
Onions	10

NOTE: The use of the soil fumigant, methyl bromide, accounts in part for the high ranking of such crops as strawberries, carrots and potatoes.

Source: Pesticide Action Network

The Environmental Protection Agency has identified more than 55 pesticides that can leave carcinogenic residues in food. While pesticide residues can turn up in some surprising places, a common source is the fruits and vegetables on our plates. California is known for growing produce that is consumed across the country. A study by the Pesticide Action Network found that more than 50 million pounds of fungicides, herbicides, insecticides, and soil fumigants were applied to farmland in that state in 1998. Meanwhile, growers of some crops there—namely of grapes, oranges, peaches, nectarines, and cauliflower—are attempting to use less chemicals and more compost and beneficial bugs. To the left is a chart indicating the California produce that is grown with the heaviest dose of chemicals.

DDT is an example of a pesticide that we have tried to eliminate from our diet. It was banned for use in the United States three decades ago. Still, American manufacturers have persisted in exporting it to other countries around the globe. Now we are seeing DDT residues coming back to us in the foods we import. Each year, the EPA performs a study of the chemicals found in human fat tissue samples. DDT continues to be found in 100% of the tissue examined.

- Do you work or live near a highway?
- Is your home in close proximity to a working farm where pesticides are used?
- Have you applied pesticides in your house or on the lawn and garden?
- Are pesticides regularly sprayed around your apartment building or neighborhood?
- Do you work or live beside a dry cleaner?
- Is your home cleaned with traditional household products?
- Does the paint on the walls of your home contain lead?
- Have you recently installed new carpet?
- Do you sleep near a TV that you keep on overnight?
- Are there high voltage power lines near your home?
- Are you being exposed to geopathic stress?
- Are fluorescent lights used in your home or office?
- Are you confined for many hours each day to an office with little air circulation?
- Do you spend significant time during your workday near office equipment, such as a computer or Xerox machine?
- Are you often exposed to cigarette smoke from others while working, traveling, or dining out?
- Is there a nuclear power plant near your home or office?

Although it is impossible to eliminate all the toxins in our environment, we can reduce some of them and work toward balancing out the rest. You'll find more on the balancing process later in this chapter. If you answered yes to three or more questions, your environment may be having a significant impact on your health.

▪ Habits

Ironically some of our own habits, choices, and routines can contribute to our toxic load. The good news is that this can be one of the easier areas in which to make changes. Altering our habits begins with becoming alert to what we are actually choosing to do. Because many

WHAT IS GEOPATHIC STRESS?

Is the term *geopathic stress* new to you? Geopathic stress (GS) is a disturbance of energy fields caused by subterranean streams or piped water, mineral concentrations, underground faults or cavities, and other elements. The distorted energy has been known to seep up into homes and buildings. Occupants are most strongly affected if they sleep or tend to sit in an area where this energy is more concentrated. Some of the reported symptoms of GS include fatigue, depression, irritability, frequent colds, allergies, body pain, back problems, headaches, and insomnia. One extensive study by the U.S. government even found geopathic stress to be a factor in 40 to 50% of all human cancers.[2]

of us have been involved in the same routines for so long, it's easy to run on "automatic" and ignore the fact that we can make new decisions. After going through the following questionnaire, you may think of a few other areas to add to your list.

Habit Questionnaire

■ Do you smoke cigarettes or cigars?

■ Are there recreational drugs in your life?

■ Do you wear clothing that has been traditionally dry-cleaned?

■ Do you use standard cosmetics rather than ones made with natural, nontoxic ingredients?

■ Do you wear perfumes rather than essential oils?

■ Do you use commercial antiperspirants rather than nontoxic alternatives?

■ Do you swim in a chlorinated rather than ozonated pool?

■ Do you sit at a computer for a long period of time each day?

■ Are your clothes washed with regular detergent?

■ Are you a daily TV viewer?

■ Do you watch TV before you go to bed at night and first thing in the morning?

- Do you spend long hours on the Internet rather than in nature or with friends?

- Do you rarely exercise?

- Do you stay inside all day without taking a break to go outside?

If yes was your answer for three or more, your habits may be adding to a life that feels more stressful instead of joyful, contributing to low energy and a susceptibility to illness.

You may wonder why television watching is included on this list. In this case, it's not because of your possible exposure to electromagnetic fields (the reason TV was mentioned on the last questionnaire). The concern here is for the people who may be using television as a sort of numbing electronic drug. Actually, watching too much TV can *add* to emotional stress and instability due to its overstimulating nature. (You don't necessarily notice these effects while watching television, as you are vegging.) Many people consider television relaxing, unaware of the stimulatory effects on the brain. Also, too much TV watching can steal time you could be using for more satisfactory creative expression.

Some alternative activities to being "glued to the tube" can be taking a bike ride, listening to music, developing your inner life through meditation, engaging in a hobby, taking a dance class, or enjoying a walk in the park. There are many ways to be more aware of your real needs and feelings. While it is easy to become hooked on external stimulation to keep yourself going, life is a lot more satisfying and fun when you tune in to you. By connecting inside, you can identify and work through feelings that are causing you to feel anxious and stressed. You can also contemplate goals that truly suit you and pastimes that you would sincerely enjoy.

Think of all the hours that you have spent in front of the TV over the course of your life. What if you were able to recapture all that time? Imagine some fun, creative, and soulful ways you might choose to use those hours. What would make you laugh? How could you nurture yourself? What activities would be fulfilling? Keep these ideas in mind for alternatives to be used in the future.

▪ Stress

Toxins of all types are stressful because they are destructive to the body, mind, and spirit. For the purposes of the following questionnaire, let us define stress as a feeling of tension that interferes with our ability to be at peace with ourselves. Often this particular type of stress comes from a *perception of lack*—a lack of time, money, support, ideas, fun, creative outlets, resources, etc. Since stress is a major factor in the formation of many diseases, it is important to find ways to transform stress. The following questions will help you become more aware of your level of stress as well as some of the areas that are causing tension in your life.

Stress Questionnaire

- Do you feel like you're always in a hurry?
- Do you become irritated easily?
- Do you find it difficult to sit still and relax?
- Do you have trouble falling asleep and/or wake up during the night?
- Are you judgmental of yourself and others?
- Are you envious of the things others have and what they are able to accomplish?
- Do you worry about having enough money to meet your needs?
- Do you stay in relationships even though they offer more distress than nurturance?
- Do you have a hard time accepting yourself the way you are— the good and the bad?
- Do you feel a lack of purpose in your life?
- Do you dislike your job?
- Do you feel overworked?
- Do you often feel like a victim?

If you had three or more yes answers, then your relationship with and perception of the stressors in your life could probably use improvement. You would likely benefit from replacing these toxic stress patterns with alternatives that support the life you were created to live.

Like other toxins, lack of sufficient stress management is on the increase in modern life. Many of us find ourselves juggling multiple responsibilities in an environment that is busy, chaotic, and ever changing. What can be important in managing stress is getting back in charge by realizing that we *do* have control over how much we take on. It is important to learn to set limits with others and to become conscious of when and why we are attempting to do too much.

▪ Emotions

The questionnaire below highlights a number of emotional patterns that can be considered toxic. You may be in a healthy place emotionally and not relate to any of them. Or you might find yourself identifying with several items. No matter how many seem to ring true for you, it is important to realize that part of detoxification is growing out of negative emotional patterns that are not serving you. Instead, you can develop ways of responding that reinforce your well-being. You'll find an in-depth discussion of emotional health in Chapter 13.

Emotions Questionnaire

- Do you hold in your emotions or feelings and tend to not share them?
- Are you troubled by guilt over past experiences?
- Do you obsess over problems that come up in your life?
- Do you turn to food, drugs, or alcohol instead of dealing with your feelings?
- Is it difficult for you to forgive others?
- Is your view of life pessimistic?
- Do you feel that it is not OK to cry?
- Are you more likely to sit in feelings of loneliness rather than reaching out to others?
- Do you feel helpless to change yourself or others?
- Is it easy for you to become nervous?
- Are you judgmental about yourself?
- Do you delay decisions and as a result worry about the potential outcomes?

- ▪ Do you lack love and joy in your life?
- ▪ Are you uncomfortable with your sexuality?
- ▪ Is it difficult for you to accept your body the way that it is?
- ▪ Are most of your thoughts self-destructive rather than self-supportive?

If you answered yes to three or more questions, you would most likely benefit from learning how to use your emotions to support you. There are healthy alternatives to feeling that your emotions control you or contribute to the destruction of your happiness.

Part of the growth process as a human being is learning to feel, express, and utilize your emotions in healthier ways. For instance, sitting in negative feelings for too long without taking action or gaining perspective only results in getting yourself upset. Without appropriate expression and action, there's not likely to be a satisfying resolution to the initial problem. Fortunately you can find healthier ways to respond. If you feel some anger, be aware of it, but find a way to forgive. Talk out the problem in a calm manner. If you instead just dwell on your anger, it can taint your physical and emotional health. Research is finding that toxic emotional patterns contribute to various disease processes, including cancer, heart disease, and autoimmune conditions.

▪ Spirituality

Cultivating a spiritual life is essential to navigating through the world we live in today. The disappointments and challenges we all face can be transformed and have meaning and purpose when we learn to live connected to our true nature. Spirituality is a potent method of detoxifying that which does not serve our highest good and the good of all around us. Reclaiming our Spirit reminds us of the magic and beauty of the world, our intimate connection to all of life, and the joyful wonder of our own existence.

Spirituality Questionnaire

- ▪ Do you feel a connection with a higher power, whether you call it God, the Creator, Spirit, or your Higher Self?

- Do you trust that there is a larger plan and that things are not always as they appear?

- Do you take time to just "be" rather than always "do"?

- Do you smell the roses and know that there doesn't always have to be an external reward connected to how you spend your time?

- Do you go inside yourself to find the answers to your problems rather than only asking others for solutions?

- Do you feel supported by God/Life/the Universe?

- Do you trust your inner guidance?

- Do you operate out of a spirit of receptivity rather than fear?

- Are you grateful for the many blessings in your life?

- Are you kind to others and yourself, offering simple acts of kindness throughout your day?

- Do you cultivate the best that is within you and in those around you?

- Do you greet life with a playful, joyful spirit, welcoming laughter, pleasure, and fun?

- Are you open to the many things that life has to teach you?

Take some time to reflect on the questions included in this particular list. Do you see a need for expansion in this area of your life? Everyone can benefit from support on a spiritual level. Spiritual activities range from practicing meditation, prayer, breath work, yoga, Tai chi, or Qi Gong. You might attend a church or temple service, a 12-step program, and/or spiritual workshops. Journaling thoughts and feelings or being in nature brings us back in touch with our spirit. It is deeply rewarding to be open to the highest levels of creation in your life.

CHANGING OUR RESPONSES

The introduction to the Stress Questionnaire presented the idea that all toxins create some type of stress because they negatively impact the body. In fact, we could exchange the word "stress" for "toxin" because they basically mean the same thing. Both indicate something that is not supportive of wholeness.

In the course of a day, each of us encounters a number of stressors/toxins. How we choose to respond to them does influence how much they impact us. Remember that you always have the power to choose how you respond to things. So if you find that it seems to be impossible right now to remove a toxin/stressor in your life, you can make a point of finding a way to balance it. Again, our attitudes toward things will either bind us to our current patterns or free us to make appropriate choices in any circumstance. Below are some examples:

Toxin/Stressor	Balancer
■ I work 80 hours a week.	■ I schedule a regular Saturday massage.
■ I'm always on the go and eat quickly.	■ I select foods that are easy to digest.
■ I have many stressful job responsibilities.	■ I meditate daily.
■ My workday is spent in a sterile office environment.	■ I start my day with a brisk morning walk.
■ I feel isolated as I spend a lot of my time at home, even though my children are with me.	■ Twice during the week, I hire a baby-sitter and go to classes at the yoga center.

By beginning to make these kinds of changes, we empower ourselves. No longer do we feel powerless to external forces. We see that by taking action—positive action—we can restore *balance* in our life and in our bodies.

Supporting our body's natural detoxification is part of achieving balance. As you are learning, your body is working continuously with the toxins it is attempting to process and remove. Since there is an increased load of toxins in our modern world, we must balance this by increasing the attention and assistance we give to detoxifying. You can take charge by reading this book and learning how to detoxify at an optimal level.

THE BROADER PICTURE

Taking the idea of balancing toxins/stressors a step further, it can be helpful to begin to view the world in terms of what supports your energy and what depletes it. Know that every choice you make is either a deposit or withdrawal from your body's energy account. This perspective will help you move away from toxins and towards the things in life that will support you. Below is a list to get you started.

Drains Energy	Supports Energy
■ Tap water	■ Purified water
■ Packaged/processed/ nonorganic foods	■ Whole, fresh, organic foods
■ Heavy proteins/excess red meat	■ Easily digested proteins/fish, tofu
■ Excessive dietary protein, carbs, and/or fats	■ Balance of dietary protein, carbs, and fat
■ Stimulants/caffeine	■ Tonifying herbs/ "superfoods"
■ Being overweight/ underweight	■ Maintaining ideal weight
■ Fluorescent light	■ Natural light/full spectrum light
■ Constant activity/busy mind	■ Meditation/quiet mind/spiritual practice
■ Noise pollution	■ Healing sounds/nature/music
■ High intensity exercise	■ Yoga, walking, swimming
■ Working too much	■ Playing more often
■ Watching the news/violent movies	■ Choosing media that supports values
■ Holding grudges	■ Forgiveness
■ Impatience	■ Trust in the Perfect Timing of Life
■ Too little sleep, or tossing and turning	■ Deep, restful sleep

Drains Energy	Supports Energy
■ Expecting the worst/ pessimism	■ Looking for the best/ optimism
■ Limited beliefs about your abilities	■ An openness to your possibilities
■ Focusing on what one doesn't have	■ Gratefulness for all of life
■ Thoughts of despair, doubt	■ Knowing at your deepest core that all is well
■ Feeling disconnected from others	■ Developing an awareness of our connection and need for each other
■ Wanting to control	■ Letting go and being open
■ Feeling unlucky and victimized	■ Seeing obstacles as opportunities for transformation
■ Imbalanced relationship with money	■ Trust in the flow of money/provision
■ Being out of touch with your life	■ Being present, aware in the moment
■ Judgmental, conditional love for self and others	■ Unconditional love for self and others
■ Operating out of fear and doubt	■ Operating out of love and harmony

This is your life, and there will be no moment in it that is more significant than right now. Why not make the most of this moment by taking measures to become more self-supporting? You do not have to wait until you accomplish certain external goals before you can take care of yourself. You can begin today to make at least one change toward enjoying life more and living in healthier ways.

LOOKING AHEAD

In the next chapter, we will take a closer look at the toxic elements that we began to explore in this chapter. You'll find many creative solutions for clearing toxins from your world or lessening their impact.

THREE

Toxins in Your World:
Simple Solutions

We are part of the earth, and it is part of us.

The perfumed flowers are our sisters; the deer,
the horse, the great eagle, these are our brothers.

The rocky crests, the juices in the meadows,
the body heat of the pony, and man;

All belong to the same family.

—Chief Seattle

The increasing amount of toxicity on our planet is truly astounding. For example, let's look at pesticides. According to the Natural Resource Defense Council, the use of pesticides has risen more than tenfold since the 1940s. Today, in the United States alone, over 1.2 billion pounds of pesticides are used in agriculture a year[1]. That is an average of 10 pounds of these toxic chemicals per person in the U.S. When you consider all commercial chemicals, the numbers become even more staggering. According to the eye-opening book, *Toxic Deception: How the Chemical Industry Manipulates Science, Bends the Law, and Endangers Your Health,* at least 70,000 chemicals are used in commerce today, with about *six trillion pounds* produced annually to be used in plastics, glues, fuels, dyes, and other products.

Although the problem of toxicity may seem overwhelming—since these products appear to be everywhere, the point of this chapter is not to dwell on how bad things are. It is to bring to your attention the many simple choices you can make to reduce the impact of toxins. The truth is that there's an abundance of "green" products you can choose to replace those that are having a negative impact. The tide is turning. One of the more obvious ways you can see this positive current is in the increasing amounts of organic food that are appearing in our grocery stores and farmers' markets.

In the last chapter, you began to determine many areas where you can reduce the toxins that you are taking in. *If you have not completed the questionnaires in Chapter 2, go back and do so now.* Having identified the sources of toxicity in your daily life, you will be able to move forward by educating yourself further about them and by becoming familiar with the earth-friendly replacements you can select instead.

Sources of toxins can be divided into two basic categories. First, there are those that come from outside of our bodies—from the foods we eat, the water we drink, the air we breathe, etc. These are called *"external toxins"* or *"exogenous toxins."* The second type actually comes from within our own body and is produced through various metabolic and mental processes. They are known as *"internal toxins"* or *"endogenous toxins."* This chapter will focus on the external toxins. The following chapter will cover how toxins are produced internally, as well as how to minimize those occurrences.

The ground we will cover in the current chapter relates directly to our basic paradigm, the theoretical framework for the detoxification process that you are beginning to explore. *Remember that it is important to first evaluate what you are currently taking into your body before you begin any herbal cleansing regimen. By taking this step, you will decrease your toxic load by locating its sources.* This initial process will allow you to reduce the negative influences on your health and energy level while increasing the positive ones. *Only then will you be ready to clean out the residues that your previous exposures to toxins have left behind.* Taking both steps will vastly increase your daily energy—an ultimate goal of *The Detox Solution!*

Thanks to the "progress" of the past century, a massive volume could easily be written on the sources of toxins—instead of a sole chapter. Levels of toxicity in the human body, as well as on the planet, have been higher in the past 20 years than in the entire history of the world. In this chapter, we will cover the basic sources of toxins and address the areas mentioned in the questionnaires of Chapter 2.

As you learn more about toxins and begin to identify them in your world, please do not become discouraged. You can begin by making changes in one area—such as the purity of the water you drink—and then gradually move on. After you make changes to reduce the influence of the external toxins as well as improve your nutritional intake, you will be ready to begin the herbal cleansing regimen outlined in Chapter 11.

WATER

Necessary for virtually every bodily function including circulation, digestion, absorption, and waste elimination, water has long been touted for its remarkable healing abilities. In fact, the body weight of the average adult is made up of approximately 60% water. We also rely on water to cleanse ourselves, our children, our pets, our dishes, and our environment. Throughout Earth's history, sparkling pure water has been gathered from sunlight-drenched flowing rivers and streams, but now such pristine sources are dwindling. The basic nectar of life is being tampered with in a major way.

For example, industrialized progress in the Western world has resulted in huge amounts of chemical wastes that threaten our water supply. Much of this **industrial waste** is highly poisonous and carcinogenic. In 1992 alone, the EPA received official notice from companies that 273 million pounds of toxic waste had been dumped into surface water. We can only wonder how much additional discharge into our waters went unreported. Another 338 million pounds of toxic waste were deposited on land that year, and 726 million pounds illegally injected underground. Runoff from these land sites also reduces the quality of water supplies and underground waterways.

Alarmingly, **pesticide residues** are also turning up in drinking water samples, specifically specimens taken from farm areas of the Midwest, California's Central Valley, and the East Coast's Chesapeake Bay region. In 1999, the Environmental Working Group (*www.ewg.org*) found the pesticide DBCP—which they describe as "one of most potent carcinogens known"—in the drinking water that's delivered to 1 million Californians of the Central Valley. That same year, Aztrazine—the country's most widely used pesticide—was reported by EWG to be in tap water used by 800 midwestern communities.

As municipal water authorities are relying more and more on recycled water from waste treatment plants, questions are being raised about what might remain in the water after processing. Now more than 100 published reports on tap water worldwide show that **pharmaceutical drugs** can be detected even following treatment. Initially these drugs were discovered accidentally in drinking water by researchers looking for pesticide residues. Substances identified have included cholesterol reducers, painkillers, chemotherapy drugs, antibiotics, beta-blockers, and anti-seizure medications.

For these reasons and more, people are becoming increasingly concerned about the safety of their tap water. The EPA estimates about 30 million Americans each year use public water systems that violate at least one health standard.[2] The agency has identified more than 700 pollutants that regularly occur in drinking water taken from the tap or springs and wells. The Environmental Working Group and Natural Resources Council have jointly estimated that one-fifth of the U.S. population drink tap water containing **lead, fecal material, toxic waste, and/or other pollutants.**

■ What You Can Do

In seeking cleaner water, it is a good idea to broaden your perspective. The most obvious move is to improve your drinking water. However, in a study done by the Massachusetts Department of Energy and published in the *American Journal of Public Health*, it was reported that 50 to 70% of exposure to water pollutants in adults occurs *through the skin!* The figure was 29 to 46% for children. This means that we need to look at the water we use for bathing and showering as well as drinking. Another often-overlooked area is the water used for cooking.

Here are some ways that you can boost the quality of the water you use:

Have the water you are drinking analyzed for contaminants – A drinking water analysis that tests for 17 toxic heavy metals (such as arsenic, lead, mercury, and the chromium contaminant exposed in the film *Erin Brockovich)* can be obtained from Doctor's Data (*www.doctorsdata.com*), a fully licensed clinical laboratory specializing in testing of toxic materials.

Invest in a high-quality water filter – Some of the best filtration systems combine reverse osmosis (RO) with activated charcoal and screen filters. Other units use just one of these methods—such as RO or activated charcoal. You are safest if you install a system that cleans all of the water in your home. A whole-house unit is attached to your incoming cold water line and provides filtered water for all purposes. Another approach is to install a filtering system near the point of use, such as directly on the kitchen faucet or under the sink. Countertop filters are another option. They allow you to filter water by pouring it directly through a device that is similar to a coffee filter. For specific products, check your local home improvement store, *www.gaiam.com*, and *www.real goods.com*. Additional companies are provided in the Resources section.

If you cannot install a whole-home system, don't forget to filter the water you use for showering – Taking a shower exposes you to as much as six times the chloroform (a toxic compound in chlorinated water) through steam as you would absorb from drinking treated water. A New Jersey study showed elevated breath levels of chloroform in subjects even hours after they had taken a shower. Companies who carry water filters usually supply shower filters.

Another option for the kitchen: Purchase bottled water for drinking and cooking – If a filtering system in the kitchen is not feasible for you right now, use bottled spring, mineral, or purified water instead. It is best to purchase it in glass containers, as plastic can pass chemicals into the water. Consider a water delivery service that packages water in glass bottles, such as Mountain Valley Spring Water. Their website (*www.mountainvalleyspring.com*) has extensive information about bottled water as well as great links to water safety sites.

When out of the house, drink bottled water – To insure the best quality water, order bottled water when you're dining out, and carry your own pure water along with you during your travels in the car or by foot.

Consider using ozone in your pool – Many pool services have ozone available as an alternative to chlorine.

CHLORINE & FLUORIDE:
Here's to Your Health?

Two inorganic chemicals—chlorine and fluoride—are routinely stirred into America's public water supplies. The rationale for mixing in chlorine is to destroy waterborne disease-causing organisms, such as bacteria, viruses, and protozoa. Fluoride is seen as a method of reducing tooth decay in a population. Though these practices are widespread, there is rising debate over the effectiveness of each chemical, as well as growing concern about possible side effects of ingesting the substances on a life-long basis.

Certainly chlorine has helped to assure us that we can drink our water without ingesting dangerous microorganisms—such as those responsible for typhoid or cholera. Yet along with harmful organisms, chlorine also destroys "friendly" bacteria that are essential for human health. Also, bacteria that would fight off common communicable diseases in water are destroyed. In addition, some critics assert that certain harmful microorganisms, particularly viruses, are not adequately eliminated by chlorine.

One of the most compelling arguments against adding chlorine to drinking water is the risk of cancer. Studies conducted jointly by Harvard University and the Medical College of Wisconsin have linked the consumption of chlorinated water to 15% of all rectal cancers and 9% of all bladder cancers in the U.S. This equates to 6,500 additional cases of rectal cancer and 4,200 of bladder cancer.

Studies are finding that consuming glasses of fluoridated water may increase both the risk of cancer and of osteoporosis. In a classic study, John Yiamouyiannis, Ph.D., compared cancer death rates in the largest fluoridated and nonfluoridated cities in the U.S. The rates were similar in both cities before fluoride was first introduced in 1953, but then rose noticeably in the study areas where fluoride was used. Indeed, a researcher at the National Cancer Institute has concluded that fluoride *causes* more cancer deaths than any other chemical—blaming it for an estimated 61,000 cases of cancer in 1995. Other scientists warn that additional sources of fluoride (toothpastes, pesticide residues, etc.) in combination with treated water can result in toxic levels of exposure and a weakening of the teeth and bones.

Stay informed about safe water issues – One useful website (*www. fluoridealert.org*) is sponsored by the Fluoride Action Network (FAN). It provides updates on breaking news about fluoride—such as possible Congressional hearings on its safety—as well as historical and general background and links to other advocate groups. The Environmental Working Group's site (*www.ewg.org*) deals with chemical pollution of drinking water among other matters.

AIR

Air pollution is usually obvious during an extreme exposure. When walking into a printing shop, factory, or smoke-filled bar, one can immediately sense the toxicity in the air. Seeing a layer of smog over a city is another easily discernable indication of the presence of toxins. Unfortunately, if we are continuously exposed to such polluted environments, our body's natural awareness can become desensitized. We may begin to breathe more shallowly in order to compensate, and each breath of that oxygen-depleted toxic air we take in compromises our health in some way.

▪ Outdoor Air Pollution

The condition of the outside air is usually what we think of when we hear the term "air pollution." Outdoor pollutants come from a wide range of sources, but two of the major ones are **industry** and **motor vehicles**. The statistics related to these two sources are mind-boggling. In 1992, U.S. companies reported to the EPA that they had released 1.84 billion pounds of toxic chemicals into the air. And a 1999 government study on air pollution in Los Angeles found the risk of cancer in that city to be *426 times greater* than health standards established by the 1990 Federal Clean Air Act. The primary pollution source in L.A. is motor vehicles, with diesel exhaust from trucks and buses having a significant share of the detrimental impact. Certainly we are seeing increased cancer risk from vehicle exhaust in other cities as well. Additional sources of outdoor air pollutants include **dry cleaners, vehicle refueling operations, gas-burning lawn mowers,** and **agriculture.**

Early symptoms of an exposure to outdoor air pollutants include irritation of the nose, eyes, and/or throat. Living in cities with toxic air can lead to respiratory conditions such as emphysema, bronchitis, asthma, and lung cancer. Air pollution poisons the whole body, not just the lungs, and such toxicity has been noted as a factor in allergies, cancer, heart disease, and premature death. Air pollution affects everyone's health to some degree.

▪ Indoor Air Pollution

In many instances, indoor pollution can be more harmful than outdoor pollution because there is not as much space for contaminants to dissipate. This problem has worsened with the trend toward creating more energy-efficient, airtight structures. The Environmental Protection Agency reports that levels of indoor pollutants can be two to five times, and sometimes even a hundred times, worse than levels outdoors. Yet many families are inhaling numerous toxins in their homes without being aware of the impact on their health. Some common toxins that affect the air in the home are **cigarette smoke, dust, pet dander, lead, outgassing from carpets, formaldehyde from particleboard, chemicals in aerosol sprays, unclean air ducts, fumes from cleaning products, asbestos, the solvent benzene, carbon monoxide,** and **flame retardants.**

Due to exposure to a brew of concentrated toxins in poorly ventilated offices, "sick building syndrome" and other work-related environmental illnesses are on the rise. People may simultaneously experience extreme fatigue, lowered immune response, and occasionally flu-like symptoms. The immune systems of these people are basically overcome by toxicity. In the typical office setting, workers may inhale **outgassing from carpets** as well as toxins from **building materials, office supplies, fax machines, photocopiers, synthetic furniture,** and **recycled air.** Even fellow workers can contribute, with **solvents from dry cleaning, chemicals from personal care products,** etc. More than 250 toxins have been identified in indoor office "smog."

A surprising contributor to indoor air toxicity can be the use of **candles.** Most candles are made with paraffin, a petroleum by-product. Also, many contain metallic wicks that contain lead. *The Journal of the American Medical Association* reported that burning the lead-containing candles for three hours would result in toxic levels ten to thirty-six times the U.S. Environmental Protection Agency standards.[3]

■ What You Can Do
Outdoor air pollution

Many people feel helpless when it comes to doing something about outdoor air pollution. They don't realize that there are concrete steps you can take to reduce the effects these toxins have on your health. In Part Three, ways to remove toxins that polluted outdoor air has left in your lungs and body will be presented. Here are some other simple steps you can take that relate to outdoor air pollution:

Do your part by planting trees in your environment – Besides adding beauty to a landscape, trees assist us in other ways. They help improve the quality of our air by absorbing pollutant gasses and releasing oxygen. Trees also provide surfaces that trap airborne particles that can harm human lungs. Shade created by trees and water evaporating from their leaves cool the temperature and reduce the need for air conditioning. This cuts the air pollution generated by power plants. Groups, such as TreePeople in Los Angeles (*www.treepeople.org*) and The Green Environmental Coalition of Yellow Springs, Ohio, are committed to planting trees to help improve air quality. Check with local environmental groups to see if there is such activity in your area.

Bike or walk during light traffic hours and in locations where you are away from the congestion – These choices will reduce the amount of toxins you take in as you exercise. Locate nearby parks, woodlands, or waterfront trails for a more natural environment. When going to these spots is not possible, select quiet residential areas rather than hectic business centers as sites for bike rides and strolls.

When moving to a new residence, consider air quality to be an important factor on your relocation checklist – Living in a clean environment can be worth putting up with a commute to your job. Also, even in urban environments, there are areas where the natural terrain is more likely to disburse airborne toxins. If you are considering a move, look for reports of air conditions on your local TV weather segments or in the newspaper. And when you are hunting for a new home, be alert for commercial and industrial sources of outdoor air pollution such as freeways, dry cleaners, gas stations, paint and autobody shops, or industrial plants.

Indoor air pollution

You have more control over the air quality in your home than at work, but there are also steps you can take on the job. Here are some ideas for both locations:

Purchase a top-notch air purifier, especially if you are a city dweller – There are three basic types for the home—portable models, those that run through your central heating and air conditioning system, and purifiers that can operate both independently or with your central unit. Among the indoor pollutants that these units filter are smoke, bacteria, mold, toxic fumes, hydrocarbons from cooking, pollens, odors, dust, dander, and static electricity. You can find excellent units at most home improvement stores, as well as *www.gaiam.com* and *www.realgoods.com*. For additional companies to contact, see the Resources section.

Expand your "clean air" zones by installing air purifiers in your office and car – For the office, you'll find units quiet and compact enough to set up on your desk. The Roomaid 7" x 8" Tabletop HEPA Filter, which offers a three-step purification system is one example. This unit is also suitable for use in your car. To make the adjustment for your car, you can purchase a two-piece accessory kit that includes a 12-volt adapter and seat belt clip. For various products, visit *www.selfcare.com*.

Don't overlook the cleaning of the ducts and vents in your central heating and air-conditioning system – They need periodic attention just as much as the rest of the house. These air passages can collect dust mites, bacteria, mold, fungi, smoke, cooking gases, toxic chemical vapors, and more. Local services will come to your home—often for reasonable rates—to periodically vacuum and clean these areas. To find a contractor near you, ask neighbors for referrals or visit the National Air Duct Cleaners Association website at *www.nadca.com*. Supply your own nontoxic cleaning products if necessary.

Allow your home to "breathe" by opening windows and creating ventilation – Air flowing through open windows supplies fresh oxygen and helps clean out toxins deposited from cleaning products, smoke, and other sources. Even in cold weather, you can keep a few windows open just a crack to permit airflow. One good habit to adopt is opening doors and windows in the morning to refresh the air captured in the house all night long. During winter, you could close most of them after several minutes.

Enlist the aid of houseplants known to be toxin fighters – Plants are known for their ability to clear carbon dioxide from the air, but they have the ability to remove dangerous man-made pollutants as well. Dr. Bill Wolverton and other NASA scientists spent 25 years investigating plants that would gobble up air pollutants in closed environments; this research was part of preparations for setting up livable outposts on other planets. In the process, they discovered that certain houseplants absorb airborne toxins such as formaldehyde, benzene, and trichloroethylene. To promote further work in this area, the Plants for Clean Air Council was founded in 1989. And now, Wolverton is sharing what the NASA experiments revealed in his book *How to Grow Fresh Air*. The chart on the following page shows some plants that NASA found to be efficient in removing three of the major indoor air pollutants.

For furnishings, "go natural" rather than synthetic – Many of today's furnishings are made from materials that give off toxic fumes. Bookcases made from particleboard and plywood release formaldehyde, a suspected carcinogen. Fabrics used in upholstery are often treated with formaldehyde resin to prevent stains. Your stuffed furniture and synthetic mattresses may be made with polyurethane foam plastic that has been treated with chemical fire retardants. As alternatives, look for natural furnishings made of such materials as wood, cotton, and wool without harsh chemical treatments. One source is the website *www.healthyeverything.com*. Click on "furniture" on the main page. *Natural Home* magazine (*www.natural homemagazine.com*) is a wealth of resources for natural furnishings and building materials, as well as nontoxic products for the home.

Find new choices to replace wall-to-wall synthetic carpeting – Many cases have been reported over the years of ill health effects after the installation of new synthetic carpets. One famous incident occurred right at the Environmental Protection Agency in 1987! At the EPA, more than 10% of employees got sick after they were exposed to the new floor coverings. Synthetic carpeting is made from acrylic, polyester, and nylon plastic fibers and treated with a formaldehyde-based compound. This type of carpeting has been known to give off toxic gasses including benzene, formaldehyde, toluene, zylene, and styrene.

LIVING PLANTS:
Nature's Air Cleaners

Research conducted by Dr. Bill Wolverton and NASA reveals that plants are effective toxin fighters.

Chemical toxins studied include trichloroethylene, benzene, and formaldehyde. The sources of these toxins include household cleaners, particle board, clothing, detergents, carpeting, insulation, paper, plastics, inks, paints, plastics, dry cleaning, and adhesives.

Conditions caused by these toxins include allergies, dizziness, headache, blurred vision, cancer, dermatitis, respiratory diseases, irregular heartbeat, tremors, kidney and liver damage, and psychological disturbances.

The plants studied that protect against effects of these toxins include:

- Bamboo palm
- Boston fern
- Chrysanthemum
- Dwarf date palm
- English ivy
- Ficus
- Gerbera daisy
- Golden pothos
- Peace lily
- Philodendron
- Poinsetta
- Spider plant

For more information, visit Dr. Wolverton's site at *www. wolvertonenvironmental.com.*

Instead of wall-to-wall carpeting, consider using area rugs made of natural fibers such as cotton or a cotton/wool blend. Select ones without the latex backing. One source is the Allegro Rug Weaving Company (*www.earthnet.net/~allegro*). Natural wall-to-wall carpets are also now on the market, such as an all-wool product from Colin Campbell & Sons (*www.colcam.com*). Ceramic tile, marble, hardwood, and natural linoleum are other good choices for flooring.

Switch to the nontoxic cleaning products now widely available in the marketplace – Commercial cleansers are among the most toxic substances used in the home. Not only do many of these products give off fumes as you use them, their vapors can also remain in the air for days! Toxic ingredients include lye, chlorine, ammonia, and petrochemical solvents. Many ingredients are suspected carcinogens, yet manufacturers are not required to list the contents on labels. The Consumer Products Commission believes that the higher percentage of cancers among homemakers may be due to the toxins they are exposed to while sprucing up the house.

Fortunately there are now a lot of natural and nontoxic alternatives; you just need to know where to look for them. Manufacturers include Orange Glow Products (*www.greatclean ers.com*), Soapworks (*www.soapworks.com*), Seventh Generation (*www.seventhgen.com*), Ecover (*www.ecover.com*), and Earth Friendly Products (*www.ecos.com*). Web shopping sites include Ecomall (*www.ecomall.com*), Green Market Place (*www.green marketplace.com*), and Healthy Environments (*www.healthy environments.com*). When natural products are not on hand, a precaution you can take is to select commercial products that require the least number of warnings on the label.

Choose cloth diapers over disposable ones – What could your choice of diapers have to do with air quality? According to a study in the *Archives of Environmental Health,* plastic-coated disposable diapers give off an array of chemicals including toluene, xylene, and styrene.[4] These were found to cause eye and lung irritations as well as breathing difficulties in laboratory mice. No such symptoms were seen with cloth diapers. So take care of your baby and yourself by using quality cloth diapers.

Reject commercial air "fresheners" – These products are marketed as an easy way to cover up unpleasant odors with more appealing ones; however, you will be getting more than you bargained for.

DID YOU KNOW?

Much of the oxygen that humans breathe is produced by plants as a byproduct of photosynthesis. "Plants are the central pivot, without which the world outside would gasp for breath." T'ai Hsuan, 10 B.C., in a companion text to the *I Ching.*

HEAVY METALS: Not a Rock Concert

Over the years, you have probably heard about the problem of heavy metals, though you may not be sure of the specifics. In the modern world, our environments, food, and water regularly expose us to metals that are toxic to our systems, and over time, they can accumulate in our body. They are referred to as *heavy metals* because most are five times heavier than water. A build-up of heavy metals interferes with the normal functioning of the body and can result in an array of symptoms such as fatigue, headaches, depression, diminished memory, and anemia (see metal-specific symptoms below). An estimated 25% of the U.S. population suffers from some form of heavy metal toxicity.[5] Below are the major culprits.

Mercury – This highly toxic metal tends to concentrate in the nervous system. In fact, the saying "mad as a hatter" comes from the 19th Century when hatmakers used mercury, lead, and arsenic to stiffen their construction material. The toxic metals were absorbed by hatters in the process, and some developed mental dysfunction and psychosis.

Note: Today a major source of mercury exposure is amalgam tooth fillings. All fillings that are referred to as "silver" actually contain a high percentage of mercury. Your dentist may not know this. Most fillings used today have significant amounts of mercury. Every time a bite is taken with mercury in the mouth, this toxic metal outgases and invades your entire system. Demand to know what goes in your mouth (and consequently your bloodstream).

Autopsy samples have demonstrated that higher mercury levels do settle into the central nervous systems and kidneys of those with this type of dental work. Other symptoms of mercury toxicity consist of cognitive problems, immune depression, muscle weakness, allergies, fatigue, and gastrointestinal disorders. While mercury fillings are a very direct source of this poisoning, additional sources are contaminated fish, inks, laxatives, paints, cosmetics, fabric softeners, plastics, and solvents.

To find dentists using alternative materials, contact the Environmental Dental Association at (800) 388-8124. For more detailed information on mercury and health, visit the website *www.holisticmed.com/dental/amalgam* for excellent research and links to other related sites.

Aluminum – While not specifically a heavy metal, aluminum is the most abundant mineral on earth, and its accumulation is a major cause of concern. One of the problems is that exposure to this metal can bring about free radical damage in the brain. This is a condition often seen in Alzheimer's patients. Workers from an aluminum smelting plant who were examined displayed the symptoms that can occur with overexposures—including neurological disorders, loss of balance, memory loss, lack of coordination, and depression. Other common complaints of sufferers have been headache, ringing in the ears, heartburn, compromised digestion, and frequent colds. Sources of aluminum include antacids and other over-the-counter drugs, aluminum cookware, cans, and foil, antiperspirants, carbonated sodas, baking powders, and contaminated water.

Lead – Children are particularly vulnerable to lead toxicity, because they absorb more of this metal than adults do. A 1994 government study found that almost 1.7 million children had excessive levels of lead in their blood.[6] Attention deficit disorder, hyperactivity, and juvenile delinquency have been tied to excessive lead buildups in youngsters. Because lead is so prevalent, overexposures in adults are also rampant. Symptoms of lead toxicity are immune depression, irritability, decreased concentration, and tremors. Some of the sources to be aware of are paint chips and dust, water piping, cigarette smoke, canned goods, pottery, contaminated food and water, air pollution, and insecticides.

Cadmium – Though lesser known, cadmium toxicity is widespread and comes from many sources—including first- and second-hand cigarette smoke. Exposures also result from industrial contamination, auto exhaust, metal food containers, pesticides, medications, instant coffee and tea, batteries, polluted water, soft drinks, processed grains, and plastics. Cadmium buildups have been linked with lung and prostate cancer, heart disease, kidney damage, and hypertension. Symptoms include anemia, fatigue, hair loss, dry skin, depressed appetite, joint soreness, and back pain.

Other Heavy Metals – Additional heavy metals also amass in the body, including **arsenic** (from wood smoke, cigarette smoke, polluted air and water, coal dust, weed killers, paints), **nickel** (from jewelry, cooking utensils, cigarettes, hydrogenated fats), and **copper** (from plumbing, cookware, water, birth control pills, amalgam fillings, fungicides).

The detoxification plan in *The Detox Solution* will help to prevent heavy metals from collecting in your system. Five specific steps you can take are: (1) avoid the listed sources above, (2) drink high-quality water, (3) eat organic foods, (4) exercise frequently, and (5) decrease the toxic chemicals in your environment. Ideas from Chapter 12 on improving circulation are also relevant. Information on heavy metal testing and removal is provided in Chapter 15, a guide to working with health professionals.

Dr. Robert Cass, a physician with over 28 years' experience treating patients with heavy metal toxicity has noticed that a large majority of degenerative conditions such as multiple sclerosis, Parkinson's, cancer, fibromyalgia, and chronic fatigue significantly improve when the heavy metal problem is addressed. He states, "More often than not, these conditions are exacerbated (if not created!) by mercury amalgam fillings, dental appliances, and root canals. It should also be noted that candida and other fungal overgrowth toxicities have an affinity for heavy metals, particularly silver mercury amalgams." Dr. Cass adds, "Heavy metal toxicity is finally beginning to be seen for the epidemic it is. Enlightened and discerning physicians will need to become increasingly skilled in identifying and cautiously treating this very serious problem."

Supporting the comments of the pioneering Dr. Cass, many colleagues and I have witnessed countless patients improve dramatically from the removal of these highly toxic (and unfortunately too common and usually undetected) metals. *If you have a significant health issue, testing for heavy metal toxicity is highly recommended.*

Instead of purifying the air, most simply introduce more toxins—including propellants, formaldehyde, colors, ethanol, phenol, and xylene. If you want to "refresh" your air, try better ventilation and essential oils such as eucalyptus, citrus, lemongrass, sandalwood, rose, geranium, or vanilla. (More on the use of essential oils later in this chapter.) There are also natural air freshener products made exclusively from pure essential oils. My personal favorite is a product called Air Therapy from Mia Rose (*www.miarose.com*). Made with 100% natural ingredients, it comes in three scents—orange, key lime, and spearmint. It is truly a miracle product in that it instantly replaces foul odors with a pleasant and nontoxic scent.

Use candles made from nontoxic materials – Look for candles made from plant wax or beeswax. Make sure they are scented with 100% pure essential oils, not synthetic fragrances.

DAILY SURROUNDINGS

Other factors in your physical environment expose you to toxins every single day. Everything from artificial lighting, to electronic equipment, to the paint on your walls, to the pesticides you use in your home and garden can add to the toxic burden your body is forced to cope with.

The problem with most **artificial lighting**—both fluorescent and incandescent—is that it does not contain the full spectrum of wavelengths that exists in sunlight. For most of human existence, the body has had adequate access to sunlight (full-spectrum light) throughout the day. Today many people spend the majority of their hours indoors. As a result, people can suffer from a toxic deprivation of sunlight or *malillumination*. Scientists believe that we are not receiving as much full-spectrum light as our biology requires. Fortunately, full-spectrum artificial lighting is available for purchase. And you can also judiciously expose yourself to more natural light as well. You'll find more information on these options in the "What You Can Do" section starting on page 58.

The effects of malillumination are multiple. One reason full-spectrum light is needed by humans is that it triggers the secretion of chemical messengers in the body that regulate many automatic functions. Thus bodies deprived of full-spectrum light do not run optimally. Also, a lack of full-spectrum light can deter the full absorption of dietary nutrients. In addition, full-spectrum light is an important source of Vitamin D. I have seen many cases where the health of patients improved with an increased exposure to full-spectrum light.

Depressed moods are among the various consequences of malillumination. This is seen in people who experience Seasonal Affective

Disorder (SAD), a type of depression that occurs during the winter season when there is less daylight. An estimated 12 million people suffer from SAD in the United States. Studies have shown that the likelihood of experiencing SAD increases the farther you are from the long and sunny days at the equator.

Wherever there is artificial light, there is electricity, and wherever electricity flows, **electric and magnetic fields (EMFs)** are created. "Electric fields" are generated when an appliance is plugged in but is not in use; "magnetic fields" occur when electricity passes through the wires. Though some claim the radiation from these invisible fields is too low to have a negative effect on health, others are linking EMFs with sleep disorders, mood changes, stress syndromes, suicide, susceptibility to infections, allergies, brain tumors, and particularly cancer and leukemia. An EPA study is among the research that has been establishing the role of EMFs in increased cancer risk.

It is interesting to note that the human body and its individual organs radiate EMFs; however, electromagnetic changes in the environment appear to affect the delicate natural balance. Several lab experiments have shown that outside sources of EMFs can create changes in the body on a cellular level.

Another energy-field-related problem was highlighted in the last chapter—**geopathic stress,** also referred to as "GS." Geopathic stress is a distortion of earth energy caused by subterranean streams, piped water, mineral concentrations, underground faults, and additional elements. Residents or workers can be impacted if they spend long periods in the path of the distorted energy. In Germany and Austria, this phenomenon is widely acknowledged and building sites are routinely tested for its influence. However America seems to be just waking up to the issue. Two common symptoms of geopathic stress are extreme tiredness and depression. Other indicators include frequent colds, lowered immunity, nightmares, migraines, body pain, headaches, anxiety, and insomnia. Geopathic stress is also a factor in cancer.

A controversy pitting convenience versus safety is whether or not it is wise to use **cellular phones,** based on the potential dangers of microwave radiation. Some 80 million Americans now carry these devices, and the numbers are growing. Yet, in late 1999, researchers at the University of Washington turned up study results that are troubling. As part of the study, 100 rats were taught to swim a prescribed course around barriers in a water tank. Later, half of the rats were exposed to microwaves similar to those emitted by cell phones. Remarkably all the exposed rats forgot the route, while the other group remembered it. The microwaves appear to have affected the exposed rats' spatial memory. Earlier studies have suggested a link between the use of cell phones and brain tumors. As further studies are conducted, manufacturers are trying to work around the problem. More on this under "What You Can Do."

Commercial **paints** contain a cocktail of toxic chemicals that can enter the body through the skin, eyes, and respiratory system. These include cadmium, mercury, chlorine, benzene, sulfur, formaldehyde, and xylene, among others. The danger from the toxicity is clear when you look at the experiences of people who paint frequently for work or pleasure. Toxic reactions are common in both house and canvas painters. For instance, house painters have a 40% higher cancer rate than average, and they are also more susceptible to allergies and skin eruptions.[7] However, paint professionals are not the only ones who are taking in these toxins from our environment. The federal government reports that measurable amounts of common paint chemicals can be found in the bodies of an estimated *90% of Americans.*[8]

Another concern about paint is the lead contained in old mixtures sold before 1975. In rooms with flaking and peeling old paint, this lead can be ingested as dust or eaten in chunks of the veneer by children.

Another deadly source of toxins are the **household pesticides** you use to get rid of critters in your garden and home. Designed to kill tiny pests, many of the active ingredients are quite strong and are known to cause immune suppression, cancer, birth defects, and liver damage in humans. An applied pesticide can remain active for days, weeks, or even years. As human beings, we become especially vulnerable when chemicals from pesticides build up over time in our fatty tissue. In one study, childhood leukemia was found to be four to seven times greater when store-bought pesticides had been used in the home and garden.[9]

Finally, we are often exposed to **radioactive wastes** that we may not be aware of. Also, living near a nuclear power plant appears to raise your cancer risk. This increased risk may be due to the **radioactive gases** that are released each day at levels permitted by the U.S. government. This radiation returns to us in rainfall. A University of Pittsburgh radiation physics professor found high breast cancer rates among women in 268 countries who lived within 50 miles of a nuclear plant. In the United Kingdom, a higher rate of leukemia was discovered in children who reside in the vicinity of such a facility.

▪ What You Can Do

If your home is to truly be a refuge for you, you'll want to make sure that it's as toxin-free as possible. Changes are likely to also be in order at the office. Here are some ideas:

Brighten your world by installing full-spectrum lighting in the areas where you spend the most time – This might be by your desk, favorite reading chair, living room sofa, or in the kitchen. These lights can be purchased at many hardware stores or ordered if they are not in stock. Other sources include *www.gaiam.com* and *www. realgoods.com.*

Enjoy the great outdoors – Make a point of spending some time outside each day in natural light. Go for a walk after lunch, sit outside and eat dinner on the porch, read a book under a shade tree, bicycle in the mornings or on weekends. When inside, sit by a sunny window when you can.

If you experience Seasonal Affective Disorder (SAD), consider switching on a light box for longer hours of full-spectrum light exposure. One reason SAD occurs is that the daylight hours are shorter in winter. You can counterbalance this by extending those hours with your own source of full-spectrum light. Full-spectrum light boxes are also available at *www.gaiam.com.*

Make it a top priority to reduce the electrical devices and cords in your bedroom – Most of us spend about one-third of our time in bed, so it is wise to keep your exposure to EMFs especially low in this room. Use a battery-operated clock. Move radios and answering machines away from the head of your bed. Watch TV in the living room.

Get smart about turning off electrical devices and even pulling the plug when they are not in use – Why leave the TV on all evening if you're not watching it? And if the television is still in the bedroom, don't keep it on all night while you sleep. Unplug electrical devices you use only occasionally.

Choose down comforters or layers of wool spreads instead of electric blankets – Sleeping with an electric blanket can expose you to as

FOR EMFS,
THERE'S NO PLACE LIKE HOME

Listed below are the levels of magnetic fields generated by some common household appliances. While EMFs from appliances drop off at about 4 feet, most people stand or sit closer than this distance. If you feel you cannot live without a certain appliance, try to put as much space between the two of you as you can. Also, limit the amount of time that you use the appliance.

	1.2" away	12" away	39" away
Microwave Oven	750 - 2,000[*]	40 - 80	3 -8
Clothes Washer	8 - 400	2 - 30	0.1 -2
Electric Range	60 - 2,000	4 - 40	0.1 - 1
Fluorescent Lamp	400 - 4,000	5 - 20	0.1 - 3
Hair Dryer	60 - 20,000	1 - 70	0.1 - 3
Television	25 - 500	0.4 - 20	0.1 - 2

[*]Measurements are in milligauss.
Source: Adapted from Gauger 1985

As you can see, your hair dryer can produce one of the highest exposures to EMFs, yet this is one appliance you need to keep close to use effectively. This exposure can be minimized by simply allowing your hair to dry naturally on most days.

many as 10 continuous hours of EMFs. Avoid this long exposure by using other types of bed coverings to keep yourself warm.

Reduce your EMF exposure by selecting computer monitors with lower emissions – One way to accomplish this is to use a laptop computer with a LCD screen instead of a traditional desktop computer. (To cut back on radiation exposure, operate the laptop on battery energy and recharge the battery overnight.) Or look for low radiation PC screens, signified as such by a TCO emblem. Those who need to work on regular computers should install a grounded screen guard or at least turn off the screen when possible. Keep the monitor about an arm's length away from you. Unplug a regular computer when it is not in use. Also, put some distance between you and the CPU drive box and the computer printer rather than setting them up right beside you. Products to help counteract the effects of EMFs are available at *www.clarus.com*.

Suspect geopathic stress? Try moving your bed, desk, and favorite chair to new spots in the house – It's not unusual for just one person in a family to be affected by GS. Rearranging the furniture in the spaces where that person spends most of their time can help bring relief. Laying cork tiles under the furniture can also reduce GS's impact. If the problem persists, consult a professional to check the building. Search the web under "geopathic stress" for more research, details, and referrals. One interesting website is *www.geopathicstress.com*.

Think twice before making lengthy unnecessary calls on your cellular phone – Besides the expense of cellular minutes, recent health questions call for caution. They center on possible changes in the brain from microwave radiation. While you may want to have a cellular phone at hand for emergencies and making arrangements, it appears wise to save those longer chats for a regular phone.

Reduce the effects of cell-phone radiation with the use of diodes – Products specifically for this purpose are available through Ener-G-Polari-T (*www.energpolarit.com*).

Is house painting on your "to do list"? Find sources for the least toxic products – For instance, check out the Auro organic house paints at *www.dcn.davis.ca.us/go/sinan/auroinfo.html* and the solvent-free products offered at both *www.healthyeverything.com* and the resource directory in issues of *Natural Home* magazine.

Use safe alternatives to harmful home and garden pesticides – A wide range of natural-based techniques have been developed for ridding your environment of unwelcome critters in the home or garden. Natural products to eliminate pests indoors can be found in health food stores. You can use boric acid or borax to discourage ants and cockroaches. Termites can be eliminated with special microwaving or freezing techniques (*www.tallontermite.com*) rather than with the harmful chemicals typically used. Replace pesticides applied directly to skin that contain DEET (very toxic) with safe alternatives found at sport shops and health food stores; the safer options include Gone by Aubrey Organics (*www.aubrey-organics.com*) and All Terrain Herbal Armor Insect Repellent (1-800-2-INSECT).

Outdoor defenses against unwanted insects include fatty acid soaps, sulfur, horticultural oils, and nontoxic bug traps. Sometimes a periodic flushing of plants with water from the garden hose will do. There is a brand called Safer that offers nontoxic pest control formulas. For a regular supply of ideas, check out *Organic Gardening* magazine (*www.organicgardening.com*). For organic seeds and plants along with gardening tools and additional nontoxic pest control strategies, visit *www.naturalgardening.com*.

FOOD

Consumer demand for both a wide variety of fresh foods and easily prepared meals has vastly altered the foods we eat. Pressured to generate high yields per acre, our farmers are using an ever-increasing number of pesticides as well as genetic engineering. Produce is being exposed to radiation to kill pests and extend shelf life. And, in order to deliver "convenience," manufacturers are overprocessing our foods and stripping them of nutrients while adding harmful ingredients, such a preservatives and artificial colors and flavors. As a result of these developments, we are losing the wholesomeness of the foods we eat. The changes are affecting even what we serve at our own kitchen tables.

Smarter choices are available but will only be made by informed consumers. Let's take a look now at the major areas of concern.

■ Produce

The government is encouraging us to eat five servings of fruits and vegetables a day so we can reduce our risk of cancer and improve our health. Underlying this advice is the recognition that these foods are excellent sources of vitamins, minerals, and fiber. But it is important to also be aware of the hidden dangers of produce when it has been grown or processed in certain ways.

At the top of the list of concerns are **pesticides.** Although the international best-selling book *Silent Spring* by Rachel Carson exposed the dangers of pesticides in 1962, the life-saving information has been highly ignored. Each year in the U.S., over 1.2 billion pounds of pesticides are applied to the land. Now residues of pesticides can be found in the fat tissues of most Americans. Even the EPA has listed pesticides in our foods as one of our nation's most pressing health and environmental issues.

One especially alarming area of discovery concerning pesticides is their ability to mimic natural hormones. In the early 1960s, researchers at Syracuse University discovered that roosters treated with DDT were feminized. This occurred because the DDT affected the roosters' bodies as if it were the female hormone estrogen. Unfortunately we have learned over the years that pesticides are just one of many synthetic chemicals that act as hormone imposters. This issue was recently exposed in the groundbreaking 1996 book, *Our Stolen Future*, by Theo Colborn, Dianne Dumanoski, and John Peterson Myers (with a Foreword from Al Gore). These authors and others warn that such hormone-like chemicals are lowering sperm counts in men, increasing premature hormonal expression in young children, and increasing cancers of the reproductive organs.[11]

A curious development in the processing of produce is the use of **irradiation**. Foods are zapped during this procedure with an amount of radiation that is equal to 10 million X-rays (100,000 rads).[12] The rationale given for this processing centers on the need to kill bacteria and insects, as well as to increase shelf life. However it appears that beneficial food enzymes are also destroyed, levels of vitamins A, C, E, and B are reduced, and chemical toxins called "unique radiolyptic products" (URPs) are created. Irradiation of produce by food processors has been somewhat limited due to the public's concern about its safety, however both fruits and vegetables are on the FDA's irradiation approval list. Other foods that have received the FDA nod of approval include spices, wheat, wheat flour, nuts, beef, poultry, and pork.

PESTICIDES ARE NOT A PAL TO KIDS

Consumption by children of foods containing pesticides has been receiving particular attention recently since their health risks are greater. The reasons for their special vulnerabilty? A five-year, $1.1 million federal study of children and dietary pesticide residues gave the following reasons why the risks for youngsters differ from adults: youngsters tend to eat a smaller range of foods, their food consumption is greater pound for pound than an adult's, and their bodies are moving through critical stages of development.

The Environmental Working Group (EWG) reported that one-third of a child's exposure to, and cancer risk from, pesticides appears to occur *by age five!* In fact, EWG stated that by his or her first birthday, the average American child has already been exposed to more than the lifetime threshold set by the government for certain carcinogenic pesticides. Some health advocates charge that these exposures are tied to learning disabilities and hyperactivity in children.[13]

The good news is that nearly 50% of all mainstream U.S. groceries now carry some organic produce, and the number of natural foods stores is also on the rise. So it is becoming easier to serve organic fruits and vegetables to your children. Americans are now spending an estimated $4.5 billion a year on organic produce. Not only are organic consumers reducing their family's pesticide intake, they are also providing more nutritional bang per bite. A study published in the *Journal of Applied Nutrition* found the nutritional value of organic foods to be about twice that of commercial fare.[14] This additional nourishment can benefit both you and the children in your world.

Concerned parents can contact Mothers and Others (*www. mothers.org*), an organization founded by Meryl Streep and other parents committed to improving food safety. The group lobbies to reduce pesticides and genetic modification in food. Their website is very educational and helpful in the transition to a more "green" diet.

Approval for irradiation of deli meats, frozen foods, prepared fresh foods, fresh juices, seeds, and sprouts has been requested by food processors and is now under consideration by the FDA.

Currently the FDA requires that any *non-meat foods sold in their whole form in a package* (such as wheat flour or oranges) must be labeled if irradiated. Labeling is also mandatory for *fresh whole fruits and vegetables.* The United States Department of Agriculture demands labels for *packaged or unpackaged meat products irradiated in their entirety.* The USDA also says that *any irradiated meat product included in a packaged food* must also be identified as such in the ingredient list. If other individual ingredients in a processed food were irradiated (for instance, spices), notice is not mandatory. At this time, labeling is not required for foods served in restaurants, salad bar fare, hospital or airline meals, items prepared by delis or supermarket take-out departments, spices or herb teas, or supplement ingredients.

Genetically altered produce was sanctioned by a FDA policy paper in 1992. The result is that "genetically engineered" crops are now on the market without special labeling—including those with transplanted genes from fish, toads, etc.! Since the results of ingesting engineered products are unknown, we are all serving as human guinea pigs. Currently legislation requiring labeling for GMOs (genetically modified organisms) is being considered in Congress, and the FDA is holding hearings on the topic. However, the U.S. government's basic position has been that claims of dangers from GMOs are thus far "unfounded" and "unwarranted" and will not stop the marketing of these products.[15]

In the U.S., there are currently more than 50 genetically altered crops and plants that have been approved for use, and the FDA estimates that within the next few years another 150 will be added. *Genetically altered produce includes varieties of soybeans, yellow corn, Russet potatoes, canola, tomatoes, and papaya.*

Research published in *Nature* magazine has already shown that genetically engineered corn designed to ward off insects has killed neighboring monarch butterflies. The monarchs died from ingesting milk thistle that was covered with pollen from the corn. The development has critics worried about other effects that might be taking place in our environment from genetically engineered products.

EUROPEANS JUST SAY "NO" TO GENETICALLY ENGINEERED PRODUCE

Some European nations are resisting the importation of crops that have been genetically engineered by Americans. They are questioning the need for such modifications when weighed against the many unknowns about using the technology. In response, the U.S. is now involved in a boycott of some European products in an attempt to force countries to purchase the genetically engineered foods.

Meanwhile, in England, the British Medical Association called for a moratorium on GMOs until their safety is determined through research. A concerned Prince Charles commented, "Isn't there at least a possibility that the new crops (particularly those that have been made resistant to antibiotics) will behave in unexpected ways, producing toxic or allergic reactions? Only independent scientific research, over a long period of time, can provide the final answer."

■ What You Can Do

Some consumers have increased their intake of fruits and vegetables without considering the special concerns listed above. The following tips can help you make sure that you are making the best choices when purchasing produce:

Don't panic about pesticides; go organic – Look for produce that is certified as coming from an organic source. This means that it was produced without herbicides, insecticides, fungicides, synthetic fertilizers, artificial ripening processes, or growth stimulators. Foods that are irradiated cannot be labeled organic.

Support your local farmers' market or food co-op – These are the places where you are most likely to find the freshest organic produce at the best prices.

Remember the strategies that can help you save money on organic foods – These include watching for in-store specials, buying store brands, shopping in season, and noticing shelf tags designating items that the store has selected for "everyday low prices." *However, when considering the additional expense of organic foods, keep in mind that health is your wealth.* Your investment can pay off in the form of an improved sense of well-being, as well as a lowered risk of cancer and other health concerns tied to absorbing pesticides residues.

Thoroughly wash any regular produce you buy, using some of the new natural products designed for this purpose – Nontoxic products include Environné's (*www.vegiwash.com*) and Fit's (*www.tryfit .com*) Fruit and Vegetable Wash.

Skip the imported produce – It is possible that these fruits and vegetables were grown using pesticides—such as DDT—that have already been banned in the U.S. As an alternative, look for locally grown fruits and vegetables that are in season. Farmer's markets are good places to find produce that has been harvested in your region.

Scan labels for an indication that a food may have been irradiated— and avoid them. You might find a line such as "this product has been treated with ionizing radiation" or "this food has been irradiated." You could also find the irradiation symbol. (See graphic below.) Keep in mind that a single irradiated ingredient (an exception is meat) need not be described as such on the label of multiple-ingredient food products.

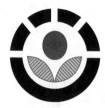

The Irradiation Symbol

This wholesome-looking symbol indicates a food that has been irradiated.

Add fresh, organically grown spices to your shopping list – This is one way to avoid ingesting both pesticide residues and an irradiated food.

Be on the lookout for labels that specifically say the product was *not* irradiated – McCormick, one of our country's largest suppliers of spices, has decided against irradiating its consumer products. This is a rare exception as most spices are irradiated.

Stay tuned for developments in the genetically engineered foods debate and avoid such products whenever possible – Two excellent sources of information are the websites of the Union of Concerned Scientists (*www.ucsusa.org*) and Mothers for Natural Law (*www. safe-food.org*).

Some innovative food manufacturers have already been marking their products as GMO-free options. An extensive listing of GMO-free foods as well as foods that have genetically-modified ingredients can be found at Greenpeace's True Food Shopping List (*www.truefoodnow.org*).

EVEN GOD IS NOT A FRIEND OF GMOs

In November 2000, Pope John Paul II addressed an audience of 50,000 farmers in Italy, reminding them that using genetically modified organisms was contrary to God's will. He urged the farmers to "resist the high temptation of high productivity and profit that work to the detriment of nature," adding that "when (farmers) forget this basic principle and become tyrants of the earth rather than its custodians . . . sooner or later the earth rebels."

Make an impact by writing or calling public officials regarding your concerns about genetic engineering, irradiation, and pesticides – Government policy can be changed through public opinion. Let your thoughts be known! You can reach the national Capitol switchboard by dialing 1-888-449-3511. Find contact information for your state representative at *www.house.gov/writerep* and your senator at *www.senate.gov*. To keep informed, visit the following websites: Organic Consumers Association (*www.purefood.org*), Center for Food Safety (*www.centerforfoodsafety.org*), Pesticide Watch (*www.pesticidewatch.org*) and the National Coalition Against the Misuse of Pesticides (*www.pesticides.org*).

▪ Refined Foods

It was only in the 20th Century that our diet began to include an array of refined food items, including grains, sugars, and fats. This refining process removes important nutrients, and alters the once-natural state of these staples making them toxic to our systems. Today, in our supermarkets, most of the products offered contain refined ingredients instead of whole ones. Our nourishment has been sacrificed for the sake of shelf life and profit. In fact, in America, the largest manufacturing industry is food processing. This powerful lobby attempts to keep the status quo, but fortunately consumer demand is slowly filtering in more wholesome choices.

Eating **refined grains**—for instance, in products made with white flour—deprives us of life-nourishing components, including vitamins, minerals, oils, and fiber. These empty calories deplete the body's reserves of essential nutrients. Over the years, this toxic aspect of our diet can result in premature aging and chronic health concerns. Bread is a good example of a product whose nutrient value has been depreciated. One hundred percent whole wheat bread is only minimally processed. It contains the grain's original amount of fiber, along with B vitamins and the minerals chromium, iron, magnesium, manganese, selenium, and zinc. In contrast, "enriched" white bread—made with grains from which the heart and coating of the wheat is removed—offers significantly less fiber and nourishment. Enrichment adds back only a small amount of the nutrients that were taken away.

Refined sugars—such as table sugar—enter our bloodstreams in a rush, upsetting our internal balance. When consumed habitually, some aspects of our systems remain in constant high drive, while others become worn out from overstimulation. However, in their natural form, the sweet foods from which sugar is manufactured—sugar beet, sugar cane, and corn—contain nutrients that play important roles in maintaining healthy sugar metabolism. These nutrients include B vitamins, magnesium, and chromium.

There has been a shocking increase in our sugar consumption in America. In 1821, the average sugar intake in America was only 10 pounds per person a year; today, this has gone up to 170 pounds—making up over one-fourth of our calories. One reason for this increase is that food manufacturers often add sugar to make processed foods taste more appealing.

Like its cousins, overly processed grains and sugars, **refined oil** is de-mineralized, de-vitaminized, fiberless, and nourishment-empty. In the 1920s, large oil-processing presses using heat technology (rather than the old cold-press methods) were developed. These produced depleted refined oils, contaminated with pesticides and chemical solvents. Oil refinement also changed the fatty acid composition of the oil; oils low in essential fatty acids became common in our groceries. These manufacturing changes took place, in part, to slow the rancidity of oil that naturally occurs. Today most of the oils sold in supermarkets are refined and have undergone some solvent extraction. Healthy alternatives are fresh expeller-pressed oils found in health food stores and virgin olive oils.

About one-third of the oil produced is either *hydrogenated* or *partially hydrogenated* to prevent spoilage. This involves treating the oil with hydrogen gas at high temperatures. The artificial saturation of refined oils with hydrogen hardens them and creates spreadable products. Oils that undergo hydrogenation include coconut and palm, as well as canola and cottonseed oils. Complete hydrogenation removes the essential fatty acid content, and it leaves altered molecules behind, which can be toxic. Partial hydrogenation is used to produce margarine, shortenings, shortening oils, and partially hydrogenated vegetable oils. These contain toxic trans-fatty acids and other altered fat substances. Hydrogenation has been linked to high cholesterol and heart disease.

▪ What You Can Do

Read labels on bread packages carefully to insure that you are really buying an unrefined product – Many breads in supermarkets just add food coloring to make them look like they're made with whole grains. However, when you scrutinize the label, you will see that enriched flour is often the first and main ingredient. Note that sometimes white flour is labeled as "wheat." The word "wheat" used alone describes the refined, nutritionally depleted flour, which is sometimes misleading to consumers. "Wheat" is often confused with "whole wheat," the latter being the unrefined grain that is more nutritious. Unrefined bread usually only contains whole wheat and/or other whole-grain flour, water, yeast, salt, and perhaps honey, nuts, and seeds.

When eating whole grains, such as brown rice, soak them overnight before cooking – This predigestion process neutralizes phytic acid, a substance that otherwise would bind with iron, calcium, phosphorus, and zinc and prevent the absorption of these minerals.

Choose stevia (see "Sweeten Up with Stevia" on page 71), raw honey, date sugar, dehydrated cane sugar juice, or maple syrup over white table sugar – These sweeteners have natural vitamins and minerals. Still, be sure to limit your intake to small amounts.

Avoid refined sugars – This includes table sugar, raw sugar, brown sugar, corn syrup, and fructose.

Be on watch for hidden added sweeteners in processed foods – You might notice any of the following mentioned on food packages: corn syrup, sucrose, honey, malt syrup, high-fructose corn syrup, dextrose, maple sugar, and the artificial sweeteners aspartame (Equal and Nutrasweet) and saccharin.

Satisfy your sweet tooth by eating fruit – Select the varieties that are in season. Enjoy both whole fruit and fruit juice, but in small quantities.

Pass on food products containing hydrogenated or partially hydrogenated oils – How do you know? Look at the label, of course! You will find these highly processed oils in baked goods such as crackers, rolls, muffins, cookies, pies, and doughnuts among other processed foods. Hydrogenated and partially hydrogenated oils are also widely used at fast food restaurants.

Stock up on organic unrefined oils such as extra virgin olive oil and flax seed oil – Other healthy oil choices include coconut, walnut, and sunflower. These unrefined products and others are available from Omega Nutrition (*www.omeganutrition.com*), and can usually be found in most health food stores.

Choose organic butter over margarine – Butter has received a bad rap because of concerns about consumption raising cholesterol levels, yet studies show the increase is minimal. Not so for margarine, which has been tied to high cholesterol levels. Additionally, margarine seems to increase the risk of cancer and heart disease. Use butter moderately.

■ Convenience Foods

Most health experts agree that the poor state of many people's diet today is caused by dependence on "convenience foods." Walking down the aisle of the average supermarket and taking an inventory of what is offered on the shelves is an easy demonstration of this fact. Along with nutrient-stripped refined products, packaged convenience foods can also contain a long list of **additives**. *More than 3,000 additives and preservatives can be found in our food supply today.* Many of these additives are synthetic and toxic. Ingredients not found in nature can be difficult for our bodies to process or may cause health complaints in the short term and disease over time. The health effects are compounded when various additives interact with each other in the body.

SWEETEN UP WITH STEVIA

What if there was a natural sweetener that was delicious, had virtually no calories or toxic side effects, did not adversely raise blood sugar metabolism, and was easy and safe to use? Hard to believe? Think again! Stevia is such a sweetener, and it has been in use for over 100 years.

Very popular and consumed in most industrialized nations, stevia is used in over 40% of soft drinks as a sweetener in Japan. Although not legally approved by the FDA for commercial use as a sweetener or flavoring agent, stevia is available as a dietary supplement on a retail basis. The website *www.stevitastevia.com* has more information on stevia and products made with this wonderful sweetener.

Artificial sweeteners (Equal, Nutrasweet, and saccharin) have many dangerous side effects. See the website *www.holisticmed /com/aspartame* for detailed information on this important topic. Make Stevia your safe choice for sweetening your favorite foods and beverages.

Some noted short-term ill effects of consuming additives are depression of the immune system, an irritation of internal tissues, ADD (attention deficit disorder) and ADHD (attention deficit disorder with hyperactivity). Cancer has been cited as one of the long-term consequences. *Among the more troubling additives are monosodium glutamate (MSG), aspartame, sulfites (sulfur dioxide, sodium sulfite, potassium bisulfite, metabisulfite, bisulfite), nitrates, BHT and BHA, brominated and hydrogenated vegetable oils, propylene glycol, and such artificial colors as red number 40 and yellow number 5.*

A certain subcategory of additives has been identified and termed **excitotoxins.** These ingredients are dangerous combinations of amino acids and can cause an overstimulation of the nervous system. *Particular excitotoxins include MSG, aspartame (Equal or Nutrasweet), L-cysteine, and hydrolyzed vegetable protein (HVP).* Though amino acids are naturally occurring components of food, they are normally consumed in combination with other amino acids and thus easily processed by the body. However when amino acids are taken in the form of excitotoxins, the proper mix is absent and our systems can become overwhelmed. Consumption of excitotoxins by children has been linked with hyperactivity and other behavioral problems. Some believe that eating excitotoxins over a lifetime can contribute to brain disorders such as Alzheimer's. You can find more information on excitotoxins in Chapter 9.

■ What You Can Do

The average American eats an amazing 150 pounds of additives in just one year! Here are some steps you can take to start cutting back:

Review the ingredients on the label before you buy any food – Pass on food products with ingredients that are unpronounceable or unfamiliar to you.

Take note of how you feel after you have eaten foods that contain additives – Are you tired? Disoriented? Do you get headaches? Are you agitated? These are all likely signs that these additives are toxic to your body.

Start cutting back on the number of convenience foods you buy – By dropping these items from your diet, you will eliminate a wide array of toxins.

Be selective. Find foods that are in their natural state or have only been minimally processed – Look for whole grains, fresh fruits and vegetables, nuts and seeds. Consider only lightly processed foods that contain natural ingredients.

In particular, stay away from foods sweetened with aspartame, which is sold under the brand names Equal and Nutrasweet – An estimated 80 to 85% of all complaints registered with the FDA comment about problems with aspartame. Symptoms contributed to aspartame use include dizziness, headache, loss of equilibrium, and eye trouble[16]. Studies have also found aspartame to be addictive.[17]

■ Meat and Dairy

Currently, there are four major questions to have on your mind when you shop for meat and dairy products. First, were antibiotics used in raising the animals? Second, were hormones administered on the farm? Third, was the feed that was provided to the animals organic? And last, have the cuts of beef, chicken, or pork been irradiated? Let's take a closer look now at each of these issues.

THE NAME GAME & HIDDEN MSG

Monosodium glutamate (MSG) is a controversial additive that is used in many foods to enhance the flavor. Because reports of adverse physical reactions have been widely circulated, consumers often attempt to avoid MSG by scrutinizing labels. Unfortunately, looking for the words *monosodium glutamate* is not enough, as manufacturers often play a name game that camouflages the presence of MSG. Some other ingredients that often contain MSG include the following:

- Autolyzed yeast
- Calcium caseinate
- Gelatin
- Glutamate
- Glutamic acid
- Hydrolyzed protein

- Hydrolyzed soy protein
- Monopotassium glutamate
- Sodium caseinate
- Yeast extract
- Yeast food
- Yeast nutrient

Reactions to MSG can be dose-related, wherein some people have noticeable symptoms within 48 hours to a small amount and others to more. Because MSG is highly toxic both in the short and long run, it should be avoided. Symptoms of MSG sensitivity run the gamut from headache, dizziness, nausea, diarrhea, burning sensation of the skin, changes in heart rate, and difficulty in breathing. Ingesting MSG over the years has also been linked with Parkinson's and Alzheimer's. One way to abstain from MSG is to pass on processed foods and to make your own meals from whole, organic ingredients. When eating out, select restaurants that feature cuisine prepared with pure natural foods. For more information on the MSG labeling issue, visit the Truth in Labeling website, *www. truthinlabeling.org.*

Antibiotics are often overadministered to livestock (many animals take in antibiotics in some form every day of their life); thus unhealthful residues are left in the meat that is sold in our markets. Other animal drugs also leave traces behind. Critics warn that some residues have carcinogenic effects.

Hormones are given to both beef cattle and dairy cows, yet the International Agency for Research for Cancer has listed such hormones as known carcinogens. Another danger of eating meat or dairy products with hormone residues is possible resulting abnormalities in the reproductive systems of humans. Beef cattle receive hormones to stimulate their growth and dairy cows to boost milk production.

Note: In January 1999, the Canadian government refused to permit Monsanto Corporation from marketing its Bovine Growth Hormone (rBGH) in their country. The drug is injected into dairy cows to make them produce more milk. A Canadian panel questioned the scientific validity of the FDA's 1993 approval of rBGH.

Additives are not only found in food produced for humans, many are also part of the *commercial feed* given to farm animals. Reasons given for augmenting the feed include disease prevention and growth promotion. Both antibiotics and hormones are added to animal feed. In fact, over 31 million pounds of antibiotics manufactured in the U.S. are mixed into the feed manufactured for cows, pigs, and chickens each year. If the feed is not organic, pesticides are likely to be present. Residues from these chemicals can remain in the meat and dairy products we eat.

Concerns over E. coli and other bacteria were cited as the reason the FDA approved the **irradiation of red meat** in late 1997. Irradiation had already been sanctioned by the agency for fresh and frozen pork and poultry products. Immediately after the 1997 approval, advocacy groups protested by arguing that irradiation depletes nutrients and creates toxins in foods. Recognizing that meat contaminated with bacteria is a serious health threat, protesters called for more sanitary conditions on farms and meat processing plants. They also suggested that new technologies such as probiotics and enzyme treatments for cattle be considered. Groups also pointed to the potential radiation-related dangers that could result from creating irradiation facilities around the country.

▪ What You Can Do

As with all products, a demand for organic meat and dairy will increase their availability. Here is how you can do your part.

Expand your organic shopping to include meat and dairy products –
    Start by visiting these departments in your local health food store. You may find meat available there that was raised by organic

farmers. At the very least, there will probably be "natural meat" sold, which means it is from animals that were not treated with antibiotics or hormones *but were given commercial feed*. Organic dairy products such as Horizon Organic (*www.horizonorganic .com*) and Alta Dena Dairy (*www.altadenadairy.com/organics*) can be found in many supermarkets as well as health food stores.

Spend your dollars on brands of poultry supplied by companies that do not use antibiotics and/or hormones – Shelton's Poultry (*www. sheltons.com*) is one company that distributes their natural free-range poultry to health food stores and supermarkets across the country. Another source is Petaluma Poultry (*www.healthychicken choices.com*), which supplies free-range and organic chicken lines to health food stores, including both the Whole Foods and Wild Oats markets. You'll find more information on the natural chicken issue on both company's websites.

If only nonorganic meat is available at your market, at least make sure it wasn't irradiated – If you see an irradiation symbol and/or notice on the label, buy something else. Packaged and unpackaged meat that has been irradiated are required to be labeled.

Speak up at your markets about your desire for organic meat and dairy – Tell employees and managers at the markets where you shop that you want these products, and reject the irradiated meat. Let the people who supply you with your food know your preferences. Public response has and will make a difference.

■ Fish

Many are increasing consumption of fish as a healthy source of protein. Benefits include the omega-3 fatty acids it contains. However it is wise to shop selectively, as fish can hold **concentrations of industrial pollutants and pesticides.** (Industrial chemicals that accumulate in fish include PCBs [polychlorinated biphenyls] and methyl mercury.) Fish is also a medium where **bacteria** can flourish if this food is not stored properly or is kept for too long before using.

■ What You Can Do

Fish can be so beneficial to your health yet may contain toxins, so be smart about the way you shop for it. The following tips will help:

FISH:
THE BEST TYPES TO BUY

Some varieties of fish are less likely to contain concentrations of toxic chemicals. In his book *Diet for a Poisoned Planet,* author David Steinman provided two lists—one naming the best and safest choices and the other noting those items that are better to skip (because of possible chemical residues). Here are the seafood selections he noted which you're most likely to encounter:

Your Best Buys	Seafood to Avoid
Abalone	Bass (freshwater)
Dungeness crab	Bluefish
English sole	Carp
Flounder	Catfish
Haddock	Cod
Halibut	Lake trout
Mahimahi	Maine lobster
Orange roughy	Mackerel
Pacific salmon (wild)	Norwegian salmon
Scallops	Ocean perch
Sea bass	Shark
Shrimp	Striped bass
Sole	Swordfish
Yellowtail	White perch

In general, pass on most freshwater fish and select deep-water ocean dwellers instead. It is likely that these deep waters are less polluted.

Buy fresh fish only from reputable sources and have it wrapped specifically for you in butcher paper – Some communities have fish markets that have been open for years because of their reputation for having the freshest, cleanest product available. These can be excellent places to shop. If you buy fish from a supermarket, use one that allows you to pick product that is on ice behind the counter.

When you shop at a fish market or grocery with a fish department, ask questions about your possible purchases – Find out which fish might be the best choice that day and where a particular type of fish was caught. Select fish from the most pristine waters possible such as deep-sea locations.

Pick up tips on selecting fresh fish – For instance, the scent of fresh fish is mild and ocean-like. In contrast, rancidity is indicated by a strong smell. If you are buying a whole fish, the scales and fins should cling to the skin and be shiny and translucent. If you select fillets,

---

TROUBLE AT THE FISH FARM

More and more, the United States and other countries are increasing their dependence on farmed fish and harvesting less from dwindling wild sources. In fact, so-called "aquaculture" is one of the fastest expanding segments of American farming. And about 25% of the fish consumed around the world is now farmed.

At first thought, farming may appear to be a good solution for bringing a wider, more affordable array of fish to our kitchen tables. Unfortunately, conservationists and scientists are warning that such facilities can actually be harmful to ocean habitats.

Most fish farms now consist of floating nets or pens. Critics charge that these structures leech microbe-containing sewage into nearby waters, adding to coastal pollution problems. And because of the close quarters, diseases can spread quickly among the farmed fish. Vaccines and antibiotics have been administered to handle such outbreaks, but are also said to be affecting the surrounding environments. Herbicides that are used to control algae travel elsewhere too. Other drugs are also given to the fish as they are raised.

Ironically, more fish may be fed to these farmed fish than is eventually produced! Many of the fish being farmed (such as salmon and trout), are wholly or partly carnivorous. In such cases, roughly three to five grams of fishmeal protein can be used for every gram of fish protein that is produced.

the fish should appear firm and moist and show no brown edges. Discoloration, flakiness, and sliminess are all signs of an aging product. Ask the clerk for more tips on freshness as you develop your knowledge.

Eat wasabi (Japanese green mustard) and ginger with any sushi you consume – These condiments have natural antibacterial and anti-parasitic properties that can destroy unwanted microorganisms in the raw fish.

■ Beverages

Water can be the healthiest drink available, if you use the guidelines described earlier in this chapter to filter or select it. However too many people are in the habit of slugging down **sodas** all day long and are not meeting their basic daily requirements of water. Among the troubling ingredients in sodas are *caffeine, aspartame, sugar,* and *phosphoric acid.* Although the concerns about the other three ingredients have been well publicized, phosphoric acid is a lesser-discussed ingredient. Research is emerging that too much phosphoric acid can affect mineral deposits (particularly calcium) in bone, leading to weaker bones and osteoporosis. In fact, a Harvard University study found that teenaged girls who drink sodas had three times as many bone fractures as those who passed on pop. The researchers speculated that both low milk intake and the high soda consumption had contributed to the higher numbers.

Coffee and some teas are also potent sources of *caffeine*. While caffeine is a naturally occurring substance in plants, it has been associated with cardiovascular disease, fibrocystic breast disease, cancer, and behavioral problems in humans. Coffee itself has been linked with ulcers and heartburn.

Coffee can be hard to avoid, for cups of java seem to be offered everywhere. More than 10 pounds of coffee are consumed per person annually in the United States.[18] Most people drink two or more cups daily.

In addition to its caffeine content, the alarming amount of pesticides used is another concern with java. Most coffee is grown in third world countries, where highly toxic chemicals that are illegal in the States, such as DDT and BHC, are used. Also, the farming methods used to grow nonorganic coffee are rapidly altering ecosystems, especially in the rainforest.

Alcohol—aside from having addictive qualities—often contains a variety of toxins. These include *pesticides* (from the vineyards) and *lead* (from the foil around the corks). Drinking alcohol also strains the body's detoxification capacity, as the liver becomes focused on processing the alcohol in one's system at the expense of other functions. Since excess alcohol is stored in the liver, binge drinking can lead to cirrhosis of the liver and hepatitis. Research has also shown an association between alcohol consumption and cancers of the mouth, esophagus, liver, and breast.

■ What You Can Do

On an average day, your body loses about 10 cups of water through various bodily functions including perspiration. And on a hot or particularly rigorous day, the amount can be much higher. As human beings, we need to be sure to take in enough liquids to keep our systems running smoothly. Here are some ideas for meeting your needs for fluids without taking in those pesky toxins:

Make it easy to sip pure water all day by setting a full glass on your desk each morning – Select a glass that is appealing to you, and refill it during breaks.

Instead of indulging in soda, make a refreshing drink yourself – Pour a glass half full with sparkling water and fill the rest with the organic fruit juice of your choice.

If you cannot live without your java, choose organic regular or decaffeinated coffee – Coffee from Urth Café, Allegro, and the Thanksgiving Coffee Company are several brands committed to sustainable growing techniques.

For variety, try different herbal teas—both hot and iced – You can find some natural brands, such as Celestial Seasonings, on the store shelves. Watch out for and avoid brands that mix caffeinated teas with herbal. Celestial Seasonings offers a natural fruit tea line that is refreshing iced; try Wild Cherry Blackberry, Raspberry Zinger, Cranberry Cove, or the Country Peach Passion flavor. Organic tea lines can be found at most health food stores and some supermarkets.

Go organic when it comes to selecting wine too – Avoid the high concentrations of pesticides sprayed on the grapes used to make wine. Try organic wines sold at health food stores, liquor stores, upscale supermarkets, or via the Internet. Companies that sell organic wines include Chartrand Imports (*www.midcoast.com/~chartran/index. html*), Frey Vineyards (*www.travelenvoy.com/wine/organicwines .htm*), the Four Chimneys Farm Winery (*www.travelenvoy.com/ wine/organicwines.htm*), and the Organic Wine Company (*www. ecowine.com*).

Take the lead off – Wipe the top of wine bottles thoroughly after removing the foil at the top and before pouring. This will help get rid of lead residues. Use a moist, clean, cotton dishtowel and toss it in the clothes bin afterwards.

Consult Chapter 9 for nutritional tips if cutting back on caffeine and/or alcohol – Since nutritional imbalances often contribute to cravings of addictive substances, proper nutritional support is a valuable aid during the detoxification process.

■ Packaging

Another way toxins get into our foods is from packaging. Unfortunately substances from **plastic, aluminum foil, aluminum cans, product boxes,** and **takeout containers** can migrate. For instance, cling film wrapping—used to cover cheese as well as packaged fruit, vegetables, meat, and fish—may transfer DEHP or DEHA (both carcinogens) into foods. Its cousin, plastic wrap, might add vinylidene chloride, another identified carcinogen. These toxins in plastic wrap have the hormone-mimicking properties that are believed to be linked to reproductive cancers. Aluminum bowls or foil wrapping enable aluminum to move into stored food. Chemical components in microwave packaging also leaches into many foods such as popcorn, pizza, French fries, and fish sticks. If the microwave package is designed to also be used in a conventional oven, it may transfer even more chemicals there. Polystyrene ("Styrofoam") also transfers toxins and alone contributes about 4 billion pounds of trash a year.

■ What You Can Do

Frequently you can make choices about the packaging you use yourself or endorse with your purchasing dollars. Though it will take some effort in the beginning, you will be consciously building a new and more health-supportive routine:

Avoid plastic bags and wrapping on such items as fruits, vegetables, meat, or fish – For produce, buy the items loose and place them in paper bags. For meat or fish, buy these foods fresh and have them wrapped in butcher paper.

Select eggs in cardboard containers – Protect the environment at the same time that you are reducing toxins by selecting cartons made of recycled cardboard.

Opt for waxed paper to cover your stored food – This is a much better choice than aluminum foil or plastic wrap. Store larger quantities of leftovers in glass bowls with accompanying glass covers.

Favor glass bottles for your beverages if available – Reach past the plastic bottles and aluminum cans.

Watch for canned goods with protective enamel linings at the health food store – Some brands sold at health food stores use cans that are lined to prevent tin or lead soldering from entering the food.

Pass on Styrofoam products whenever possible – Reusable dishes and mugs are safer for you and kinder to the environment.

■ Food Preparation

Part of clearing your life of toxins is being aware of the ways undesirable elements can enter our meals during food preparation. What is the point of making the effort to buy nontoxic food if it is then tainted during the cooking process?

Half of the **cookware** that is sold today contains **aluminum**, even though this metal can migrate into our foods while they are on the stove. Ingesting aluminum can lead to neurological changes in the brain, a gradual mental deterioration, and eventually contribute to the development of Alzheimer's disease. Even in the short term, people have reported symptoms shortly after they switched to a set of aluminum pots and pans. Some researchers believe *fluoride in water* increases the leaching of aluminum from such cookware.

Nonstick cookware can emit toxins from the *synthetic lining*. A demonstration of this is the fact that bird lovers have learned that polytetraflouethylene (PTFE) fumes from overheated nonstick pans can actually kill their feathered friends. The birds' smaller size and lung capacity make them more susceptible to these toxins. However, the fumes are not good for people either. Usually these pots and pans also have *aluminum* as their base, which adds to their toxic contribution.

FIGHT BACK AGAINST TOXINS FROM PLASTICS WITH CALCIUM D-GLUCARATE

Some toxins in our foods—including chemicals that migrate from plastic wraps and plastic bottles—can mimic the estrogens that are linked to breast cancer and other hormone-related illnesses. In addition to avoiding beverages and foods delivered in plastic containers, you can also supplement with Calcium D-Glucarate to remove this dangerous estrogen buildup. A daily dose of three 500 mg. capsules is recommended. Calcium D-Glucarate is quite effective. When given to rats bred to have a 100% chance of developing cancer, this supplement reduced the rate to just 56%.

As an alternative to stovetop cooking, many people have become dependent on their **microwave ovens** because of the speed and convenience. However, there are growing suspicions that microwaves may cause chemical changes in foods as a result of the intensity of the electromagnetic waves that move through items during the cooking process.

Also, depletion of nutrients caused by microwaving appears to be higher than from cooking on the stove. The concerns about the changes caused by microwave ovens have been given focus around the issue of microwaving milk for infants. In the *Journal of Pediatrics*, researchers at Stanford University found that immunoglobulin-A antibodies (which provide passive immunity for infants) were destroyed in milk during microwaving. The destruction of the immune factor resulted in an abundance of E. coli, a potentially harmful bacteria that is usually kept in check by the immunoglobulin-A.[19] This concern led to a decision by the school's medical center to stop warming breast milk in microwaves.

A common but toxic method of cooking is deep-frying. **Fried foods** are so popular in America, in fact, that more than 400 million pounds of commercial frying oil are used each year. Despite a growing awareness about cutting down on fat intake, deep-fried foods (such as french fries) remain popular fare at fast food restaurants. In fact, french fries have unfortunately become one of the favorite "vegetable foods" eaten by children in the U.S. While the fat content is high in fried foods, that is not the only danger here. Another problem is that the cooking oil breaks down with repeated use, forming a nasty mix of toxins. Also, frying creates free radical damage in the food, which is another form of toxicity.

An additional food preparation technique that has come under scrutiny is **barbecuing.** The high temperature cooking involved can create mutations in the food, especially if items are charred. Some of the resulting "mutagen" compounds have been linked to cancer and birth defects. Studies have found that when PhIP (a substance produced in high-temp cooked meat) was fed to lab rats, tumors developed in the animals' mammary glands. Also, a German study of 900 women showed that those who ate lots of charred and grilled meats had a two-fold greater risk of breast cancer than female participants who rarely or never consumed these foods.[20] On a related note, drippings from chicken, beef, or fish can splash down on hot coals during barbecuing and create a carcinogen called benzopyrene. This chemical is returned to the food through smoke.

A last area of concern is actually part of the serving process—that is, the **dishes and glassware** you use at home. Particularly dangerous can be items *purchased while traveling in other countries.* These glasses, pots, mugs, and plates may contain cadmium and/or lead. Craftware and older dishes may also leach toxins. The FDA put limits on the cadmium and lead levels allowable in ceramicware in 1980 and lowered the amounts in 1991. Most U.S. manufacturers now meet the U.S. standards. Note that crystal glassware can be a source of lead and should only be used on an occasional basis.

■ What You Can Do

When it comes to the concerns related to food preparation, there are many things you can do to protect yourself from toxins.

Switch to stainless steel cookware – Stainless steel appears to be one of the safest materials for cooking. To prevent food from sticking, use a natural olive oil spray.

Use your microwave oven sparingly, if at all – Microwaving may be a little faster than some other cooking methods, but are the risks really worth it? If you do occasionally use a microwave, limit its use to briefly heating up foods instead of high-heat cooking.

Choose fried foods only on rare occasions and try broiling instead – Foods to avoid include french fries, donuts, and tempura. Note that some restaurants are discovering alternative cooking methods such as creating a french fry-like food by baking the potatoes. If you eat fried foods once in a while, increase your fruit and vegetable intake to supply your body with free-radical-scavenging antioxidants.

Cut back on barbecuing and do not use it as a regular cooking technique – If you like the barbecued taste, one way to reduce toxins is to precook foods and set them on the grill for shorter periods.

Acquire dinnerware from U.S. manufacturers who assure their safety – Most American manufacturers have 800 numbers that you can call to check if their dinnerware contains lead. There are also testing kits available. The Environmental Defense Fund lists the lead content of 8,000 china patterns on their website at *www.edf.org/pubs /Brochures/LeadinChina*.

■ Eating Out

In response to the ever-increasing pace of society, Americans are relying on restaurant food more then ever before in our history. According to the National Restaurant Association, sales at U.S. eateries reached over $336 billion in 1998—up by more than 4.5% over the previous year. Fast food restaurants also experienced an upswing, with sales of over $105 billion that year. In fact, it is estimated that over 200 fast-food hamburgers are eaten every second in this country!

In order to eat healthy while dining out, you must be knowledgeable about the hidden dangers of restaurant food as well as what items to just generally avoid. As you become more informed about good nutrition, some of this will simply involve common sense. Other decisions will require some deliberate self-education.

Note that restaurant food is another potential source of toxic **food additives**. Though you may be aware of asking the waiter if they add *monosodium glutamate* (MSG) to their food at a Chinese restaurant, did you know that it is already in many prepared soups and gravies that are supplied to eateries? While dining away from home, also watch the *salt* intake. Some Chinese dishes, such as Kung Pao Chicken and Orange Beef, are loaded with it.

The tendency to serve **huge portions** at restaurants can also deliver too much of a bad thing. Realize that although the price looks cheap for larger sized meals at fast foods joints, what they deliver is really no bargain when considered from a health viewpoint.

■ What You Can Do

The good news for consumers is that restaurateurs are taking notice of the demand by consumers for healthier choices. In a report on industry trends, the National Restaurant Association mentioned a growth in requests for organic foods, locally grown produce, and vegetarian entrees. Though it may be difficult or impossible to find restaurants serving organic entrees in your area, most menus will feature at least a few healthier choices. How do you continue to avoid toxins when you eat out? The following ideas can help.

Frequent restaurants that promote healthy eating – Some restaurants make a special effort to serve nutritious and clean meals. Look for ads in local publications geared toward alternative health and ask friends where they dine. If you discover such an eatery on your own, spread the word.

Scan menus for specialty items that emphasize good nutrition – If you find this missing, ask the waiter how they accommodate health-conscious patrons.

When at fast food joints, ask for broiled or roasted sandwiches – Chicken breast sandwiches and salads are healthier choices. Mexican fast food can be healthy—emphasize beans, rice, lettuce and tomatoes, and skip the fried options.

Remember that you can always take food home – That is what doggy bags are for. Restaurant portions are notoriously large in the United States.

Develop a taste for the finer things in life - Learn to enjoy the real flavors of food. Our tastes buds are so desensitized that we have been led to believe that the over-salted, over-sugared, microwaved junk we call food actually is enjoyable. Have you noticed when people return from a trip to Italy, after eating food prepared from fresh ingredients as well as passion and love, they have to "adjust" back to the "taste" of devitalized American food? Never in the history of humankind has a culture viewed eating as something to be done as fast and conveniently as possible.

To the contrary: throughout history, in most cultures sharing meals has been considered a sacred ritual – breaking bread – "holy communion." There is nothing like enjoying meals with friends, especially when they are well-prepared.

Whether eating out or at home, choose a relaxing environment to enjoy your meals - Rushed eating in noisy, chaotic environments is one reason that indigestion and heartburn are at epidemic levels in this country. It is important to make a conscious effort to support your body as it digests the healthier foods you are taking in. Take the time to find a quiet space for your meals, relax and thoroughly chew your food, and savor all the delicious flavors. If you find that you are upset at mealtime, take some time out before you eat to sort through your feelings and calm down.

■ Personal Care Products

It's natural to want to look your best, but many people fail to realize their primping could be causing a toxic overload. Makeup, perfumes and colognes, hair colorings, deodorants, toothpastes, shampoos, and dry cleaning all can deliver toxins that your body could well do without. The story really isn't so pretty!

One benefit of detoxification is that you will have less of a need to enhance your appearance with toxic personal care products. Actually, personal care products are often used to cover up the effects of toxins, such as pimples and wrinkles. Over the years, I have seen many patients' coloring and skin condition improve dramatically through detoxifying. With time, you'll achieve a natural healthy glow that is very attractive. Note: The use of nontoxic personal care products can enhance your natural beauty.

There are many reasons to avoid toxic personal care products. What follows are some of the major concerns.

Commercial cosmetics are severely underregulated and undertested for safety. Over 850 toxic chemicals are available for use in makeup; two particularly potent ones are *diethanolamine (DEA)* and *triethanolamine (TEA)*. These commonly used chemicals can combine with others to produce carcinogens known as *nitrosamines*. Of the makeup products that are tested by the FDA, 37% contained nitrosamines. Another concern about makeup is that the carcinogen, *formaldehyde*, is released by preservatives added to these products.

Though **perfumes and colognes** bring up images of flowering meadows and forest sanctuaries, the truth is that many of these products are made from petrochemicals and other toxic synthetic ingredients. *A shocking 95% of the chemicals used in perfumes and colognes come* *from petroleum!* Adverse reactions to scents can include headaches, allergies, skin rashes, asthma attacks, nausea, irritability, and memory loss.

The record of **hair dyes** is deadly. People who use them over their lifetime significantly increase their risk of non-Hodgkin's lymphoma, multiple myeloma, leukemia, and Hodgkin's disease. In fact, the National Cancer Institute has determined that as many as 20% of cases of non-Hodgkin's lymphoma are related to the artificial coloring of hair. The risk for negative health effects is highest for those who use dark or red shades rather than light colors.

Certain ingredients in **shampoos** should also be avoided, because of their carcinogenic and other ill health effects. Formaldehyde is a possible by-product of some substances including *polyethylene glycol* and *DMDM hydantoin.* Other toxic elements are *DEA, propylene glycol, sodium lauryl sulfate (SLS), sodium laureth sulfate (SLES), coal tar, polysorbates 60 and 80, quaterium 15,* and *numerous coloring agents such as FD&C Blue 1 or D&C Red.*

Mass-market **toothpastes** also contain questionable ingredients. Manufacturers may add *saccharin, FD&C Blue 1,* or *polysorbate 80.* All three are suspected carcinogens. *Fluoride,* which is in wide use in this industry, is also under scrutiny as a contributor to increasing cancer risk.

One of the major issues with commercial **deodorants and antiperspirants** is that many contain *aluminum,* which has been associated with Alzheimer's disease. A study in the *Journal of Clinical Epidemiology* verified that risk of the disease could increase along with lifetime use of such products when they contain aluminum. Many *colorings* used to enhance the appearance of these products are suspected carcinogens. Other problem ingredients include *triclosan* (linked to liver damage) and *zirconium-based products* (linked to inflamed nodules of tissue with prolonged use). Chemicals in deodorants and antiperspirants are instantly absorbed into the body when applied under your arms.

Feminine hygiene products, such as tampons and sanitary pads, are usually bleached with toxic chemicals and contain dioxin, a carcinogenic material. Dioxin has been linked to reproductive cancers, endometriosis, as well as other immune disorders. The rayon also found in commercial tampons seems to enhance the absorption of dioxin.

Though you take your garments to the dry cleaners to purge them of dirt and odors, you are actually bringing home toxins that were not in your clothes to begin with. **Dry-cleaning** solvents include such toxic ingredients as *benzene, chlorine, formaldehyde, toluene, naphthalene,* and *perchloroethylene.* The impact from fumes is at its worst if you leave slightly damp dry-cleaned clothes hanging encased in plastic bags; such items can take a week to dry. These chemicals are so toxic that if you are going to buy a house near a dry-cleaning facility, many cities require that the prospective buyer sign an acknowledgement of the toxicity prior to closing escrow.

▪ What You Can Do

More and more nontoxic brands are becoming available in the area of personal care products. Some even include organically grown or wildcrafted ingredients. Here are alternatives you can try to what's described above:

When it comes to makeup, skip the fragrance – Unscented cosmetics are now sold that contain little or no petrochemical derivatives. These cleaner products can be found in health foods stores and some department stores. Makeup with organic ingredients includes Jurlique (*www.jurlique.com*), Dr. Hauschka (*www.drhauschka.com*), and Aubrey Organics (*www.aubrey-organics.com*).

Pick essential oils from plant sources in place of perfumes and colognes – These are the oils that are used in aromatherapy. You can use a single oil or a blend. They come in sprays, roll-ons, or dropper bottles.

Talk to your hairdresser about Igora Botanic or other lines of natural or less-toxic hair colorants – Semi-permanent products, Igora Botanic colors are plant-based and biodegradable. Other nontoxic brands include VitaWave Creme Color Sets and the Antica Herbatint/ Vegetal Color lines. Or try a natural henna, such as the 100% organic Rainbow Henna product.

Shop for a mild, high-quality, natural shampoo – Jurlique (*www. jurlique.com*) has an interesting line, including their Lavender Essence and Sandalwood Essence Shampoos. Aubrey Organics (*www.aubrey-organics.com*) and Aveda (*www.aveda.com*) are two other nontoxic brands.

Pick antiperspirants/deodorants and toothpastes made from nontoxic ingredients – Two such products are Tom's of Maine's Stick

Deodorant (*www.tomsofmaine.com*) and Jurlique's Deo Spray Deodorant (*www.jurlique.com*). Toothpastes include Tom's of Maine's Natural Fluoride-Free and Weleda (*www.weleda.com*).

Choose tampons and pads made from 100% organic unbleached cotton – Companies such as Organic Essentials, Natracare, and Terra Femme carry a wide range of safe feminine hygiene products.

Scale down your dry cleaning pile and look for cleaners using nontoxic solutions – Even though a piece of clothing comes with a label "dry clean only," this does not mean it is necessarily so. Many items you take to your dry cleaners could be washed with care at home. Also, some areas have dry cleaners that purposely use an alternative to the toxic chemical perchloroethylene or various petroleum cleaning fluids. One such progressive company is Cleaner By Nature of Southern California, which utilizes a new technology called "wet cleaning." A list of other firms using "wet cleaning" is available on a Greenpeace site at *www.greenpeace usa.org/media/factsheets/wetcleanlist.htm*. The organization also provides background on the wet cleaning process.

■ Toxic Habits

As you are now quite aware, every day we make choices that either bring beneficial elements into our lives or toxic ones. When it comes to our personal habits, we sometimes identify closely with something that is toxic. We might see it as part of who we are. It's important to ask yourself whether you really want to continue the same behavior or if there is an alternative you would enjoy just as much or more. The following are some areas for you to evaluate.

Even with all the media reports and campaigns about the dangers of **smoking**, new customers start lighting up every day—most of them teen-aged or younger. Though reports of possible health effects began surfacing in the 1950s, we are now seeing the legacy of a lifetime of lighting up—related increases in lung and other cancers, heart disease, stroke, and chronic lung diseases such as emphysema and bronchitis. It has become so bad that *the American Cancer Institute estimates that one in five deaths in the United States today is the result of the use of tobacco.* And over the past 20 years, we have also been learning of the very serious dangers of "second-hand smoke" or "passive smoking." Underlying all of this is the fact that cigarettes contain over 4,000 known toxins.[21]

ESSENTIAL OILS – Nature's Fragrance Does More Than Just Smell Good

Inhaling perfumes and colognes pulls toxins into our bodies. What's the solution? Pure essential oils from plants.

Try this experiment to experience the oxygenating effects of essential oils vs. the toxic, oxygen-depleting effects of synthetic fragrances. The next time you walk through the cosmetic section of a department store, ask yourself if you feel like breathing deeply. Probably not. Next, locate a health food store that stocks essential oils, find a fragrance you like, and inhale the scent deeply. Notice how much you want to breathe in the natural scent. If you have ever visited a spa, you may have had a similar aromatic delight.

Aromatherapy is the name for the use of pure essential oils derived from plants. These oils can be inhaled or applied directly to the body. In addition to their pleasant scent, essential oils have various health benefits such as mood balancing, reduction of anxiety and depression, immune support, pain relief, circulation improvement, and energy enhancement. Essential oils increase oxygen availability in the body and provide antioxidant protection—unlike synthetic perfumes, which contribute to free radical damage in the body. Essential oils are detoxifying and good for you – synthetic perfumes add toxins.

At the Santa Monica Wellness Center, we use essential oils throughout the day, different ones with different patients. People walk in and say, "Oh, it smells so wonderful in here, what is it?" What they're smelling is actually a blend of the oils that were used that day. This is kind of like when you walk into a great restaurant and it smells so good, you say, "I'll take whatever I smell," but it's really the combination of the delicious foods that have been prepared all day.

When choosing essential oil products, look for those made with organically grown plants, such as Jurlique (*www.jurlique.com*) and Simplers (*www.simplers.com*). Be aware that aromatherapy is a buzzword now and many brands are actually completely or partially synthetic. The fancy labeling of the synthetic products can lead you to believe they are natural when they are not.

Like smoking, **recreational drugs** have been glamorized in film and on television. Yet many of these drugs deliver potent toxins. There are suspicions that active agents in *marijuana* can decrease immune function and fertility and strong evidence that smoking pot contributes to lung disease and cancer. *Cocaine, amphetamines, hallucinogens,* and *narcotics* all put extreme stress on the body during use and leave toxic residues that linger. Research has linked the destruction of brain cells to the use of the currently popular party drug, *ecstasy.*

Though doctors write the prescriptions, have *you* given deep thought to the real necessity of the **medication** you are currently taking? Could one or more of them be overkill or a wish for a quick solution without any effort on your part? Many prescribed drugs are just as hard on the body as recreational ones, despite the relief they may bring. *Nontoxic, natural remedies are often available, which are friendlier to the body but just as effective.*

Surveys show that 20 to 25% of Americans do not **exercise** and another third aren't moving enough to receive a health benefit. Yet *research is proving that the health gains from regular exercise are impressive.* In the short term, you begin to feel less stressed, have more energy, lose weight, and sleep better. And in the long run, you have less risk of developing many of the most common serious diseases, have greater mobility and flexibility, sharpen your mental capabilities, and experience higher levels of health in old age. *Exercise also enhances the body's natural detoxification process.* For instance, the largest excretory organ that the body has is our skin. Through physical activity, you will flush out toxins through skin oil and sweat. In addition, regular exercise will improve the circulation in both your cardiovascular and lymphatic systems, which fosters the removal of harmful toxins from your cells.

Note: You want to be careful not to engage in physical activity in such a way that would add to the toxic load your body already endures. For instance, in the air pollution section, it was suggested that you walk at times and in areas where traffic is at its lowest. If you swim in a chlorinated pool, you may want to vary your routine with other types of exercise to reduce your exposure to chlorine.

▪ What You Can Do

Most of us could benefit from cleaning up our habits in some ways. It is easy to get locked into practices that do not serve our highest good.

They became part of our routine; something we seem to do without even thinking. What's important is to bring unhealthy habits into our conscious awareness so we know once again that we have a choice. Here are some of the new choices you can begin to make in place of the toxic habits described above.

Develop strategies for relieving tension besides smoking – In a way, smokers are on the right track when they attempt to relax by puffing on a cigarette. Deep breathing can be quite relaxing—on its own. You don't need to add in the nicotine and the other toxins contained in cigarettes. If you smoke, begin to pay attention to when you reach for the pack. Then instead of smoking, choose to practice some relaxed breathing or even a bit of meditation if it's possible to take a little break. The reward may be that you find your need for cigarettes decreases. If you are really having difficulty breaking the habit, seek professional help. Acupuncture and hypnotherapy are two therapies with excellent track records in aiding smoking cessation.

Spend some time journaling or meditating to discover the feelings you may be escaping through recreational drugs – Ignoring or pushing down uncomfortable feelings only gives them more power. Make it a point to have some quiet time with yourself for reflection and renewal. Other strategies for emotional balancing are presented in Chapter 13.

Turn to prescription and over-the-counter medications only when really needed – Avoid the knee-jerk reaction of popping a pill every time you have a physical problem. Seek natural alternatives first, and only take synthetic medications as a last resort. To reach this goal, you will want to seek counsel from a practitioner who understands both the traditional and complementary approaches to medical care. *Of course, never make any changes in your medication without guidance from your health care practitioner.* Two sources for ideas to discuss with your health care professional include the books *Natural Alternatives to Over-the-Counter and Prescription Drugs* by Michael T. Murray and *Prescription Alternatives* by Virginia Hopkins and Earl Mindell.

If recreational or prescription drugs have become an addiction, it is crucial to seek professional help – Although *The Detox Solution* can be a valuable aid during a drug detox process, it is not enough.

Professional help is essential. There are usually treatment facilities in most cities.

Make getting regular exercise a priority; even 20 minutes three times a week brings benefits – If you are not exercising, begin with small blocks of time and work up to more. In this way, you'll avoid injury and it will be easier to get started. Research has shown that just 20 minutes of working out three times a week for one year will add five extra months to your life. Five years at that level will add more than two years. Longer stretches of regular exercise will extend your life even further. And you'll be healthier longer too!

▪ Getting Started

By now, you probably have a long list of toxins that you'd like to avoid in the future. Although toxicity is a reality of today's world, you *can* put a positive twist on the process of removing them. Place your emphasis on recognizing the vast resources for nontoxic and supportive items you can add to your life! In fact, by discovering the sources of toxins, you have opened the door to a whole new world of positive possibilities.

Proceed with the changes at a comfortable pace and don't be hard on yourself for not being able to make them overnight. Even small changes make a difference! If you just switched to pure water and continued this habit, it would have a significant positive effect. And as you progress further, you will see even greater results as the drain on your body's resources is reduced. You'll be rewarded with greater energy, a brighter outlook, improved health, and a higher quality of living!

FOUR

Toxins in Your Body:
How Using Enzymes, The Detox Superstars, Can Help

**Man is not nourished by what he swallows,
but by what he digests and uses.**

— Hippocrates, Greek physician known
as "the Father of Medicine"

n Chapter 3, we explored how toxins from the outside get into our systems and the many ways that we can prevent this from happening. In this chapter, we will look at how toxins are actually created *inside* our bodies. These *"internal"* or *"endogenous toxins"* are the by-products of imbalances in the digestion system. As you will learn, their presence can have some uncomfortable and dangerous effects.

Lack of enzymes in food contributes to poor digestion and the resulting internal toxicity. One way to promote good digestion, and therefore avert the formation of these internal toxins, is to supplement your diet with digestive enzymes and eat foods that contain them in rich supply.

What is an enzyme, and why are they so important in preventing autointoxication and facilitating detoxification? Enzymes are catalysts to every chemical reaction in your body, and are extremely important in the digestive process. They facilitate optimal nutrient delivery and the efficient excretion of wastes at the cellular level. Yet facilitating complete digestion is only one of the many duties that enzymes are responsible for. Over 3,000 types of enzymes responsible for a multitude of duties have been identified in the human body so far by researchers, and thousands more are believed to exist.

When enzymes are in ample supply, their work keeps your body running at an optimal level. In this high state, more effective detoxification can take place. Because enzymes can play such a crucial role in keeping you in an excellent state of health, much of this chapter is devoted to the topic. You'll also read about the success of enzymes used to treat numerous chronic health conditions.

First, let us delve into the issue of internal toxins and the part enzymes play in warding off their appearance. To understand how internal toxicity is produced, you will need to become acquainted with the main stages of digestion—both what should occur and what actually takes place in most cases today.

Reminder: Do you recall the Alexis Carrell experiment on page two that showed that in order for organisms to thrive, they must properly digest their nutrients and eliminate their toxic waste products? The information in this chapter is based on this basic health principle.

DIGESTION STEP-BY-STEP

As you learned in the last chapter, food is one area that is most emphasized with respect to avoiding toxins. This makes a lot of sense when you consider the volume of food (and the load of possible accompanying external toxins—additives, pesticide residues, etc.) that the digestive tract handles. Over a lifetime, *more than 25 tons of food moves along its passageways!*[1] This food also has the potential to produce a debilitating amount of toxicity internally. To avoid the creation of internally generated toxins, good digestion must be maintained. A large proportion of the toxicity contributing to chronic illness, low energy and weight problems comes from poorly digested foods and the subsequent internal toxins that are generated.

The following two scenarios for digestion—the ideal versus the real—will help you become more aware of the many factors involved in processing the food you eat, as well as the numerous ways that you can support the health of the digestive tract.

STEP 1. **Ideal: Whole food enters the mouth.** This is food of superior quality that has not been refined, irradiated, sprayed with pesticides, etc. This ideal food is loaded with vitamins, minerals, enzymes, etc.

Reality: With the availability and popularity of processed foods, most of what we are actually eating does not deliver optimal nourishment. Instead most of the food has been sprayed with chemicals and stripped of its nutrients. If it has been irradiated or heated above 118 degrees (enzymes cannot live above this temperature), the food has absolutely no enzymes—those substances essential for optimal digestion.

STEP 2. **Ideal: Food is chewed well.** Saliva provides the enzymes amylase (for carbohydrates), lipase (for fat), and a little protease (for protein), which are released during the chewing process. These enzymes initiate digestion. Food is thoroughly masticated in the mouth until it becomes as liquefied as possible. Protein molecules are tagged by saliva for more efficient digestion later.

Reality: Many people tend to eat in a hurried, rushed manner. The ever-increasing popularity of fast food testifies to this development. If food isn't thoroughly chewed and soaked in saliva, digestion will be compromised.

STEP 3. **Ideal: Enzyme-rich food enters the upper part of the stomach where the enzymes from saliva and the food do some of their best work on digestion.** Keep in mind that *there must be enzymes in the food* for this to be accomplished at a desirable level.

Reality: Most of the food we eat today contains absolutely no digestive enzymes. The only foods that contain digestive enzymes are those that come from plants or animals and are uncooked (not heated over 118 degrees). This is the only time in history in which people have attempted to live on a diet consisting mostly of enzyme-depleted foods. If Step 3 is skipped or incomplete in the upper part of the stomach due to a lack of enzymes in the food, digestion will be further compromised. Proteins should be predigested here, and if this process is incomplete, by-products of compromised protein digestion are likely to show up as toxic residue in the stool. The toxic by-products have been linked to various health conditions, such as depression, anxiety, cardiac arrthymia, headaches, and cancer.[2]

STEP 4. **Ideal: Food enters the lower part of the stomach where hydrochloric acid (HCl) is secreted.** HCl aids in the conversion of pepsinogen (an inactive enzyme form) to pepsin (a protein-digesting enzyme). The acidic environment created by HCl is crucial to the assimilation of certain minerals, such as calcium and iron, as well as to prevent an overgrowth of unwanted parasites and bacteria. At this stage, there is a small amount of lipase (a fat-digesting enzyme) secreted to initiate some fat digestion.

Reality: With the onslaught of antacid commercials, it is easy to forget that *we actually do need acid in our stomach for proper digestion.* For instance, people suffering from osteoporosis (a disease marked by brittle bones) often lack enough stomach acid.[3] Since bone-strengthening *calcium needs an acidic environment in the stomach to be absorbed*, it is ironic that certain commercial antacids market themselves as a great source of this mineral! Antacids compromise the absorption of calcium and other minerals and also interfere with the digestion of protein. Adequate protein digestion is also essential for a healthy stomach lining.

STEP 5. **Ideal: Now the food moves on to the small intestine where more digestion and absorption takes place.** Enzymes are secreted from the pancreas. Bile is secreted by the liver, emulsifying the fats. In the small intestine, individual components of food—amino acids (from the protein), simple sugars (from the carbohydrates), fatty acids (from fats), vitamins, minerals, etc.—are absorbed into the bloodstream. These materials are further metabolized and are used by the body for repair, energy, and the maintenance of health.

Reality: If the food is deficient in digestive enzymes, the pancreas is forced to dispense huge amounts of these biochemical catalysts. This is stressful to the gland. Research shows that animals that receive adequate enzymes in their diets are likely to have healthy pancreases, whereas animals fed an enzyme-depleted (cooked food) diet develop enlarged pancreases. In order to create extra digestive enzymes, the pancreas must "steal" metabolic enzymes meant to be used by other parts of the body. The body then chemically remodels them into digestive enzymes. Because the enzymes were not in the food as Nature intended, the whole body suffers from this deprivation.

STEP 6. **Ideal: The remaining liquid and undigested food move into the large intestine** (also called the colon). Here fluid and minerals can be absorbed into the body. The large intestine is where the beneficial bacteria (such as acidophilus) manufacture some vitamins, such as vitamin K. They also keep harmful bacteria at bay, and prevent the overgrowth of fungi, such as candida albicans.

Reality: Often food has not been completely processed because of a lack of enzymes, so the partially digested material (chyme) putrefies (if it was protein), ferments (if it was carbohydrate), or rancifies (if it had been fat) in the large intestine. Poor digestion, along with a lack of fiber, contributes to slow bowel transit time. The waste stays in the colon longer than is healthy, causing toxins to be absorbed into the bloodstream to poison the entire system. Slow bowel transit time has been linked to colon and breast cancer and other diseases. This scenario creates a perfect environment for the growth of fungus and harmful bacteria, while discouraging the presence of beneficial bacteria. The use of digestive enzymes is often helpful in establishing regularity and normalizing bowel transit time without an undesirable laxative effect.

ENZYMES—THE FOUNDATION OF LIFE

"Enzymes are substances that make life possible. They are needed for every chemical reaction that takes place in the human body. No mineral, vitamin, or hormone can do any work without enzymes. Our bodies, all of our organs, tissues, and cells, are run by metabolic enzymes. They are the manual workers that build our body from proteins, carbohydrates, and fats, just as construction workers build our home. You may have all the raw materials with which to build, but without workers (enzymes) you cannot even begin."

— Edward Howell, M.D., a physician who researched enzymes for over fifty years

FOOD FOR THOUGHT:

Will the food you choose to eat turn into nutrients or poisons? When you eat foods that are depleted of enzymes, vitamins, and minerals, you set the stage for noxious toxins to be created inside your body.

THE BOOMING SALES OF DIGESTIVE AIDS

Today digestion and elimination problems are epidemic in this country. Many people are taking antacids, laxatives, and other "digestive aids." In 1995, Americans spent $1.7 billion on antacids like Tums, Mylanta, and Maalox, and the following year, U.S. purchases tripled as new products were introduced to the marketplace. The situation has become ridiculous because many of these products simply mask problems without getting to the root cause.

In 2000, an estimated 200,000 people died because of conditions related to their digestive tracts, most alarmingly cancer. Yet while the statistics have become appalling, many people accept digestive troubles as normal and natural, which they are not. Commercials on TV even encourage us to eat all and anything we want, promising that an over-the-counter remedy will resolve any subsequent discomfort or trouble with digestion.

My own father is an antacid convert. I remember when I was a little girl, his Christmas stocking was always filled with Rolaids at the holiday. My Dad was never without antacids until I discovered natural enzyme therapy. Now Dad faithfully takes his enzymes, and he has delightfully noticed how his digestion has actually improved with age.

Most digestive aids and medications sold today do not really assist in improving the functioning of your body. In fact, some of them can even have negative effects, such as reducing nutrient absorption and neutralizing the stomach acid that you actually require for complete digestion. You may need to take enzymes with your meals instead. Because our foods are deficient in enzymes, it often helps to take an enzyme supplement to support your digestion to replace what was supposed to be there in the first place.

The body's basic requirements are water, protein, carbohydrates, fat, minerals, vitamins, *and enzymes*. The first six are the building materials for a healthy body, and enzymes are the workers that turn the materials into a finished product. Enzymes put together and take apart the materials. This includes taking apart the components of food and converting them into substances the body can use.

These precious enzymes facilitate hundreds of thousands of reactions. They are present in the raw plant or animal foods that we consume, and are also produced in the body. Raw organic foods contain optimal levels of enzymes.

Every function of your body relies on a chemical reaction, so as catalysts, enzymes are crucial. In addition to their digestive functions, enzymes are involved in movement, hearing, smelling, tasting, breathing, thinking, dreaming, and even having sex! Enzymes are required for the functioning of all of your organs. They rebuild and regenerate tissues, break down and digest your food, and enhance your body's natural detoxification efforts. Enzymes are essential for a healthy metabolism as well.

When enzyme activity stops, death occurs. So without enzymes, you would not exist! Yes, enzymes are the very foundation of life.

DIGESTIVE ENZYMES

Like following a recipe, success with digestion requires the right ingredients and efficient processing. Among these needed ingredients are enzymes specifically designed to work with digestion. These digestive enzymes help the body break down and absorb nutrients, as well as preventing undigested foods from turning into toxins.

The body needs about 22 different digestive enzymes. Below are the major ones. The suffix "*-ase*" indicates that the substance is an enzyme.

Protease digests dietary protein into subunits called amino acids. Amino acids are the basic building blocks of the thousands of different enzyme systems in the body. They also contribute to the manufacturing of metabolic enzymes in the liver. Protease has the ability to engulf and destroy viruses, bacteria, and other toxic materials as well.

Amylase digests carbohydrates into simpler forms to be utilized for energy. Since this digestive enzyme also has natural antihistamine properties, it can also assist in relieving allergic, asthmatic, and inflammatory reactions.

Lipase breaks down fats into smaller more usable units, including glycerol and fatty acids. Insufficient levels of lipase in the diet may result in difficulty losing weight, dry skin and hair, liver and gallbladder concerns, and high cholesterol or triglycerides.

Lactase digests the milk sugar commonly known as lactose. (You have probably heard of lactose-intolerant people—they lack the enzyme lactase.) Most milk sold in stores has been pasteurized and homogenized. These processes destroy 100% of the naturally occurring lactase. Breast milk, being a "raw" food, is loaded with lactase and other enzymes. In contrast, infant formulas contain absolutely no enzymes (including lactase).

Cellulase digests plant fibers. This enzyme processes the usable part of some fibers so they can be converted into energy. The human pancreas has absolutely no ability to make cellulase, so this is a digestive enzyme that must come from the diet or supplements. Cellulase is helpful in treating yeast overgrowths, acute food allergies, and heavy metal poisonings that affect the nervous system.

Invertase helps to digest sucrose found in cane or beet sugars.

Maltase breaks down maltose (the sugar in grains that can contribute to bread and carbohydrate cravings). Gas can be caused by a lack of the enzyme maltase.

Alpha-Galactosidase assists in the digestion of beans by breaking down melibose, raffinose, and stachyose. Incomplete breakdown of these starches can also cause gas. In addition, this enzyme supports the processing of cruciferous vegetables such as broccoli.

Since the ability to absorb nutrients is a fundamental requirement for optimal health, eating an enzyme-rich diet and enhancing your food intake with digestive enzymes can clear up a wide range of physical problems. One great source of enzymes is raw organic foods.

THE BODY HAS A LIMITED CAPACITY TO PRODUCE ENZYMES

Each person is born with a certain "enzyme potential"—that is, the number of enzymes their body can make over a lifetime. You can think of your enzyme potential as similar to a bank account. Every time you eat food that is enzyme deficient, you must use enzymes from your metabolic potential, draining your lifetime supply. People in the most developed countries tend to make more withdrawals than deposits in their enzyme bank accounts, and the degenerative diseases that result are astounding.

RESULTS OF ENZYME DEFICIENCIES

Remember how you felt that you could eat almost anything as a kid? Your enzyme supply was at an all-time high when you were a youngster. As most of us were raised on refined, enzyme-depleted foods (white bread, table sugar, pasteurized dairy, etc.), many of us have exhausted our precious supply of enzymes. When the body ingests foods that are lacking enzymes, it is stressful to our whole system. The following conditions are the various results of tampering with Nature's original plan:

"With heavy withdrawals of enzymes needed to digest an almost all-cooked diet, it's not hard to see how we would become metabolically enzyme poor, even in middle age. Heavy withdrawals and skimpy deposits of enzymes lead to eventual bankruptcy. Unfortunately, the glands and the major organs, including the brain, suffer most from the unnatural digestive drain on the metabolic enzyme potential."

— Edward Howell, M.D., enzyme researcher for over fifty years

■ Leukocytosis (White Blood Cells Responding to Trauma-Like Condition of Enzyme-Depleted Food)

Research by Paul Kouchakoff, M.D., shows that whenever cooked, enzyme-depleted food is eaten, the white blood cells increase as part of an immune activation, as if you were sick with a viral or bacterial infection.[4] Instead, the body is reacting to the burdensome digestive needs of the enzyme-depleted food. This reaction, which occurs within 30 minutes of eating cooked food, does not occur when raw foods are consumed. Leukocytosis (this white blood cell increase) is very stressful to the immune system.

■ Pancreatic Hypertrophy (Swelling of the Pancreas)

The enlargement of the pancreas is a result of the continual burden on the gland to supply enzymes for digestion that should have been in the food in the first place. When the pancreases of laboratory rats (fed on cooked food) were compared to those of wild rodents (living on raw food), the pancreases of the lab rats were found to be 2 $\frac{1}{2}$ times larger, an observation clearly indicative of digestive stress.[5]

■ Dysbiosis (Lack of Beneficial Bacteria)

Dysbiosis refers to a condition in which the bacteria in the intestines are out of balance, resulting in a vulnerability to the overgrowth of yeast, fungi, parasites, and harmful strains of bacteria. Poorly digested food alters the pH in the intestines, creating a perfect environment for dysbiosis.

■ Autoimmune Response/Leaky Gut Syndrome

When digestion is compromised due to an enzyme deficiency, undigested food particles seep into the bloodstream and can become circulating immune complexes (CICs), which can create an autoimmune response. Inflammation, allergies, fibromyalgia, arthritis, and asthma are some of the conditions that result from this situation.

■ Autointoxication/Intestinal Toxemia

When foods aren't completely digested, they often turn into toxic by-products and enter the bloodstream, another burden on the health of the body. A method of identifying this condition is a urine test that measures indican (see Chapter 15).

■ Sugar Cravings

Undigested proteins contribute to sugar cravings. When protein isn't completed digested, blood sugar levels can tend to be unstable, resulting in an overwhelming desire for sugar.

■ Insufficient Nutrient Delivery

Without adequate digestive enzymes, nutrients from the food cannot be completely released into the system. Enzymes are a crucial part of nutrient absorption. Research shows that vitamins and minerals are absorbed better when digestive enzymes are plentiful.

INCREASING ENZYMES IN YOUR EVERYDAY LIFE

Over the years, I have asked many people, "Are you tired after eating?" Most of them respond with an emphatic "Yes!" Certainly, there are many factors involved in feeling fatigued after meals (type of food, time of day, etc.). A common reason for this, which can be rectified, however, is the lack of enzymes in the food. The right nutrients + sufficient chewing + enzymes = energy, health, and healing.

In order to supply ourselves with adequate amounts of enzymes, we need to include some raw foods in our diet. The answer, however, is not to eat raw foods exclusively. That diet is not for everyone. Remember, our early ancestors ate a diet that was high in enzymes, yet included some cooked foods.

One easy way to incorporate raw foods into your eating plan is to increase your intake of organic fruits and vegetables. For instance, add fresh raw fruit to your breakfast. (Raw papaya, mango, pineapple, and figs are especially enzyme-rich.) Eat salad with your meals. Snack on raw vegetables such as cauliflower, carrot, celery, cherry tomatoes, avocado, or zucchini.

Here is a list of some other foods that are particularly rich in enzymes:

- Raw yogurt
- Kefir (a type of fermented milk)
- Sauerkraut
- Raw honey
- Fresh soy sauce
- Miso
- Sprouts
- Soaked seeds and nuts

Some readers might be interested in exploring raw foods gourmet cooking. A great guide is *Raw: The Uncook Book, New Vegetarian Food for Life* by Juliano. The author is a raw-foods guru in Los Angeles. His recipes include Butternut Squash Soup, Mock Salmon Sushi, seven varieties of burritos, nine types of pizza, and nine unique smoothies.

More ideas for raw eating can be found at *www.rawfood.com*. Remember, previous cultures always included substantial amounts of raw foods in their diet.

SUPPLEMENTING WITH ENZYMES

Over the years, I have spent countless hours keeping up with the research and fascinating breakthroughs in the field of nutrition. There are thousands of wonderful supplements that are available today, such as vitamins, minerals, herbs, and amino acids. However, I have observed that the use of enzymes has resulted in the most dramatic benefits for overall health in all types of people. The use of enzymes also enhances the benefits of other supplements by facilitating greater assimilation.

Enzymes are one of the substances that the body needs at all times. While herbs and many other supplements have become popular and can be helpful, the body is not always deficient in them. For example, although the herb *echinacea* can be quite powerful in enhancing immunity, there is no such thing as an *echinacea deficiency*. Enzymes, on the other hand, are a universal necessity and are often deficient. As enzymes improve the nutritional value of food, people who take enzymes notice that over time they need less food and have more energy. Cravings, which often come from nutritional deficiencies, also go away.

There are a lot of enzyme products on the market today. One thing to be aware of is the variance in quality. The units listed on the labels are not standardized, so it is important to make sure you are using a good quality enzyme. Quality varies with the sources of the ingredients and manufacturing methods. I have researched many brands over the years, and I have found some particular products that I think are the most helpful. See the Resource section for suggested brands. A plant-based, broad-spectrum product that includes the enzymes described earlier in the "Digestive Enzymes" section is best.

Broad-spectrum enzymes, those that include enzymes to digest protein, fats, carbohydrates, and fiber, have been safely used by people of all ages. The only caution associated with broad-spectrum enzyme products is for those with gastritis and/or ulcer conditions. These individuals will need to use an enzyme supplement that does not include protease (the enzyme that digests protein), but does include the other enzymes as well as gastric soothing herbs. After the inflamed lining is healed by the use of these special enzyme products, the individual will eventually be able to use the broad-spectrum enzyme—which is the enzyme of choice. If you have suspicions that this might be the case for you, one way to tell if you can take the broad-spectrum enzyme is that there will be no burning in the stomach upon use. Of course, if you are suffering from gastritis and/or an ulcer condition, it is best to work with a health professional experienced in enzyme therapy.

Many supplements on the market that claim to be "energy" supplements are actually stimulants. In contrast, enzymes, whether in food or supplements, provide the body with the support it needs for its natural energy production. While enzymes will not give the "quick fix" associated with stimulant products, they do contribute to long-term sustainable energy. Therefore we must make sure that we take in enzymes by eating raw foods, and also complement this by taking enzyme supplements. I suggest taking plant-based digestive enzymes with each meal.

Of course, all of the enzymes in the world will not help if the food being digested is of poor quality. Taking enzymes to assist in digesting donuts isn't using these enzymes in an optimal way. You will learn more about devising a healthy individualized food plan in Chapter 9.

ENZYME MISCONCEPTIONS

It has been wonderful to hear countless success stories for almost two decades regarding the importance of enzymes. Colleagues, patients, friends, and readers love to share how their health has improved with the use of this foundational substance. Replacing something that has been missing for a while is bound to have dramatic effects.

The basic enzyme concept seems to make sense to most people, but here are some of the concerns that have been presented:

Doesn't the body make its own enzymes? Yes, the body does make its own enzymes. It makes metabolic enzymes from *properly digested* protein, which supplies the raw material to the liver to manufacture enzymes. The problem is that often protein is incompletely digested (due to a lack of digestive enzymes in the food), and instead of contributing to the enzyme-making process, the protein is turned into toxic substances that end up circulating throughout the bloodstream.

Although the pancreas does supply enzymes during the digestive process, it was not designed to supply all of the enzymes. The Divine Design was to have the food itself supply some enzymes for digestion. As you have read, research supporting this shows that animals eating enzyme-depleted food have weaker pancreases than those eating enzyme-rich food.

Aren't enzymes destroyed by stomach acid? No. Enzymes are temporarily inactivated in the acidic pH of the lower part of the stomach and then reactivated in the small intestine.

FOR FELINES TOO, ENZYMES MAKE ALL THE DIFFERENCE: The Famous Pottenger Cat Study

One of the most well-known and dramatic studies concerning food enzymes and health was conducted by Francis M. Pottenger, Jr., M.D., in the 1930s and 1940s. Pottenger ran a sanitarium in Monrovia, California, for the treatment of tuberculosis. He was interested in the importance of nutrition in achieving better states of well-being.

Over a 10-year period, Pottenger oversaw an experiment involving over 900 cats that were divided into two groups. The first set of felines was fed raw milk and raw meat. The second cluster of kitties dined on pasteurized milk and cooked meat. Of course, the pasteurized milk and cooked meat diet did not supply any enzymes, while the raw food regimen was rich with them. Those cats fed raw food stayed in much better health, and the results were even more marked for later generations of felines. Examples of a higher state of health included a greater resistance to infection, fleas and parasites; fewer allergies; and more positive behavior patterns. The cats fed the cooked food diet experienced ill health in the form of allergies, brittle bones, frequent infections, skin diseases, endocrine disorders, and frequent miscarriages.

Pottenger's classic study is frequently cited today. It is clear evidence of the importance of including enzyme-rich foods in our diets. Other researchers have found the colons of wild animals that are surviving on enzyme-rich raw foods to lack the harmful bacteria and toxins commonly found in the human large intestine.

The Pottenger study clearly contrasts the results of eating a cooked diet compared to consuming raw foods. Since the time of his work, numerous experiments have been conducted in which researchers studied the effects of these two diets on wild mice and rats. The researchers discovered that captured rodents fed a raw foods diet stayed sleek and trim, exhibited more energy, and looked better than those fed animal kibble (a cooked food like dog food). Fed food similar to what we give our pets, the wild critters also became overweight and developed similar degenerative diseases and cardiovascular problems as domesticated animals (and as also seen in humans consuming cooked foods). What makes the difference? The diet! When autopsies are conducted, enlarged pancreases are found in animals that lived on cooked foods. These enlarged glands are an indication of the physiological stress imposed on the pancreases due to a continuing lack of enzymes in the diet.

Does adding more enzymes to the diet cause the digestive system to become lazy? That is like asking if breathing clean air every day will cause a dependency on clean air. When you supplement cooked food with enzymes, you are simply replacing what was eliminated from the food through cooking and processing. Likewise, clean air allows the body to operate without having to deal with airborne toxins. Giving the body what Nature intended supports optimal health.

I have yet to observe or hear about any problems with the proper use of enzymes, whether in food or supplemented. It seems as if the research keeps mounting in support of these precious catalysts.

HOW AND WHY ENZYME AVAILABILITY CAN APPEAR LIMITED

To optimize your body's enzyme stores, it is beneficial to have an awareness of the many reasons enzyme availability can be compromised. Some of these factors relate to the way our foods are managed; others involve our personal habits.

Depleted Soils: Overused, worn-out farmland produces crops that are lower in health-supporting enzymes. Less crop rotation is used today which contributes to this problem.

Genetic Engineering: One of the many concerns about genetically modified produce is that the body can deal with it as a foreign substance. This diverts enzyme activity that could be put to much better use.

Food Processing: Refining exposes foods to heat, destroying precious enzymes and vital nutrients. Chemical preservatives, as well as coloring and flavoring agents, block the effectiveness of the enzymes that actually do manage to arrive inside your body.

Irradiation: This process is being used in hopes of keeping harmful organisms from reaching your kitchen table. Unfortunately, we are also losing vitamins A, E, K, the B family, important fats, essential amino acids, and last, but certainly not least, *enzymes!* Avoid irradiated foods whenever possible.

Pasteurization: When it comes to pasteurization, enzymes are certainly something of the past. Success of the process is actually measured by the absence of active enzymes! During pasteurization, milk is heated to extremely hot temperatures in order to kill bacteria. Enzymes also are completely destroyed. In contrast to pasteurized milk, certified raw milk provides many enzymes along with beneficial bacteria.

Cooking: When foods are heated above 118° F, the enzymes are deactivated. Any type of heating of foods above this temperature will stop enzyme activity—baking, boiling, frying, or stewing. Including some raw foods in your diet (such as certified raw dairy and sushi, in addition to fresh produce) as well as eating fermented foods will help you take in the enzymes you need. For more ideas, see the list of recommended foods in the section, "Increasing Enzymes in Your Everyday Life."

Microwaving: While a microwave oven may seem to be a convenience, using one to prepare your food at home is robbing you of both enzymes and nutrients. Their use also causes stress to your body by adding toxins to the foods from packaging. Lastly, there is the danger of being exposed to harmful magnetic radiation. Foods in restaurants are often microwaved without your knowledge.

Pesticides: There are more than 400 pesticides approved for use on America's food crops. Research has shown that these and other synthetic chemicals can destroy or inhibit enzymes in the body. Also, the pesticides can interfere with the original plant's functioning and produce less-nutritious and enzyme-deficient produce. For instance, they inhibit the absorption of minerals that come from the soil, which enzymes need to work properly. Pesticide studies regarding enzymes have included chemicals used in U.S. agriculture. Even more potent pesticides, such as the U.S.-banned DDT, are in our food chain as the result of imported goods from foreign countries. Eat certified organic, pesticide-free foods.

Bovine Growth Hormone (rBGH): This synthetic hormone is given to increase the amount of milk a cow can produce. When ingested, it is assessed as a toxin by the body, and uses up precious metabolic enzymes. Buy organic dairy and meat to avoid this problem.

Antibiotics: The use of antibiotics is a common beginning for the life story of internal toxins. Taking antibiotics can alter the digestive environment, creating the perfect breeding ground for internal toxicity. When the environment gets out of control, enzymes can't keep up with the workload. The healthy internal flora must be restored before enzymes can process foods effectively.

Other Medications: Many drugs are designed to inhibit metabolic enzyme activity. Along the way, appetite can be altered, digestion suppressed, and nutrient absorption hampered. These changes may place a higher demand on digestive enzymes.

Smoking: It has been clear for some time that smoking leads to lung cancer—an extreme case of toxicity! And not only are smokers themselves affected; those around them are also because of second-hand smoke. The World Health Organization estimates that 3 million people die every year because of smoking. Here is yet another reason to kick the habit. Cigarette smoke is quite toxic and creates free radical damage, destroying precious enzymes. It also depletes vitamins and minerals necessary for optimal enzyme activity. If you have recently stopped smoking, taking digestive enzymes can free metabolic enzymes to work on healing, repair, and immunity.

Your Toxic Exposure: In earlier chapters, you learned that your personal accumulation of toxins—also called your individual "toxic load"—is an issue in your detoxification. It also affects the effectiveness of your enzyme activity. For instance, heavy metals—such as lead, mercury, and aluminum—can play havoc with enzyme interactions.

Stress: Stress of any type—emotional or physical—can curtail good digestion and the adequate absorption of foods. Digestive enzyme availability is compromised during the stress response.

As you can see, the modern diet and lifestyle have had a negative impact on the amounts of enzymes that are available for digestion. Now that you know the major factors involved, you can take positive steps to prevent an enzyme shortage in your system.

CHILDREN & ENZYME DEFICIENCIES

Breast milk is an enzyme-rich food. In contrast, formula has absolutely no enzymes. I would say the majority of my pediatric cases have involved children who were not breast-fed long enough or at all. For those children who have already been weaned and are suffering from repeated ear infections, allergies, colic, and other immune challenges, I have found that enzyme formulas specifically prepared for children have been very helpful.

Here's a case example. Maria, an infant whose mother was not able to breast-feed her, could not handle any of the formulas. She was very ill, malnourished with a severely swollen abdomen. Doctors had tried "everything," with no results. The plan was to hospitalize her and feed her intravenously. Before she was admitted, her mother fed her goat's milk and supplemented enzymes and beneficial bacteria specially formulated for children. Within less than 24 hours of incorporating these changes, Maria's abdominal swelling was gone, and she started absorbing nutrients. Today Maria is a happy, active seven-year-old in excellent health.

OTHER TYPES OF ENZYMES

The enzymes emphasized in this chapter are food enzymes specifically used for digestion. However, there are thousands of metabolic enzymes used in the body for millions of functions. For example, antioxidant enzymes are crucial for the destruction of free radicals (unpaired electrons that have the potential to destroy cells). Other metabolic enzymes fight cancer, reduce inflammation, and support healthy immune function. The richer your diet is in enzymes, the more efficiently all of the enzyme systems can function.

THE CASE FOR USING ENZYMES FOR LONGEVITY

"The length of one's life is inversely proportional to the rate of exhaustion of the enzyme potential of an organism. But the increased use of food enzymes promotes a decreased rate of exhaustion of the enzyme potential, and thus, results in a longer, healthier and more vital life." — Edward Howell, M.D.

Research confirms over and over again that the conservation of enzymes is crucial to longevity—to a long, healthy life—not just living long, but living well—adding life to your years, not just years to your life.

- An experiment at Michael Reese Hospital in Chicago found that the enzymes in the saliva of young adults were 30 times higher than in persons over 69 years old.[6]

- Dr. Eckhardt in Germany tested 1,200 urine specimens for the starch-digesting enzyme amylase. In the specimens of youth, he found double the amount of amylase.

- Drs. Bartos and Groh, Charles University, Prague, Czechoslovakia, studied the pancreatic juice of both young and elderly volunteers. The pancreatic juice flow was stimulated with a drug and then pumped out and tested. Again, the enzyme amylase had much lower levels in the elderly than in the youth.

- Dr. Karl Ransberger, director of the Medical Enzyme Research Institute comments, "If you take enzymes regularly, you can arm your body with a natural defense against the aging process."[7]

- In *Enzymes in Health and Disease*, David Greenberg, Ph.D., Chairman of the Department of Biochemistry at the University of California School of Medicine at San Francisco, suggests that for optimal health, longevity, and the reduced risk of disease, the use of enzymes should commence around the age of forty and continue for the rest of the life-span.[8]

- In *Today's Health* (published by the American Medical Association), Dr. Ratcliff states, "Many research men believe that the aging process is the result of the slowing down and disorganization of enzyme activity. Might it eventually be possible to restore youthful patterns of activity by supplying those enzymes that are deficient?"[9]

- Dr. James B. Sumner, Nobel Prize recipient and Professor of Biochemistry at Cornell University, wrote in his book, *The Secret of Life – Enzymes*, that the "getting old feeling" after forty is due to lower enzyme levels in the system.[10] Younger cells contain countless more enzymes than older cells—which are loaded with toxic waste.

Basically, when you run out of enzymes, you run out of life. Just like we manage our finances, we must manage our enzymes for optimal health. Every time we eat enzyme-depleted food, we are making a withdrawal from our "enzyme bank account." Every time we eat enzyme-rich food or supplement with enzymes, we are making a deposit. Are you investing in your future or accumulating debt?

ENZYMES HEAL

"There is no other mechanism in the body except enzyme action to protect the body from any hazard. It is ambiguous to say that 'nature cures' when it is known that the only machinery in the body to do anything is enzyme action. Proteins cannot work on their own. Nature cannot work on its own either. Only enzymes are made for work. So it is enzymes that 'heal.'" — Edward Howell, M.D.

As enzymes are part of every single chemical process that occurs in the body, they naturally would be an important part of the healing process. Enzyme therapy can be a valuable part of the protocol in virtually every health condition. Research is mounting, supporting the remarkable benefits of enzymes as part of the healing process.

Cancer: There are numerous studies showing the effectiveness of enzymes in cancer treatment. Studies show that enzymes increase the activity of macrophages and natural killer cells (two types of immune cells that fight cancer). Enzyme therapy has been used very successfully in Europe for over forty years and is now being explored in the United States. Nicolas Gonzalez, M.D., a pioneer in enzyme therapy for cancer who has had success in the treatment of pancreatic cancer (a cancer that usually does not have a good prognosis), has recently been awarded a grant by the National Cancer Institute to further study this promising, safe, nontoxic cancer therapy.

Inflammation: Numerous studies have shown tremendous anti-inflammatory effects in conditions such as contusions, abrasions, sprains, strains, and various sports injuries.[11]

HISTORIC/CULTURAL USES OF ENZYMES

In the Bible's Second Book of Kings, it is believed that King Hezekiah was suffering from cancer. Isaiah was instructed to apply a fig-plaster, and he recovered. Figs are specifically high in protelytic (protein-digesting) enzymes—the ones used in cancer therapy and research today.

The Mayans, Aztecs, and Incas used poultices prepared from high-enzyme plants such as aloe vera, papaya, and pineapples to treat various diseases.

The traditional Asian diet has always emphasized foods rich in enzymes. In addition to fruits and vegetables, fermented (prepared with enzymes) soy bean products and raw fish and meat supply precious food enzymes.

Traditional Eskimos have been known to eat up to a pound of raw blubber (rich in the fat-digesting enzyme lipase) daily. They showed no signs of cardiovascular disease until they began to cook their fat. The word Eskimo means "he who eats it raw." Dr. William A. Thomas of the MacMillan Arctic Expedition of 1926 wrote: "Eskimos live on an exclusively meat and fish diet, all usually and preferably eaten in the raw. There was no unusual prevalence of renal and vascular disease. However, the Eskimos that began living mostly on cooked foods, their health changed . . . Cancer and heart disease appeared and their longevity was reduced 50%."[12]

The Standard American Diet is the first diet to emphasize cooked, dead foods. Cultures throughout history have always thrived on diets rich in raw, organic foods as well as freshly cooked ones. Ironically, the culture with the most cooked foods does not win, as evidenced by the American tendency to obesity, heart disease, cancer, and other diseases of civilization.

Lymphedema: This is an inflamed condition that usually results from breast cancer surgery. European scientists have found that the anti-inflammatory effects of enzymes can prevent this condition from developing.[13]

Rheumatoid arthritis: Studies have shown enzyme's effectiveness in reducing joint swelling, pain, and stiffness.[14]

Arterial obstruction: Enzyme therapy has been shown in several studies to be more effective than anticoagulant therapy.[15] This research points to improved prevention of conditions such as heart attacks and blood clots.[16]

Multiple sclerosis: Dr. Neuhofer has been treating MS patients with enzyme therapy since 1972. She has conducted various research studies documenting significant improvement in the majority of cases.[17]

Other health challenges: Clinical studies show the effectiveness of enzymes used to enhance treatment of sinusitis, prostatitis, allergies, urinary tract infections, pelvic inflammatory disease, recovery from surgery, post-thrombotic syndrome, ankylosing spondylitis, fibrocystic breast disease, ulcerative colitis, Crohn's disease, pancreatitis, viruses, AIDS, shingles, nerve pain, cystic fibrosis, celiac disease, and epilepsy.[18] Since enzymes are the foundation of life, it makes sense that virtually any health challenge would have a strong relationship to enzyme function.

The purpose of citing the above health challenges and their responses to enzymes is to emphasize the point that enzymes are needed for health, not to suggest self-treatment with enzymes. For more information on enzyme therapy and specific health conditions, refer to Dr. Anthony Cichoke's *The Complete Book of Enzyme Therapy.* Although it is safe for most people to use enzymes to enhance their health, if you have a chronic health condition, it is wise to see a health professional who utilizes enzyme therapy.

ENZYMES & WEIGHT LOSS

To achieve or maintain ideal weight, it is common to turn to commercial diet aids. Most of these products are stimulants; they work by temporarily suppressing the appetite or by speeding up your metabolism. Typically people who use these methods tend to be yo-yo dieters.

They move up and down the scale, never easily maintaining the weight they seek. That is because artificially controlling your weight is not the answer. Alternately, using enzymes can be part of a safe and effective weight management program. They naturally support a healthy metabolism and can reduce your cravings by providing optimal nourishment.

Research has shown that difficulty in losing weight can be linked to an enzyme deficiency. A study at Tufts University found that overweight individuals are often deficient in lipase, the enzyme that digests fat.[19]

ENZYMES IN OUR WORLD

Enzymes are indicative of a substance being alive. Think of all activity in nature as being facilitated by enzymes. You have experienced numerous encounters with enzymes that you probably were not aware of. Here are some examples of the enzyme activity that occurs all around you:

- A *raw steak* has anti-inflammatory enzymes (remember the raw steak over the bruised eye?). A cooked steak doesn't have any therapeutic value for inflammation.

- Planting a *seed* in the soil initiates powerful enzyme activity. If the seed was heated first, the seed will not sprout, for the enzymes would be destroyed. A seed is the foundation of many life forms. There would be no life without enzyme activity.

- It is enzymes that cause a *bitten apple* to turn brown and *green bananas* to ripen.

- *Raw honey* is used on wounds as a disinfectant. Cooked honey has no such therapeutic value. The enzymes in the raw honey are key for the healing process.

- Commercial *meat tenderizers* are usually nothing more than protein-digesting enzymes.

- Some *drain openers* use enzymes to "eat up" the residue in the pipes.

Edward Howell, M.D., the enzyme researcher who has been quoted throughout this chapter, found that eating food without enzymes causes stress on the endocrine glands, such as the pancreas and thyroid. Because the endocrine system is responsible for metabolic function, an overworked system often results in a sluggish metabolism.

ENZYMES & DETOX: A RECAP

Digestive enzymes ensure that food is digested completely and does not add to the toxic load. Properly digested food provides energy, nourishment, and regeneration. Conversely, improperly digested food is a burden to the body. Enzymes insure delivery of nutrients, like putting a stamp on an envelope to insure delivery of the mail. You wouldn't put an envelope in the mail without a stamp, so why choose a diet that can contribute to degeneration and illness instead of regeneration and health? Enzymes are crucial for the ongoing detoxification that happens in every cell, every second. *There is absolutely no healing process in the body that can occur without enzymes!*

The many exciting uses of enzyme therapy give us a hint of the many possibilities to come. For now, remember to optimize both your detoxification and digestion by eating enzyme-rich food and supplementing your diet with digestive enzymes.

WHAT'S AHEAD

Now that you are familiar with both the external and internal sources of toxicity, you're ready to learn how your body actually deals with toxins on a daily basis. After looking at the body's detoxification in a broad context, we'll look at each detox system in the body and what you can do to support its optimal functioning. As you fine-tune your detoxification, you will be able to achieve higher and higher states of well-being.

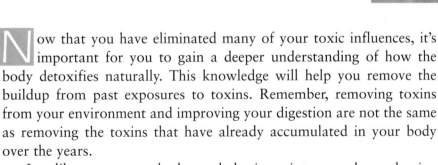

FIVE

Better Living Through Chemistry? Detoxification & Your Health

The natural healing force within each one of us is the greatest force in getting well.

— Hippocrates

Now that you have eliminated many of your toxic influences, it's important for you to gain a deeper understanding of how the body detoxifies naturally. This knowledge will help you remove the buildup from past exposures to toxins. Remember, removing toxins from your environment and improving your digestion are not the same as removing the toxins that have already accumulated in your body over the years.

Just like a car, your body needs basic maintenance beyond using wise habits on a daily basis. In addition to the habit of driving safely, few people would neglect such regular car upkeep as changing the oil every 5,000 miles. In a similar way, you should take steps to enhance your body's natural, ongoing detoxification. As you've learned, our bodies require this assistance because of the extent of our toxic load today. If you want a high quality of life in the 21st Century, it is crucial to become educated regarding your body's natural detoxification processes as well as detox techniques you can effectively use. This will prepare you to take action to move toward optimal health and the prevention of illness.

OUR BODY STRIVES FOR WELLNESS

Before we take a closer look at our body's natural cleansing mechanisms, I'd like to point out an essential truth. That is, *our body is always attempting to keep us in balance.* Its desired state is one of *homeostasis*—which basically means a body in balance and harmony.

For instance, if a thorn pricks your finger and bleeding starts, you usually don't panic. You simply clean the wound and cover the finger with a Band-Aid to slow the bleeding. Then beyond changing the Band-Aid, you don't worry because you've learned that your body's innate intelligence will figure out how to repair the small wound. And once it's fully healed, there's usually no scar! So you can see that healing occurred because you created the right environment (cleansed the wound and covered it with a Band-Aid) and did nothing to prevent recovery (such as continuing to scrape the finger as it was mending, etc.).

Samuel Hahnemann, M.D., the Father of Homeopathic Medicine, summed up the natural approach to healing in this way: "Hence the careful investigation into such *obstacles to cure* is so much the more necessary in the case of patients affected by chronic diseases, as their diseases are usually aggravated by such noxious influences and other disease-causing errors in the diet and regimen which *often pass unnoticed.*"[1]

The idea that our bodies will heal if we *remove any obstacles* and support the natural healing processes seems obvious. However, the Western medical model doesn't always *address every obstacle* that interferes with the body's natural healing process. Often we end up masking symptoms with drugs when we seek help from allopathic medicine for early signs of a developing condition. Overlooking causes of symptoms can allow the condition to turn chronic and persistent.

Dr. Howard Loomis, an enzyme expert and author of *Enzymes: The Key to Health,* offers the following description of the current situation regarding the treatment of chronic illness: "Imagine... an 18-wheeler coming down the highway right at you. You would like someone to warn you of impending danger so you can move out of the way. Unfortunately, most medical diagnostic procedures cannot do that. They can only measure the damage after the truck has hit you."

The good news is that the detoxification program outlined in this book *is* designed to work with the body and to enhance its natural functioning. It will help remove the obstacle of toxicity so that your whole system can run more efficiently, promoting optimal health and energy.

YOU ARE AS HEALTHY AS YOUR CELLS

Sometimes we need to look at our health in a less complicated way. What it all boils down to is that you are simply as healthy as your cells, because (as I remember hearing year after year in my elementary school science classes)... *Cells make tissues. And tissues make organs. And organs make systems. And systems make organisms.* You (a homo sapiens) are an organism! If your cells are healthy, your tissues, organs and whole organism will tend to be healthy as well. On the other hand, if the basic units of your life (your cells) are not getting what they need, *and are actually retaining toxic elements,* your health will be compromised. It's that simple.

Relating this to our basic paradigm, the health of a cell depends on three basic elements—(1) the quality of the nutrients that it takes in; (2) how well nutrients are assimilated; and (3) the effectiveness of its waste removal. Remember the experiment from Chapter 1, where scientist Alexis Carrell showed that these were the basic requirements for chicken heart tissue to survive? Carrell's goal was to prove that living cells thrive when their nutritional and assimilation needs are met at an optimal level and toxins are removed. Remember, after just one day of not removing the wastes, the chicken tissue died.

To properly nourish your cells, it's important that you take in a wide variety of nutrients at optimal levels *daily.* Your body will use these nutrients to maintain and repair cells or make new ones. Every cell in your body requires specific nutrients in order to function in a healthy way. Bone cells may need more calcium than liver cells, for example.

Your body is very efficient with its use of energy. Your cells will immediately attempt to eliminate waste products that result from the processing of these nutrients. *Every cell* has detoxification mechanisms to eliminate the waste. Unfortunately these mechanisms become compromised because of all the toxins that we are taking in.

TOXIC INVADERS
ERODE OUR NATURAL RESISTANCE

Toxins can gain entry into your body in a number of ways. They penetrate your *skin* (and then go into the bloodstream). They are part of the air that you breathe through your *lungs*. Toxins in your food move inside through your mouth and then travel along the *digestive tract*. In addition, repeated stress responses can be considered emotional toxins, and they affect the whole body, especially the *endocrine and nervous systems*.

Our senses have built-in sensors to protect us from toxic invaders. For instance, the first puff of cigarette smoke is repulsive. A degrading ugly environment is a turn-off. Junk food tastes like junk. But eventually our system gets desensitized, and it "settles" for second best. Refined vs. whole foods, chaos vs. mindfulness, and so on. Using the scientific term, we "maladapt." There are no more acute negative responses, just acceptance and inevitably chronic degeneration. We may no longer choke from the cigarette (an acute response), but we may be slowly developing lung cancer (a chronic condition). We no longer get sick to our stomach from eating too much sugar, but diabetes may be just around the corner.

At some point, we actually start craving the junk food, excessive stimulation, etc. And while our body chemistry is way out of balance, we think it's normal. Fortunately, detoxification offers a way out of this vicious cycle. Patients are constantly amazed that when their body chemistry is balanced through detoxification and rejuvenation, cravings for things that weren't good for them "miraculously" disappear or significantly diminish.

HOW DETOXIFICATION OCCURS
AT THE CELLULAR LEVEL

As you just read, every cell in your body has detoxification mechanisms. In other words, every cell can take in a certain amount of toxicity and either neutralize it or transform the toxins biochemically into waste products that will be excreted in some way by the body. When the cells' resources become overwhelmed by toxicity, toxins will build up in the tissue (especially in stored fat). Certain cells are more sophisticated detox factories than others; liver cells, for instance, have a heightened ability to neutralize toxins.

In all the organs and body systems, detoxification is actually taking place at a cellular level. Going back to the liver as an example, the cells of the liver work in concert to perform the detox duties assigned to that important organ. The cells are like individual singers in a choir; each cell has its part, and working together, the activity of the individual cells are blended together into a beautiful cooperative effort. When your body is detoxing at an optimal level, you might think of it as your cells singing in harmony!

Remember, your body is programmed for health. It supports you and keeps you well as long as it has what it needs and doesn't have obstacles (usually toxins) to interfere with the healing process. Your cells will constantly try to eliminate waste products that come their way to keep you at peak performance.

There are some basic ways that detoxification takes place on the cellular plane. These include:

Immune Activity – Like Pac Man, various immune cells in the body have the ability to engulf, devour, and destroy toxins. For instance, the Kupffer cells—important liver cells that are immune supporters—team up with cells in the liver called hepatocytes. While the Kupffer cells quickly swallow and obliterate bacteria and other large toxins entering the liver in the portal blood, the hepatocytes take smaller toxins to the bile to be excreted.

Free Radical Release – In certain situations, the body will release free radicals (a molecule with one unpaired electron) to clean up toxins. For instance, in cases of infection, trauma, or a toxic exposure, an effort by white blood cells may be followed by the production of free radicals. These free radicals may destroy damaged tissue, infectious agents, and toxic chemicals. The beneficial nature of the free radicals continues as long as antioxidant defenses are available. However, when the antioxidant defenses are low, free radicals can get out of control and destroy healthy tissue, cell membranes, and DNA. As a result, even more toxic substances may be created!

Phase I and Phase II Enzymatic Detoxification – This is a two-step process that neutralizes toxic chemical compounds. This two-phase system is very active in the liver, but exists in every cell. In Phase I, toxic elements are biochemically transformed into a secondary substance; in Phase II, the altered substance is neutralized or made into a form that can be easily eliminated by the body. Unfortunately, these secondary substances can be even more toxic than the original compounds. If Phase II is out of order, more damage can result than if the initial compound had never been altered! Problems with Phase II can occur in someone who has had a long-time exposure to toxins. In this case, the toxic load can be so heavy that the agents and energy needed for Phase II become depleted. Thus Phase I secondary substances increasingly get backlogged.

Bacterial Protection – Adults have about 2.2 pounds of bacteria in just their colon! Beneficial bacteria in the large intestine perform the detox function of preventing harmful bacteria, viruses, and parasites from taking over. This is accomplished by the secretions made by beneficial bacteria that create an acid pH. Pathogenic bacteria and most parasites can only survive in an alkaline environment. Unfortunately, most people don't have adequate beneficial bacteria, and as a result, their bowel ecology is a disaster. More about this in the next chapter.

An excess of toxicity can damage the extracellular matrix (material surrounding cells) and compromise the various detox efforts described above. A weakening of the matrix cripples the delivery of nutrients to the cells and slows the removal of toxic debris. Maintaining the integrity of the extracellular matrix is just one more way your body can benefit when you lessen your individual toxic load.

YOUR BODY'S SIMPLE DETOX METHODS

Besides the complex removal of wastes on a cellular level, your body has many other built-in detoxification mechanisms which are much more basic. For instance, your nostrils have hairs that trap dust. A sneeze is the body's attempt to expel germs. Sweat includes toxic bodily wastes that are released through the pores of your skin. All of this wisdom is built in. Your body is detoxifying every second.

YOUR BODY SYSTEMS & DETOXIFICATION

As you've just learned, the cells work together in a particular body system to accomplish their detox responsibilities. Though some body systems are more involved in detoxification, every system participates in some way. Some of these systems include:

The digestive system, including the mouth, stomach, liver, small intestine, and colon: This system processes the foods we eat so that nutrients can be distributed to the whole body. It must also identify toxins so they can be eliminated. When the internal flora is out of balance, internal toxins can be generated. Since the surface of the GI tract is 200 times that of our outer skin, it can be a major entry and exit route for toxins. An essential part of the digestive system, the liver is the body's most essential cleansing organ. It is being challenged with an excessive level of toxins in modern times.

The dermal system (skin), including sweat, sebaceous (oil) glands, and tears: A wide range of toxins—such as heavy metals, medications, pesticides, and other synthetic chemicals—can enter and exit the body through the skin. This is why the skin is sometimes referred to as the "third kidney." Sebaceous glands of the skin secrete sebum, which helps the body rid itself of fat-soluble toxins. Tears sometimes are created to clear the eye of sudden toxic exposures; they also assist in reducing toxic emotional responses by facilitating the release of stored emotions. When detoxification is not efficient in other systems, toxins can exit through the skin causing rashes, acne, and other conditions.

The urinary system, including the kidneys, bladder, ureters, and urethra: Waste products from the bloodstream are excreted through the kidneys. To do this, the kidneys must distinguish toxins from nutrients as they enter. The toxins are filtered from the blood, while nutrients—including amino acids and glucose—are returned to the bloodstream.

The lymphatic system, including the lymph glands, nodes, and vessels: Lymphatic fluids travel throughout your body along a network of vessels. Since this circulatory system has no pump (the heart is the pump of the blood circulatory system), its movement must be supported and enhanced through exercise, hydrotherapy, skin brushing, etc. Lymph nodes and organs filter harmful organisms and waste products from lymph fluid.

The endocrine system, including the thyroid, adrenals, gonads, etc.: The endocrine system regulates the metabolism (energy) of the body. It plays a crucial role in our detoxification efforts. If this system is operating well, toxins will be removed more efficiently. In this system, hormones are produced to regulate an array of functions—brain development, immune function, sugar metabolism, stress response, sexual drive, etc. Chemical toxins, such as pesticides, can stimulate or lower hormone production. Many diseases are related to an inadequate or excessive production of hormones.

The respiratory system, including the lungs, bronchials, throat, sinuses, and nose: Carbon dioxide, a waste product of bodily processes, is released through this system. Respiration also helps to oxygenate the cells, nourishing them to do their individual detox tasks. The respiratory system has an immune defense capability that it uses to destroy invading bacteria and viruses.

The sensory system, including the nerves/senses: As you read earlier, we often innately sense that something is toxic to our bodies during the initial exposure. However, over time, this awareness can dim as encounters become more frequent. We need to learn to listen to this early warning system, whether the toxin involved is physical or emotional. Note that the sensory system is particularly susceptible to a type of injury called neurotoxicity. One group of toxins involved in neurotoxicity is solvents, the chemicals found in paint, gasoline, cleaning fluids, etc. Neurotoxicity affects every part of the body and has been associated with many chronic health conditions.

The immune system, including white blood cells, spleen, bone marrow, and thymus: This system's basic duties include ridding the body of pathogens by either destroying or damaging them. As the body's main lines of defense against harmful invaders, our immune systems are extremely challenged in today's world. Toxins such as heavy metals, pesticides, and synthetic medications inhibit the immune system's response. Its work is further complicated by the presence of internal toxins (often resulting from poorly digested food) that build up in the bloodstream. Today, more than ever, the immune system must eliminate cancer cells generated by toxicity.

Of all the many parts of the body, people often think of the intestines when they hear the word "detoxification." This is understandable. Our daily bowel movements are one of the most obvious reminders of our body's continual detox efforts. Also, maintaining well-functioning clean intestines with a good diet and wise habits is a necessary part of a healthy lifestyle. Later, the specific cleansing of the colon will be a central element of the detox regimen described in this book.

Remember that while some of the *emphasis* of the program may be on specific organs, the whole body is always being addressed. For example, if the regimen includes detoxifying herbs that cleanse the liver, other parts of the body will also benefit as the herb travels through the bloodstream. You might contrast this benefit for your entire body to the unwanted side effects that occur from some medications. While the drug may be given to deal with a specific organ, its chemicals will be dispersed throughout your system. With herbs, this systemic distribution can be a pleasant bonus.

HOW TOXINS EXIT THE BODY

There are various exit routes that toxins might take to leave the body. Which route they will travel is determined in part by the type of substance they are. Two obvious paths would be excretion in the feces and urine. These and other common thruways are highlighted below:

Skin: When you perspire, toxins exit the body in your sweat. Toxins that use this pathway include the fat-soluble variety, including DDT and heavy metals (lead, aluminum, mercury, etc.). While this process usually does not disturb the body surface, skin-evacuated toxins may occasionally cause rashes, redness, or even skin cancer.

Kidneys: Many types of toxins escape in the urine. They are made water-soluble first by the liver before reaching the kidneys for further filtering. The urinary tract is one of the main exit routes for toxins.

Liver: The liver filters many toxins out of the blood and sends them along in the bile to be removed in feces. In the liver, toxins undergo a chemical transformation. Toxins processed by the liver include bacteria, prescription drugs, pesticides, estrogens, and histamines.

Feces: Fat-soluble toxins that have traveled out of the liver in bile are then excreted through bowel movements. Toxins that exit the body in feces also include the by-products of digestion and of processing by beneficial bacteria in the intestines.

Lungs: With every breath you release, toxins exit in a gaseous form. These include volatile organic compounds.

Mucus: When mucus is produced in large amounts, it is the body's way of removing threatening toxins such as viruses, bacteria, and irritants.

Other pathways are less heavily traveled. Toxins also leave the body in breast milk, hair and nail growth, menstrual flow, saliva, and tears. Unfortunately, not all toxins exit the body; those that are trapped inside it may even be transformed into deadlier substances than their original form.

Our bodies need support in order for these exit routes to be fully utilized. Let's look now at the factors that impact the efficiency of our detoxification processes.

FACTORS INFLUENCING OUR ABILITY TO DETOXIFY

Research has shown that our susceptibility to disease is directly related to our ability to detoxify. Each individual's ability to detox depends on multiple factors.

First, your ability to detox is dependent upon the *genetic tendencies* you inherited when you were born. If you came into this world with a weak liver, detoxification will be more difficult for you, since this is a major detoxification organ. And if lungs are not a strength in your family tree, it will be tougher for your body to get rid of the toxins you breathe in as part of city air.

On the other hand, your makeup might include some positive genetic tendencies. For example, look at the long life of comedian and cigar-smoker George Burns! Also, there are those rare people who cultivate unhealthy lifestyles but still live to a ripe old age. Don't let that less than 1% of the population be your excuse for not taking care of yourself!!!

In addition to genetic factors, we have our own particular *toxic load*. What this means is that the toxins you are exposed to will differ from people living and working under other conditions. For instance, you'd have a heavier load if you lived in a large city, worked in a toxic factory, wore a lot of perfume, and ate junk food. And your load would be lighter if you lived in the mountains, worked outdoors in an unpolluted natural setting, wore essential oils, and ate whole natural foods. Under the first set of conditions, toxins would be entering your body faster than your system would be able to process them. This is a little like storing fat if you're taking in too many calories. When your exposure level to toxins is high, you are more vulnerable to the next toxic encounter. (The sources of both external and internal toxins were presented in Chapters 3 and 4.)

Also, you also want to consider your *lifestyle stress*. Pushing yourself constantly is a strain on the body, and it will reduce the functioning of your detoxification systems. Your body needs opportunities for relaxation in order to recharge. Many people are aware of the need to eat healthier foods, yet ignore the impact of their stressful lifestyles.

Of course, there are *nutritional considerations* as well. If you're receiving optimal nutrition, then your body is getting detoxification support on a regular basis. Again I want to emphasize that your body is detoxifying every second; it must have its needs met consistently.

Once you understand these concepts, then you can work with all of the factors. Knowledge will allow you to take action to strengthen or compensate for areas of weakness. Identifying tendencies toward weakness and working to improve them is a standard approach taken by Traditional Chinese Medicine and other natural systems of medicine. If you work to support areas that are vulnerable, then you can prevent illness, add years to your life, and life to your years.

HOW TOXINS AFFECT OUR HEALTH

As you learned at the beginning of this book, toxins are often silent contributors to numerous *health challenges*. Just like a car can't run well with a clogged oil filter, the body cannot operate at an optimal level when it is overloaded with toxins. To recap, here are just some of the health problems associated with toxicity:

■ How Various Systems Can Display Toxicity

The digestive system: constipation, diarrhea, bloating, gas, yeast, parasites, hormonal imbalances, PMS, indigestion, nausea, allergies, headaches, obesity, fatigue.

The respiratory system: mucus discharge, asthma, allergies.

The lymphatic system: frequent colds, flus, cellulite, swollen lymph nodes.

The dermal system (skin): acne, eczema, rashes, allergies.

The urinary system: difficulty urinating, water retention, low back pain, kidney stones.

The immune system: autoimmune disorders, immune deficiency, cancer, heart disease.

The nervous system: poor memory, depression, anxiety, brain fog, numbness, Attention Deficit Disorder (ADD), Attention Deficit Disorder with Hyperactivity (ADHD).

The endocrine system: thyroid disorders, metabolic imbalances, hormonal imbalances, endometriosis, PMS, fibroids, cysts, infertility, prostate conditions, diabetes, hypoglycemia, cravings.

The cardiovascular system: heart disease, high cholesterol, high or low blood pressure.

The musculoskeletal system: muscle and/or joint pain, fibromyalgia, arthritis.

While considering the list above, keep in mind that since the body is a whole organism, toxins usually do not affect just one system. In most cases, multiple systems are involved in reactions to toxins. However, the main impact may be noticed more in one organ or system.

As a general practitioner who has seen many patients with the above complaints, it never ceases to amaze me how effective a detoxification program can be as a factor in their recovery. The benefits of the detoxification are further enhanced with the maintenance and rejuvenation regimen that follows.

Unfortunately *toxicity has also been linked with deadly diseases—in fact, most of the major killers in this country.* Throughout history, common causes of death were plagues, malnutrition, or poor sanitation. But now with the increased toxic load in America and other Westernized countries, our major health threats are "diseases of civilization" such as cancer. I mention cancer specifically because most people are aware that this disease is tied to toxic exposures. However, when people are treated for cancer, the actual cause or aggravating factors (toxicity, stress, and/or nutritional factors) are rarely explored or "removed" as part of the treatment. Instead, only the effect (the tumor) is addressed. The neglect in identification and removal of the cause and the failure to strengthen the immune system are believed by some experts to be the reasons why so many recurrences of cancer appear when patients have only received "effect" treatments (surgery, chemotherapy, and/or radiation).

Yes, cancer is known to be associated with contact with "carcinogenic" substances, or in other words, toxins. We've all heard the statement that "everything causes cancer." Guess what? Organically grown whole foods don't cause cancer. Love doesn't cause cancer. Relaxation doesn't cause cancer. What nourishes us doesn't cause cancer, or any other illness for that matter. But toxicity can contribute to many of today's common diseases, including cancer. A lot of the symptoms of toxicity that were listed above—if not addressed properly with a detoxification and rejuvenation program—may result in more serious disorders.

The digestion-toxicity connection was presented in the previous chapter; here are some other conditions that often have toxicity as a contributing factor:

■ Health Challenges Commonly Related to Toxicity

Allergies: It is no coincidence that we are seeing a remarkable increase in allergies over the past few decades at the same time that we are witnessing a dramatic increase in environmental toxins. When the body is overloaded with toxins, the immune system is challenged, and allergic reactions can result. The removal of toxins from the body and environment often results in a corresponding decrease in allergic reactions.

Arthritis: Arthritis pain has been linked to a toxic reaction from specific foods, especially in the nightshade family (tomatoes, bell peppers, eggplant, etc.). Intestinal toxicity has also been linked to arthritis due to a reaction that occurs in the intestinal lining which triggers an inflammatory response.[2]

Asthma: Numerous research reports have linked air pollution to asthma. A recent Harvard School of Public Health report looked at two coal-burning power plants in the Boston area and their connection to more than 43,000 asthma attacks and an estimated 159 premature deaths each year.[3]

Autoimmune diseases: Heavy metals, pesticides, and a lack of beneficial bacteria can compromise the immune system, and these factors have been linked to autoimmune diseases such as lupus and rheumatoid arthritis.[4]

Cancer: Thousands of studies have linked numerous toxic materials with cancer. Toxins contribute to malignancy by damaging the DNA, mitochondria, and membrane of healthy cells. Pesticides, heavy metals, and a host of synthetic substances have been created in the past century, many of which have been linked to cancer. Progressive approaches to healing cancer involve removing toxins (the cause) from the body instead of (or at least as an adjunct to) adding toxic chemicals (chemotherapy). Western cancer therapy at this time does not focus on removing toxic residues in the body.

Chemical hypersensitivity (multiple chemical sensitivity): This condition has been found to be the result of cumulative damage by toxic exposures. Sufferers experience a lowered threshold of tolerance to the array of human-made chemicals. Reducing toxic exposure and detoxifying the body are crucial in this condition.

Chronic Fatigue: When the body is overwhelmed by toxins, its energy production is compromised. Toxins often involved in chronic fatigue syndrome include fungi, viruses, heavy metals, and neurotoxins. The most effective treatments for chronic fatigue include detoxification protocols and nutritional therapy.

Diabetes: Studies have linked various toxins with increased incidence of diabetes. A recent U.S. Air Force study reported evidence of a connection between Agent Orange (a chemical defoliant containing dioxin which was used in Vietnam) and diabetes and possibly heart disease.[5] Other research has linked at least eight other illnesses to this powerful toxin, including Hodgkin's disease and some respiratory cancers.[6]

Fibromyalgia and pain disorders: Accumulation of heavy metals and pesticides in the tissues has been linked to numerous pain conditions. The body has built-in anti-inflammatory mechanisms that are compromised with toxicity.

Gilbert's syndrome: This disease is a result of an abnormality in the detoxification mechanism of the liver.[7] Nutritional support for the liver has proved helpful in this condition.

Gynecological concerns: Toxins accumulating in the liver often impair this organ's ability to clear unwanted estrogen from the system. Toxins tend to accumulate in endocrine glands (which dramatically affects hormone balance) and in fatty tissues such as breasts. Conditions such as PMS, menopausal symptoms, uterine fibroids, fibrocystic breast disease, and endometrosis have all been associated with the estrogen dominance that results from this compromised detoxification aspect of the liver.

Heart disease: Cardiovascular illnesses have been linked to heavy metals in the bloodstream, as well as toxic levels of cholesterol and triglycerides. A study reported in the June 5, 2000 issue of the *Los Angeles Times* linked air particulates (from diesel trucks, cars, and industrial sources) to heart attacks. Inhaling the particulates appears to affect the body's ability to regulate heartbeats. A treatment that improves circulatory health by facilitating the removal of toxins (especially heavy metals) from the arteries is called chelation therapy. See Chapter 15.

Infertility/birth defects: Heavy metals and pesticides have been directly linked to lower sperm count and other aspects of infertility. A related groundbreaking book, *Our Stolen Future*, was written by Theo Colborn and John Peterson Myers, two leading environmental scientists, and Dianne Dumanoski, an award-winning environmental journalist. Their book extensively details decades of research linking lower sperm counts, reproductive abnormalities, and birth defects to the toxins that mimic natural hormones, resulting in the interference of healthy reproductive processes.

Mental and behavioral disturbances: Numerous psychological challenges have been linked to toxicity. In Chapter 3, the history of the phrase "mad hatter" was exposed. In the past, hatmakers used toxic metals such as arsenic, lead, and mercury, and were observed to have higher levels of mental illness. Neurotoxicity can result in increased depression, irritability, and sleep disturbances. Attention Deficit Disorder (ADD) and Attention Deficit Disorder with Hyperactivity (ADHD) have been linked to food colorings, flavorings, preservatives, and refined foods. In the *Journal of Orthomolecular Medicine*, biochemist Jeffrey Bland, Ph.D., explored the link between toxins and mental illness, including schizophrenia.[8]

Multiple sclerosis: Heavy metals, pesticides, and trans fatty acids affecting the nervous system have been linked to MS.[9] Detoxification of heavy metals as well as nutritional support emphasizing essential fatty acids can be beneficial in alleviating symptoms.

Neurodegenerative diseases: Alzheimer's disease, Parkinson's disease, Lou Gehrig's disease (ALS), and seizures have been associated with neurotoxicity.[10] Toxins, especially pesticides, have an affinity for the nervous system, and many nervous system related conditions occur as a result of this exposure. *The Journal of the American Medical Association (JAMA)* reported a recent study linking pesticides to a *significantly higher risk* of Parkinson's Disease.[11]

Prostate disorders: According to the research of Larry Clapp, Ph.D, a prostate cancer victor and author of *Prostate Health in 90 Days,* prostate health is dramatically affected by toxicity. Healing of his own cancer involved an extensive detoxification program. For extensive information about the prostate-toxicity connection, visit his website at *www.prostate90.com.*

Thyroid disorders: This epidemic has been linked to the accumulation of toxins, especially heavy metals. An 11-year study in the Polish region most affected by the Chernobyl nuclear disaster found thyroid gland changes in *every second* young woman and one in ten children.[12] Environmental toxins cause a reduction in T4 and T3 (thyroid hormone) levels, depressing thyroid function.[13]

This is not an all-inclusive list—there are volumes of research on the toxicity-disease connection.

Often toxic exposures take years to develop into a disease. Meanwhile you may not realize that the toxicity you are being exposed to in your life may lead to such devastating effects. Support for our body's detoxification systems must be emphasized for good health.

While some of the research documenting the connection between these conditions and toxins might involve more extreme exposures, we can't ignore the fact that in today's world we are exposed to more chemicals than ever before in history. We also can't ignore the potential negative health effects of these exposures *or* our ability to make choices to remove toxins from our environment and bodies. It's just plain common sense to reduce our toxic exposures and remove the toxic residue from our bodies to improve the state of our health and the quality of our life.

WHAT'S AHEAD

So far, we've examined how the body detoxifies on a regular basis, what systems are involved, and how compromised health can result from inefficient detoxification. Now, let's examine what each system needs for efficient health and detoxification. The next few chapters will explore the main systems involved in detoxification, starting with the one you would probably think about when you think about cleansing—the intestinal tract.

SIX

The Intestinal Tract — Your Pipeline to Health

Bliss begins in the bowel.

—Confucius

W hen we think of detoxification, often the first thing that comes to mind is the intestinal tract. Much of our "regular" experience with eliminating toxins happens through this wonderful pathway. It is important to have an understanding of intestinal health to prevent disease as well as to improve well-being.

Most of us do not think seriously about intestinal health until there is a problem or a degenerative condition has already developed. When someone begins to experience constipation on a routine basis, it may be the first time that they become aware that their intestines might need some attention. Or they may become concerned about the development of food allergies, irritable bowel syndrome, or some other form of reoccurring discomfort associated with digestion.

There are many symptoms and conditions related to intestinal toxicity. Some of these are obviously associated with the bowels. Many of the apparent symptoms and conditions manifest in the area of the intestines themselves.

SYMPTOMS & CONDITIONS COMMONLY ASSOCIATED WITH POOR INTESTINAL HEALTH

- Constipation
- Diarrhea
- Irritable bowel syndrome
- Gas, burping, flatulence
- Colitis

- Crohn's disease
- Diverticulosis
- Diverticulitis
- Intestinal polyps
- Intestinal & rectal cancer

It does not appear that intestinal health is improving. Statistics show that intestinal degeneration is appearing in more and more Americans. For instance, in 1950, only 10% of people in the United States had numerous saclike herniations (diverticula) along the walls of their intestines. In 1987, the percentage had increased to almost 50%. The most recent edition of *The Merck Manual*, the medical standard text for diagnosis and treatment of disease, states that they are very common after the age of 40, and "essentially every 90-year-old person has many diverticula."[1] Though these bowel pockets protrude through the wall of the intestines, the person who has them is usually unaware of their presence until infection and inflammation develop. Bowel pockets appear when the intestines become sluggish and constipated, providing a perfect breeding ground for cancer and other diseases. Additional evidence of the declining health of our intestines is the fact that the two most frequent types of cancer in the U.S. are now intestinal and rectal. In fact, Americans have the highest rate of colon-rectal cancer of any nation in the world.

Less evident symptoms and conditions are usually the result of toxins that pass through the intestinal wall. Poisons from the intestines can affect the entire body when they circulate in the bloodstream and the lymphatic fluid. These migrating toxins can cause various forms of "dis-ease" and inflammation. Here are other symptoms and conditions that appear to be associated with intestinal toxemia.

OTHER SYMPTOMS & CONDITIONS NOT ALWAYS PROPERLY ASSOCIATED WITH POOR INTESTINAL HEALTH

- Allergies
- Intolerance to certain foods
- Nausea
- Bloating
- Headaches
- Breast tenderness
- Premenstrual Syndrome
- Vaginitis
- Candida albicans
- Loss of mental clarity ("brain fog")
- Fatigue
- Flu-like symptoms
- Brittle nails & hair
- Weight gain or loss
- Bad breath
- Coated tongue
- Body odor
- Dark circles under the eyes
- Protruding abdomen
- Appendicitis
- Fibromyalgia
- Other muscle and joint pain
- Acne
- Eczema or psoriasis
- Other skin problems
- Depression
- Anxiety
- Mood swings
- Irritability
- Insomnia
- Diabetes
- Cardiovascular problems
- Arthritis
- High cholesterol
- Frequent infections
- Autoimmune diseases
- Sinus problems
- Chronic fatigue syndrome
- Back pain
- Breast, colon, and other cancers

Numerous studies have supported the intestinal toxicity-disease connection. A 1981 report in the medical journal *The Lancet* dramatically links poor intestinal health with breast disease. In a study of 1,500 women, less breast disease was documented in women who had daily bowel movements. Those women who had two or fewer movements a week had more than *four times* the incidence of breast disease, including cancer.[2]

A second study reinforced these earlier findings. In January 1989, the *American Journal of Public Health* reported an increased incidence of breast cancer in women who were experiencing constipation, infrequent bowel movements, or hard stools. Over 7,000 women participated in this subsequent study.[3]

Certainly any compromised intestinal health can create challenges that may limit your efforts to achieve optimal health. But as you'll soon learn, there are many steps you can take to maintain the health of your bowel and even restore it once a certain level of deterioration has taken place. More on that later in this chapter.

FUNCTIONS OF THE INTESTINES

To understand how poor intestinal health can be connected to a seemingly endless list of health complaints, it's important to first understand how the intestines operate. The intestines are viewed by many people as just organs of elimination—the last stop before a bowel movement. However they are so much more than that! They are also essential organs of digestion. The final stages of digestion take place there. Combined, the small and large intestine measure 26 feet and cover the surface area of a tennis court!

Duties of the Intestines
- Absorption of water, minerals, and other nutrients
- Manufacturing of vitamins such as B_1, B_2, B_{12}, and K
- Breakdown of food residues via beneficial bacteria
- Formation and excretion of feces
- Elimination of poisons, toxins, and waste products
- Keeping disease-causing organisms in check with friendly bacteria

Immune Function of the Gut
Within the intestinal lining exists the Gut Associated Lymphoid Tissue (GALT). GALT is made up of lymphocytes, macrophages, Peyer's Patches, and lymph nodes. GALT can be considered the largest immune organ in the body, participating in at least 60% of immune functions.

The GALT is constantly active as it is always on guard, preventing invasion of unwanted microorganisms (bacteria, yeast, parasites, fungus) and other toxins. Secretory Immunoglobulin A (IgA) is secreted into the mucus layer in the intestinal tract to prevent pathogenic bacteria from invading.

As you can see, the intestines are more than just a hollow tube through which wastes pass. The health of the entire body depends on how efficient the intestinal tract is at absorbing nutrients and eliminating wastes.

It is important to know how to support the proper functioning of the intestinal tract not only for disease prevention, but to increase your energy, vitality, and positive emotional outlook.

ALL BOWEL TO THE KING?

In Ancient Egypt, there were seven levels of physicians. The top level was the court physician who served the royalty. This superior doctor had the highest status possible, similar to that of the Surgeon General of the United States. Intestinal health was held with such high regard in Egypt that this esteemed position of court physician was reserved for an intestinal expert. How the title for this prestigious position translates from Egyptian is *"The Guardian of the Royal Ass,"* as this doctor's major responsibility was to ensure that the royalty had proper functioning of the gut from ingestion to digestion to elimination.

CAUSES OF POOR INTESTINAL HEALTH

While well-functioning intestines work in these various ways to keep you in good health, there are many habits and actions that can cause these organs to break down. Dietary factors play a major part in the frequent occurrence of intestinal distress. Emotional upset and tension, poor bowel habits, and travel have roles as well. Unfortunately few Americans are well versed in the behaviors that support intestinal health. Thus intestinal abuse is among the factors, making cancer of the colon this country's second deadliest cancer (about 48,000 people die of this each year). Constipation alone is currently generating $825 million in laxative sales annually in the U.S., driving 40 million Americans to the store aisles each year.[4]

Let's take a closer look now at what causes health concerns that are related to the intestines.

▪ Unhealthy Eating Habits

Eating too much, forcing meals when emotionally upset, consuming food in a rush, and snacking late at night are habits that are stressful to the whole digestive system. These detrimental habits can contribute to incomplete digestion and intestinal toxicity.

Not including enough enzyme-rich foods in your diet also leads to incomplete digestion and intestinal imbalances. Since we have explored the effects of autointoxication from enzyme-poor food in Chapter 4, we know that proteins can putrefy, fats can rancify, and carbohydrates can ferment in the intestines. As these foods decay, they promote the growth of harmful fungus, parasites, and bacteria. The foods that rot quickly inside your G.I. tract are the same ones that spoil fast outside of it. This includes meat, fish, eggs, and dairy.

A diet that lacks fiber does not keep the intestines in good working order. Conversely, adequate fiber creates a bulkier stool, which can travel faster through the intestines. Speedier bowel transit time reduces your exposure to toxins. Some fiber-rich foods include bran cereals and muffins, kidney beans, lentils, peas, apples, pears, and bananas.

Not drinking enough water can dehydrate the intestines. Moist, fiber-filled waste moves much easier through your system than dry hard material. Also, among the important functions of the intestines is the absorption of water. Remember, it's important to drink at least six to eight glasses of water a day. Many people drink caffeinated beverages, which are actually dehydrating to the intestines. Add two glasses of water for every cup of caffeinated beverage you drink.

Having too many refined and processed foods in the diet can lead to constipation. These include fried foods; candies, desserts, baked goods, and sugar products; white flour; table salt; salted snack foods (potato chips, pretzels, etc.); peanut butter; processed meat products; pasteurized milk and cheese; artificially carbonated drinks; and coffee.

▪ Poor Bowel Habits

The modern toilet is not ergonomically friendly to the intestines! Throughout history, people have squatted to have a bowel movement. Squatting allows for proper alignment of the body for elimination of waste material. In undeveloped regions without toilets, there are fewer cases of rectal problems, hernias, or hemorrhoids. Incidence of bowel cancer also appears to be lower. What is the solution for the toilet-equipped? Simply place a small footstool (approximately 6 to 14 inches high) to raise your feet when you're on the porcelain throne. The height of the footstool should naturally place you in the squatting position. Many people have commented on their surprise at how much easier elimination can become with this approach! See the Resources section for information on a special stool made for this purpose.

Not answering nature's call is another poor bowel habit to break. Some people suppress the urge to have a bowel movement due to a perceived inconvenience or a level of discomfort with public restrooms. Many patients have shared with me that they will not have a bowel movement in a restroom outside their home. Oftentimes they see this as a germ issue. Let me make it clear that not having a bowel movement when you're prompted to is an unwise and unhealthy habit. It is more of a "germ issue" by holding in your bowel movements—keeping all those harmful microorganisms inside of you creates the perfect breeding ground for pathogenic bacteria.

■ Other Factors in Intestinal Distress

Antibiotics and some drugs adversely affect the intestines. When harmful bacteria are killed off by antibiotics, the beneficial ones are put out of business as well. This sets the stage for the overgrowth of pathogenic microorganisms (fungi, bacteria, etc.) in intestines. Repeated courses of antibiotics actually create *antibiotic-resistant bacteria.* Also, research has shown that amalgam dental fillings can leach mercury into your system that may alter the balance of bad to friendly intestinal bacteria! This can also be a factor in antibiotic resistance. Birth control pills, steroids, and hard "recreational" drugs can upset the delicate flora balance too. More on the effects of antibiotics and other medication later in this chapter.

Our emotions—both disturbing and uplifting—greatly impact the intestines. In earlier times, the large intestine was, in fact, referred to as "the seat of the emotions." We have learned that the brain sends messages to the bowel via the nerves in times of anxiety or excitement that can interfere with peristalsis (the movement that causes waste to travel through). Also, blood supply and muscle tension in the region can be affected by emotional upset. Emotional distress can contribute to diarrhea, constipation, and loss of bowel control. Chronic conditions that might emerge include colitis and irritable bowel disease. In the groundbreaking book, *The Second Brain,* Michael Gershon, M.D., exposes this incredible gut-brain connection, demonstrating how every type of neurotransmitter found in the brain is also found in the gut.

Lack of exercise contributes to poor intestinal health in various ways. Blood circulation to the region suffers. Muscle tone can weaken, making elimination more difficult. Lastly, less lymph is pumped through your system, so a diminished cleanup of toxicity can result.

An increase in travel can place you at risk, as you will be exposed to different strains of bacteria, viruses, fungi, and parasites. Residents at travel destinations will have developed a resistance in their internal flora to these microorganisms. Your system, however, will have a different environment, one not used to fighting off the same tiny pests.

When the functioning of your intestines goes out of whack, you can feel lousy—both physically and emotionally. So don't take the health of your intestines for granted! Your diet and routine can make a huge impact—either negative or positive. For ideas on maintaining optimal intestinal health, turn to the guidelines provided at the end of this chapter.

RESULTS OF POOR INTESTINAL HEALTH

When people think of compromised intestinal health, what usually comes to mind first is constipation. Constipation is an obvious symptom and increasingly common in our society. When the waste products are not eliminated efficiently, other health conditions occur in the intestinal lining. The following section will help you understand how the health of the intestinal tract is related to the health of the body.

■ Constipation & Slow Bowel Transit Time

Constipation is one of the most common reactions that our body has to the poor treatment described above. However most people don't think they're constipated if they consider their elimination to be "regular." Unfortunately, the true definition of regular isn't widely understood. Hippocrates, the Father of Medicine, defined it as three bowel movements a day. If that ideal is quite a bit more than you are used to, an initial goal would be to have at least one comfortable and full bowel movement daily, without straining. This often will occur first thing in the morning. The ideal frequency, however, is two to three times a day.

Sometimes patients don't indicate constipation because they are unaware of the true definition of regularity. Thus I have had numerous patients complain of seemingly unrelated disorders. It was only upon my prompting that I learned that their eliminations were every other day, once a week, etc. As soon as they underwent a detoxification program and their elimination improved, their symptoms started clearing up. Constipation can signal a need to detox.

What many colleagues and I have observed is that patients often lack information about what it really means to be regular. One woman who became my patient had previously been seen by various specialists for the treatment of chronic fatigue. She was told by more than one doctor that a bowel movement once or twice a week was normal if that was normal for her! This pattern is neither normal nor healthy. I am happy to report that she quickly recovered from chronic fatigue after experiencing a thorough detoxification and rejuvenation program. I have hundreds of similar stories regarding my patients and those of my colleagues. I can only imagine the thousands of people who have yet to make the connection between intestinal health, frequency of bowel movements, and optimal health.

Note that besides the frequency of your bowel movements, another measure of intestinal health can be your ease in passing stools. Having a bowel movement should be as easy as urinating. You go, you evacuate, you clean up, you leave. Why do some people keep reading material in the bathroom? It could be that they are suffering from difficult evacuation or slow bowel transit time.

If you're not having two to three comfortable bowel movements daily, your bowel transit time is most likely less than optimal. This basically means that it's taking longer than is desired for wastes to travel through your intestines. Leading medical journals have published numerous studies indicating that an optimal bowel transit time is an important factor in the prevention of certain degenerative diseases, such as intestinal and breast cancer. Compromised elimination has also been linked to allergies, arthritis, depression, anxiety, high cholesterol, chronic fatigue, autoimmune disorders, fibromyalgia, back pain, and a host of other chronic conditions.

It's interesting to review the difference in bowel transit times between people eating a natural diet and those consuming the typical Western fare. During his many years of practicing medicine in 20th Century Uganda, British physician Denis Burkitt studied the elimination habits of African natives versus those of the English. Burkitt found that the meals of the Africans passed through their digestive tracts and were eliminated in about 24 hours. In contrast, the English had a bowel transit time of three days!

Not only was the bowel transit time drastically different; so were the consistency of the stools. The Africans' stools were large and soft, while the English eliminated hard, small stools, which they strained to pass. Said Burkitt, "My missionary friends tell me that Africans have an expression: 'where the people have large stools, they have small hospitals.' "[5]

Burkitt was one of the first researchers to call attention to the relationship between diet, constipation, slow transit time, and disease. He observed that the dramatically different diet of the Africans and the English affected elimination and, consequently, health. The Africans were eating unprocessed natural foods high in fiber and enzymes, whereas the English were eating the typical civilized diet high in sugar, fat, and refined flour, and virtually

TEST YOUR BOWEL TRANSIT TIME

There's an easy way to check on your own bowel transit time. Eat some beets! Later you'll notice some redness in your stool as their wastes pass. If you see the redness appear longer than 24 hours after you ingested the beets, you probably have less than optimal state of wellness in your intestines. If this is the case for you, consider following the tips given in the section "Guidelines for Optimal Intestinal Health" later in this chapter. Then redo the test after a month's time. Reminder: If you regularly notice redness in your stool, you may be suffering from something more involved. If this is the case, please consult with your physician.

devoid of enzymes. The Africans also appeared to be free of Western diseases such as intestinal cancer, heart disease, arthritis and obesity. Based on his findings, Burkitt became a strong proponent of proper intestinal maintenance with diet and other measures.

■ Intestinal Dysbiosis

We know that in nature there has to be balance for the survival of the species. Inside our body, there are also microsystems where various organisms are meant to live in balance and harmony. Dysbiosis refers to a condition in which the bacteria in the intestines are out of balance, resulting in a vulnerability to the overgrowth of yeast, fungi, parasites, and harmful strains of bacteria. This can be caused by a combination of the factors noted above, such as taking antibiotics and other drugs, eating hard-to-digest protein, lack of enzymes in food, having snacks late at night, living in constant stress, and not consuming enough fiber.

The balance of friendly to pathogenic bacteria in the intestines affects the health of these organs as well as your overall well-being. This makes sense when you consider the huge number of bacteria that reside in the intestines. There are more bacteria in a gram of stool than stars in the known universe. At any time, as many as 400 different species of bacteria can inhibit the human intestines. Total microorganisms living there can number 100 trillion! While healthy intestines should contain a ratio of 85% good bacteria to 15% pathogenic bacteria, too many people host the opposite combination.

A common scenario that triggers intestinal dysbiosis is the taking of antibiotics. These drugs kill off most of the bacteria in the intestines— good and bad. Without the friendly bacteria present to fight them off, pathogenic bacteria can take control. Their growth is fostered by the presence of decaying undigested food matter that results from the lack of helpful bacteria.

Next in line come the harmful yeast and fungi. Feeding on sugars, vinegar, wine and yeast, these pathogenic critters take hold. Once established, they are very difficult to get rid of. The stage is then set for the growth of parasites, which thrive in the now abnormal, putrefactive intestinal environment. Finally, viruses arrive—among the most deadly intestinal adversaries.

Among the effects of the presence of these invaders is a decrease in nutrient absorption, possibly resulting in a Vitamin B_{12} deficiency.

INTESTINAL TOXICITY AND THE DISEASE CONNECTION

When dysbiosis occurs, it is the result of inefficient digestion and/or not enough beneficial bacteria and too much pathogenic (toxic) bacteria. Toxins resulting from the action of pathogenic bacteria on incompletely digested protein has been observed to be the result of this imbalance.

While the results of internal toxins in the intestines have been observed clinically, specific toxins generated inside the body have been identified in various research reports.[6] The following chart details some internal toxins that have been found in the bowel and their related health conditions:

Intestinal Toxin	Related Health Condition
▪ Aminoethyl mercaptan	low blood pressure
▪ Ammonia	malignant transformation of cells, mental disturbances, tremors, altered EEG patterns
▪ Cadaverine	hypotension
▪ Histamine	headache, congestion, cardiac arrhythmia, depression, nausea
▪ Hydrogen sulfide gas	irritant to intestinal lining, can cause weakness, rapid pulse rate, nausea
▪ Indole	bladder tumors
▪ Tryptamine	hypertension
▪ Tyramine	epinephrine-like symptoms, hypertension
▪ Putrescine	hypotension

■ Phenol	depressed central nervous system, poor circulation, mucosal irritation, damage to kidney and liver cells
■ Skatole	depressed central nervous system, poor circulation

Research has found that intestinal dysbiosis can also result in irritable bowel syndrome, inflammatory bowel disease, autoimmune responses, intestinal and breast cancer, psoriasis, eczema, acne, chronic fatigue, and other chronic health concerns.[7]

Constipation can also affect the friendly bacteria in the intestines. The beneficial varieties, such as acidophilus, etc., require an oxygenated, acidic environment. A constipated, alkaline bowel causes a multiplication of unwanted bacteria.

As you can see, it's not just the amount of bad stuff in the intestines that affects health, but the lack of the *good* stuff too. Caring for the intestines can be compared to tending a garden. The good bacteria residing there are like flowers growing in healthy soil. Pathogenic bacteria are like weeds. Sometimes the intestinal environment needs weeding which comes in the form of supplemental good bacteria. (We'll discuss this issue later in the chapter.) Having an adequate intake of enzymes also helps.

There are tests to determine the extent of dysbiosis and the microorganisms involved. See Chapter 15 for the tests, labs, and health professionals who treat dysbiosis.

■ Yeast and Parasite Overgrowth

Two conditions resulting from the imbalance in the intestinal tract referred to as dysbiosis are the overgrowth of yeast and parasites. These microorganisms can contribute to numerous health conditions, for they affect the entire system. As conditions that contribute to dysbiosis are increasing (antibiotics, poor diet, stress), so are yeast and parasite infections.

Yeast

One of the most commonly overlooked causes of disease and ill health is an overgrowth of a species of yeast named *Candida albicans*— and a resulting condition referred to as *candidiasis*. These organisms are basically harmless when your body is in balance. However, when the internal environment is compromised, the balance becomes disrupted as was discussed earlier in the chapter. Yeasts, being opportunistic organisms, begin to take over. Recognized as one of the most common pathogens plaguing humans, yeasts have been categorized into at least 150 species. Commonly, it's the candida albicans variety that's involved in an overgrowth.

I could write volumes on this subject alone based on how I have seen it wreak havoc in the health of thousands of patients. Candidiasis is one of the most misunderstood factors in compromised health conditions. When candida growth goes out of control, it can manifest as symptoms such as gas, bloating, constipation, depression, fatigue, and brain fog. It has been connected to countless problems from chronic fatigue syndrome to multiple sclerosis to even AIDS.

In addition to an imbalance in the intestines, a weakened immune system is an open invitation for candida to fester. In an unhealthy environment, candida typically will begin to dominate in the intestinal tract, and it can also take over in the vagina, sinuses, and surface of the tongue (a condition known as "thrush"). Left unchecked, it can migrate to various organs, including the heart, lungs, liver, brain, and uterus.

Here are some additional contributors to candidiasis:

Factors That Contribute to a Candida Overgrowth

- Antibiotics
- Excessive sugar intake
- Immunosuppressive drugs (steroids, cortisone, etc.)
- Birth control pills
- Toxic exposures, especially to mold
- High bread/wheat/yeast product consumption
- Regular alcohol intake (especially wine, beer, champagne)
- Nutritional deficiency
- Recreational drug use
- Weakened immunity
- Consumption of products containing antibiotics & hormones
- Emotional stress

- Blood sugar imbalance
- Poor diet

- Mercury "silver" fillings
- Multiple sexual partners

Parasites

Another result of poor intestinal health is a parasitic invasion. A parasite is a plant or animal that lives in or on another species, derives its sustenance from the host, and either contributes nothing to the host's survival, or actually causes it harm. Parasites, like yeasts, are opportunistic organisms. When the intestinal environment is unhealthy, parasites can become established in the alkaline environment. It is common for parasites and yeast to coexist.

Parasitic problems are on the rise due to compromised immune systems, poor nutrition, an increase in international travel, foods from all over the world entering Western countries, an increase in antibiotics, antacids, and immunosuppressive drugs, and the popularity of household pets.

According to Omar Amin, Ph.D., one of the world's leading parasitologists, "Many of us have heard about illnesses such as giardiasis or amoebiasis, but we tend to overlook the relationship between these parasites and digestive and systemic diseases and disorders. The common belief that people in the United States are free of parasites is a great illusion."

Factors Contributing to a Parasitic Infection

- Foreign travel
- Water from questionable sources
- Tap water
- Raw fruit and vegetables from foreign countries
- Poorly washed fruits and vegetables
- Sushi
- Raw or undercooked meat
- Pork

- Poor food preparation habits
- Employment in hospital, day-care, sanitation, animal care
- Ocean, lake, or stream swimming
- Multiple sexual partners
- Frequent restaurant eating
- Antibiotics
- Steroid medications

- Birth control pills
- Toxic exposures
- Excessive sugar intake
- High bread/wheat/yeast product consumption
- Regular alcohol intake (especially wine, beer, champagne)

- Nutritional deficiency
- Recreational drug use
- Weakened immunity
- Blood sugar disorders
- Poor sanitary practices
- Walking barefoot in endemic areas
- Insect bites

PREVENTION OF PARASITES

Here are a dozen simple ways you can protect yourself from a parasite infection.

- Wash hands before eating, after handling animals, and during bathroom visits.

- Cover public toilet seats.

- Drink bottled water.

- Have your home tap water tested for parasites.

- Wash fresh fruits and vegetables thoroughly.

- Avoid imported fruits and vegetables.

- Eat at home more often.

- Consider a prophylactic anti-parasitic herbal formula when traveling and/or a bismuth preparation. See a health practitioner to determine if this is appropriate.

- Employ regular use of probiotics and/or cultured yogurt.

- Reduce the sugar in your diet.

- Increase your use of turmeric, horseradish, onions, ginger, garlic, and wasabe (a condiment served with sushi). These foods have natural anti-parasitic and anti-fungal properties.

- Have your pets checked and treated for parasites, if necessary.

Symptoms of Yeast Overgrowth
(Candidiasis) and Parasitic Infection

Yeast overgrowth and parasitic infection often occur simultaneously.
They share the seemingly endless array of symptoms:

- Fatigue; unexplained, where sleep doesn't seem to remedy
- Headaches
- Brain fog; memory and concentration challenges
- Digestive problems/ abdominal pain
- Food intolerance
- Irritable Bowel Syndrome
- Bloating and gas
- Cravings for sweets/bread/alcohol
- Constipation and/or diarrhea
- Recurrent infections; i.e. bladder, sinus, vaginal yeast, respiratory
- Decreased sex drive
- PMS/Hormonal imbalances
- Inability to stay calm/ anxiety
- Depression
- Mood swings
- Irritability
- Indecisiveness
- Chemical sensitivities
- Flu-like symptoms/immune dysfunction
- Fibromyalgia
- Joint/muscle aches
- Body odor or bad breath
- Allergies
- Asthma
- Insomnia
- Numbness/tingling
- Autism
- Crohn's disease
- ADD and ADHD
- Anal and/or vaginal itch
- Jock itch
- Athlete's foot
- Anemia
- Skin disorders; acne, psoriasis, eczema, rashes
- Difficulty gaining/losing weight
- Hypoglycemia
- Thyroid conditions
- Unexplained changes in weight

How Candida and Parasites Are Diagnosed

Yeast overgrowth and parasite infections are often not diagnosed properly. I have seen many patients who have presented with many of the symptoms listed. In a large number of cases, the yeast/parasite connection was never explored, but was present.

If you suspect a yeast or parasite-related health challenge, it is crucial to find a practitioner who is familiar with this phenomena. Tip: If you find yourself craving bread, sugar, and/or alcohol and have unexplained chronic symptoms, you may be experiencing a yeast and/or parasite condition.

Chapter 15 explains some of the tests that can help further identify a fungal (yeast) or parasite problem. For more information, visit *www.parasitetesting.com*. Please keep in mind that routine tests your doctor may do can overlook the systemic yeast issue presented here. At this point, only specialty labs are able to do the advanced testing needed for the identification.

How Candida and Parasites Are Treated

Effective treatments have included anti-fungal and anti-parasitic medications and herbs; yeast-free, sugar-free diets; and nutritional supplements, including probiotics (beneficial bacteria). Detoxification is also a crucial part of the treatment.

It is important to continue treatment throughout its course as suggested by your practitioner. Sometimes patients will start to feel better and stop the treatment as symptoms initially improve. This can result in the remaining fungus and/or parasites building up again, and the development of resistance to future treatment.

The candida/parasite patient usually has nutritional deficiencies that also must be considered. If the body is only treated with anti-fungal or anti-parasite preparations, the host will not be strong enough to fight further infection. It is essential to strengthen the body's defense system with nutrition.

IS YOUR BOWEL SLUGGISH?

If so, here's an easy-to-use tip. Drink hot lemon water throughout the day. Fill up a thermos and take a few sips every few hours. This is a natural remedy to enhance digestion, relax the intestinal tract, and encourage healthy bowel movements.

It is wise to seek the advice of a health professional for a specific nutritional supplement/herbal plan. Consider the information in Chapters 9 through 11 to decrease parasite and yeast vulnerability.

Dietary Considerations for Cases of Candida & Parasites

Here are basic nutritional guidelines to minimize the effects of yeast and parasites:

1. Don't feed what you're trying to destroy. Yeast and parasites love sugar, yeast, and alcohol. Foods that encourage fungus and parasite growth also include mushrooms, peanuts, and milk products (especially cheeses, which can be moldy). Small amounts of yogurt are acceptable.

2. Follow the basic nutrition (organic whole foods) plan in Chapter 9, avoiding the specific foods mentioned above.

3. Eat liberal amounts of vegetables, both raw and steamed.

4. Be sure to include an easily digested protein source at every meal to reduce sugar cravings and balance blood sugar. Never eat carbohydrates alone.

5. Avoid foods that are difficult to digest, such as fried foods.

6. Include essential fatty acids regularly, such as flax oil and olive oil.

7. Eat foods that destroy yeast and parasites, such as garlic, onions, horseradish, and scallions.

8. Use herbs that are anti-yeast and anti-parasitic, such as basil, dill, ginger, and oregano.

9. Drink lots of water. Avoid caffeinated beverages.

10. Avoid foods you are allergic to. Many patients with candida and parasites have unknown food allergies. Consider being tested.

An excellent plan for those with candida and parasite involvement is detailed extensively in the *The Body Ecology Diet* by Donna Gates. This book might seem a bit extreme for some, but it has been very effective for many suffering from the effects of yeast and parasite infections.

Please Note: Even though parasites and yeast are included in this chapter on the intestinal tract, it is important to remember that they affect the whole body. These subjects are included in this chapter because an unhealthy intestinal tract is usually the initial breeding ground for the overgrowth of these microorganisms. It is possible to have a yeast and/or parasite problem without having classic "intestinal" symptoms.

▪ Leaky Gut Syndrome

Dysbiosis, along with yeast and parasite overgrowth, often create a condition referred to as "Leaky Gut Syndrome."

The intestines have a normal permeability consisting of small holes that allow nutrients to pass through. Toxins such as yeast and parasites can attach to the lining of the intestinal tract and increase the permeability (the holes get bigger). Toxins and undigested food can then pass through leading to inflammatory reactions. The situation in the intestines must be healed or any other detoxification attempts will be limited. This is because the toxins will continue to circulate within the bloodstream, due to the ongoing seepage from the intestines. I have seen many patients who had gone on legitimate detoxification protocols with no success because the leaky gut issue wasn't diagnosed or treated.

To further understand the permeability of the bowel, think of how drugs such as cocaine or prescription medications are sometimes absorbed through the rectum.

Symptoms of Leaky Gut

- Sinus/nasal congestion
- Joint pain, swelling, or arthritis
- Constipation and/or diarrhea
- Fatigue
- Skin disorders
- Allergies
- Poor concentration and/or memory
- Abdominal pain or bloating

Leaky gut syndrome is seen in disorders such as inflammatory bowel disease, inflammatory joint disease, food allergies, celiac disease, rheumatoid arthritis, Crohn's disease, ankylosing spondylitis, and HIV.

Leaky gut syndrome can be diagnosed with a simple test (see Chapter 15) ordered by your health care professional. There are various supplements specifically formulated to aid in healing this condition (see Resources).

■ Autointoxication

"The intestinal tract serves as an important barrier of defense between the body's internal processes and a fairly hostile external world. The hundreds of different species of bacteria and other organisms which inhabit the intestinal tract all release by-products which may be absorbed into the bloodstream and contribute to chronic health problems."

— Jeffrey Bland, Ph.D, a leading biochemist in the field
   of nutritional medicine

When conditions such as dysbiosis and/or leaky gut develop, the compromised intestinal lining can allow toxins to seep through to the bloodstream, intoxicating the liver, kidneys, and the whole body. Some toxins can cross the blood-brain barrier, affecting the brain and the nervous system. This poisoning of the system with internal toxins is known as *autointoxication.*

Toxins that escape from the bowel often also build up in the cisterna chyli, which are branches of the lymphatic vessels. This can lead to an overall congestion of the lymphatic system.

When the detoxification processes in the intestines and liver cannot keep up with the demand, the body may attempt to use the skin to eliminate toxins. Many times, a breakout or other skin condition is the result of autointoxication.

Many of the symptoms presented in Chapter 2 from asthma to allergies, PMS to prostate disorders, are often the result of this autointoxication.

GUIDELINES FOR OPTIMAL
INTESTINAL HEALTH

■ 1. Monitor Your Intake of Water

This means water! Not coffee, soda, wine, or beer. Water is a pure cleansing drink that hydrates your body. Caffeinated beverages and alcohol dehydrate your body. When you drink a dehydrating beverage, you actually *lose* fluid from your body. So pure water is crucial. Since most tap water is loaded with toxins, use purified, filtered, spring, or distilled water.

It is suggested that you drink at least six to eight glasses of pure water a day. If this seems like a lot, try gradually increasing your water intake. When your system is hydrated more efficiently, you'll notice that drinking enough water will become second nature.

There are some theories that suggest that it is only important to drink water when you feel thirsty. This might be true if our diets were more natural to begin with. A natural diet has a higher water content, and provides less toxicity. We have an increased need for water because our diets contain mostly processed, low-water-content foods, and our bodies need the extra water to help flush out all the toxins we're taking in.

It is important to sip, not chug, the water. If you chug the water, your body won't have time to absorb it and you will notice frequent trips to the bathroom and constant pressure on your bladder. Sipping water affords more efficient absorption and less stress on the system. Initially, you will notice more frequent urination. As your body adjusts to its new level of hydration, the water will be absorbed more efficiently into the tissues and you will have a healthy, not excessive, amount of urination.

You can incorporate water drinking into your schedule with very little effort. If you travel a lot, keep a liter bottle in the car or in your luggage. If you work in an office, keep a large cup of water at your desk as a constant reminder to sip. Some of my patients fill up a half-gallon (contains eight 8-ounce cups) every morning, keep it on their desks or in the car, and sip it throughout the day. That is an easy way to monitor your water intake, especially if you're not used to drinking that much.

When people begin the process of increasing water intake to the optimal amount, a common situation that comes up is that they wait until the end of the day to "get the full amount in" and then find themselves in the bathroom at night. Numerous patients and I also have found it helpful to start the drinking process as soon as you wake up. Have a full glass of water upon arising, another one before breakfast, and another one before you leave for work. This habit will make it easier for you to increase your water intake.

▪ 2. Eat an Intestine-Healthy Diet

When you see a little heart next to a menu item in a restaurant, this signifies "heart-healthy"—a designation provided by the American Heart Association. This association has continuously researched the link of poor diet to heart disease. Although the American Cancer Society has linked slow bowel transit time to increased risks of cancer, they have yet to endorse a program pinpointing "intestine-healthy" items served by restaurants. Perhaps it is because pictures of intestines on menus just aren't that attractive.

Nevertheless, cancer and other degenerative diseases are on the rise, and we have no time to waste on making our diets more intestine-friendly. To start, follow the guidelines in Chapter 9 with special emphasis on high fiber foods, especially vegetables. Be sure to include essential fatty acids, such as in the form of olive or flax oil. Try to eat your vegetables and fruit raw when possible. Eat to only slightly less than full.

The intestinal tract is especially vulnerable to emotional stress. Chew your food well. If you are eating alone, eat in peace—not in front of the television. If you are not eating alone, eat only with people you love (or at least like).

▪ 3. Use Digestive Enzymes with All Foods that are Not Raw and Organic

In this chapter, we explored how incompletely digested food is a leading cause of intestinal toxicity. Since most of our diet includes foods that are enzyme-deficient, it is wise to supplement with enzymes as often as possible. Enzymes are also a great way to enhance bowel transit time, putting an end to constipation and eliminating the need for laxatives.

▪ 4. Supplement with Probiotics

In order to maintain a healthy amount of beneficial bacteria, it is wise to supplement with probiotics daily. Bacteria that are most beneficial include:

Lactobacillus acidophilus	*Lactobacillus sporogenes*
Bifidobacteria bifidum	*Lactobacillus salivarius*
Lactobacillus bulgaricus	*Lactobacillus plantarum*

Beneficial bacteria in the body can be compared to a good defense team in sports. If harmful bacteria attempt to invade, they will be destroyed by the strong supply of beneficial bacteria.

Some benefits of probiotics include:

- Aids in digestion and elimination
- Lowers cholesterol
- Destroys free radicals with its antioxidant properties
- Acts as antagonist to h. pylori (bacteria believed to be related to stomach ulcers)
- Produces natural antibiotics, helping to destroy invading bacteria
- Controls yeast overgrowth
- Produces B vitamins
- Increases absorption of minerals, especially calcium
- Aids in immune response

You probably have read newspaper reports about *E. coli* poisoning from time to time. Did you know that *E. coli* is a normal inhabitant of the intestines? Without enough beneficial bacteria to keep it in check, however, *E. coli* can rapidly take over and be very harmful. As bacterial infections are on the increase worldwide, it is good health insurance to use a probiotic supplement.

■ 5. Exercise

The intestines need optimal circulation to function best. Exercise is crucial for radiant health, and it is specifically beneficial to intestinal health. You may have noticed how exercise contributes to better bowel transit time. If you haven't yet incorporated exercise, and feel like your time is limited, a rebounder (trampoline) is an easy place to start. See Chapter 12 for more information on the use of a rebounder and other forms of exercise.

■ 6. Relaxation

As presented earlier in this chapter, there is a definite mind-body connection in the gut. Emotions ranging from excitement and enthusiasm to anxiety and worry have a direct effect on the health of the intestinal tract.

Intestinal Advice from the Experts

An emphasis on intestinal health and its relationship to chronic illness has been recorded since ancient times in Egypt, Babylonia, Assyria, Greece, Italy, Germany, Holland, France, Arabia, Africa, Hawaii, India, and China. Hippocrates, the Father of Medicine, claimed that chronic disease came from autointoxication. In the *Essene Gospel of Peace*, Jesus Christ described the natural laws of health, with special emphasis on intestinal cleansing. Dr. John Harvey Kellogg, legendary healer and founder of the Battle Creek Sanitarium in Michigan, declared that 90% of diseases of civilization are due to improper functioning of the colon.

Below are some fascinating quotes that reinforce the importance of internal cleansing:

One should put in order the five internal organs (lungs, heart, kidneys, spleen, liver) which are remiss and cleanse and purify them. One should criticize and correct the faults in their mode of life; one should restore their bodies and open the anus so that the bowels can be cleansed and the glandular secretions will properly serve the internal organs.
— *The Yellow Emperor's Classic of Internal Medicine*,
  the first Chinese medical text

All the good food that may be eaten cannot do the body any good until you have eliminated and cleansed the body of excess acids and mucus . . . If you cleanse and nourish the body properly and leave nature to itself, it will renovate and heal the body.
— Jethro Kloss, *Back to Eden*, 1939

All maladies are due to the lack of certain food principles, such as mineral salts or vitamins, or to the absence of the normal defenses of the body, such as the natural protective flora. When this occurs, toxic bacteria invade the lower alimentary canal, and the poisons thus generated pollute the bloodstream and gradually deteriorate and destroy every tissue, gland, and organ of the body.
— Sir Arbuthnot Lane, the great English surgeon and
  physician to the English Crown

> *The intestine is the most neglected and forgotten part of the body. Intestine health emphasizes prevention rather than cure. It is the most important step in maintaining or regaining vital health. If the sewer system in your home is backed up, your entire home is affected. Should it be any different with your body?*
> — Norman Walker, D.Sc., author and health
>   expert who died at age 109

> *They are full of extortion and excess. Cleanse first that which is within, that the outside may be clean also.*
> — Matthew 23: 25-26

> *Purging the bowels eliminates the source of poisons, thereby permitting blood and energy to regenerate naturally.*
> — Chai Yu-hua, 18th century Chinese physician

> *Every tissue is fed by the blood, which is fed by the intestines. When the intestines are dirty, the blood is dirty and so are the tissues and organs. It is the intestinal tract that invariably has to be cared for first before any effective healing can take place.*
> — Dr. Bernard Jensen, America's foremost pioneering
>   nutritionist of the 20th Century

Research has demonstrated how increased stress causes a decrease in beneficial bacteria in the intestinal tract. It is important not to eat while stressed or in a chaotic environment. If you are emotionally reactive, stress reduction techniques such as meditation, breath work, guided imagery, biofeedback, and yoga can be helpful in supporting proper bowel function. These techniques can help a wide range of intestinal problems including constipation, irritable bowel syndrome, colitis, and "nervous stomach."

■ 7: Always Answer Nature's Call

Simple and basic but crucial: Whenever you feel the urge, don't delay. You would not want the garbage disposal in your kitchen to be backed up . . . .

These suggestions should ensure healthy bowel functioning in most people. If you have followed the above and are not experiencing at least one full, easy-to-pass bowel movement a day, please see a health professional who has experience with natural medicine and intestinal health.

Considering the fact that cancer, especially colon cancer, is on the rise, as well as many other life-threatening degenerative diseases, isn't it a smart idea to start supporting your intestinal health today? The steps described in this chapter are easy to incorporate into your life. Later, in Chapter 11, you'll learn about an additional step you can take—intestinal cleansing.

WHAT'S AHEAD

Now that you understand more about how your "pipes" work, you now can go on to learn about your very own "oil filter." The next chapter explores the liver, the seat of detoxification, which has often been compared to an oil filter since it accumulates toxins until they are eliminated.

SEVEN

The Liver:
Your Fabulous Filter

Good morning, how is your liver?

— Common greeting in China

Like colon maintenance, care for the liver can be found in techniques practiced throughout history. In China, the health of the liver is considered representative of the health of the whole body. Conditions such as cancer, hormonal imbalances, depression, anxiety, immune challenges, and poor digestion are treated in Traditional Chinese Medicine (TCM) by enhancing liver health. Ironically, in these toxic times when we need it most, knowledge of liver health (which used to be commonplace) is now considered somewhat obscure!

Today we tend to think of liver problems as those that are related to alcohol abuse—such as cirrhosis. And many associate liver problems with diseases such as hepatitis or liver cancer. These are simply *local* manifestations of a suboptimal liver. However when the liver isn't functioning optimally, its sluggishness can also manifest in many *systemic* complaints. Almost all diseases—i.e., cancer, arthritis, heart disease, etc.—usually involve some compromise of optimal liver function.

Why is this so? Well, the liver evaluates every substance that comes through the body. And if all goes right, it will break down and eliminate the toxic substances that pass through. However, the liver is challenged by many other toxins besides alcohol. Cigarette smoking is usually not viewed as being toxic to the liver, but it is. Pot smoking puts a burden on the liver too. Chemicals in our food do as well. And one of the most challenging burdens for the liver is the abundance of chemicals secreted as a result of emotional stress.

The liver's assessment of toxins is accomplished through the blood. As noted in the last chapter, you might think of the liver as your body's "oil filter." The liver can remove a wide range of undesirables such as allergens, viruses, parasites, fungi, unfriendly bacteria, and toxic chemicals. It detoxifies substances that might cause damage to the body's tissues, cells, and DNA. *About 2 quarts of blood are filtered through the liver each minute!* Obviously, the liver plays a major role in your body's detoxification.

The liver has proven itself to be an extremely efficient detoxifier.... that is, until the 21st Century. As you now realize, we are not living in times of ideal circumstances when it comes to the body's detox. Pesticides and other toxic chemicals are putting an overwhelming burden on the liver specifically. The liver is a filter and stores residues of drugs, vaccines, chemicals, hormones, preservatives, etc., that we have *accumulated over a lifetime.* In the clinic, we are seeing more and more conditions related to an overworked, sluggish liver. It seems like we are always talking about the liver with patients.

Because of today's barrage of toxins, the liver is dramatically thrown off balance. Scientists are discovering that some toxins are not even recognized by the liver and are stored in the body, contributing to many health challenges. We are also learning that some toxins normally processed by the liver are not getting detoxified efficiently because this organ is so overworked. Research has also found that the liver—when overloaded or exposed to man-made chemicals—may inadvertently convert a toxic substance into an even more damaging poison.

Before we delve further into the problem of a compromised liver, let's review the basics about this essential organ. It will serve you well to learn more about it, for a healthy liver is needed for a healthy life. In fact, it's no coincidence that the word "live" is in the term "liver," because you can't live without this remarkable organ!

LIVER PRIMER

The liver is very complex. If a factory were built to represent its many functions, it would cover 2,000 acres! Its workings are quite amazing, including at least five hundred *known* responsibilities, and scientists are continually discovering more. Among its many functions are the conversion of foods into life-sustaining nutrients, the transformation of toxins into harmless chemicals for excretion, and the provision of quick energy when you need it.

Located just beneath your ribs on your right side, the liver weighs approximately five pounds and is the body's largest internal organ. Its size can be compared to that of a football. This organ is usually about 8 to 9 inches long and 4 to 5 inches wide. Its texture is soft and spongy. The liver is made up of four lobes, which overlap just a bit.

This is the only one of our organs that receives a double blood supply. Oxygen-rich blood comes from the heart and lungs through the hepatic artery. This makes up about 25% of the blood the liver handles. The portal vein brings oxygen-depleted blood from the intestinal area, supplying the remaining 75%. This second supply contains nutrients. About a pint of blood can be held in the liver at one time, an amount equaling about 13% of our total blood supply!

Unique among the body's many organs, the liver can regenerate parts of itself that have been damaged due to injury or disease. However, if this occurs repeatedly, its functioning can be impaired.

Besides its major job of filtering the blood, some of the liver's other functions include:

■ Metabolic Regulation

Transforming dietary elements such as protein, carbohydrate, and fat into energy-supporting nutrients.

Constructing thousands of metabolic enzymes from properly digested protein. When there is a shortage of digestive enzymes, protein is often not broken down enough for the liver to obtain optimal amounts of material required to construct the enzymes needed for other work.

Breaking down hormones. The liver plays a key role in breaking down hormones, such as estrogen. When the liver is overloaded, estrogen-dominant conditions can occur: PMS, hot flashes, fibrocystic breast disease, difficult periods, breast and other gynecological cancers.

Converting vitamins and minerals into a form most easily utilized by the body. It also stockpiles nutrients, especially vitamins A, D, E, K, and B12, as well as the mineral iron to be used as needed. The amount of vitamins D and B12 that it can store could last four months!

Producing vital substances. The liver constructs bile, gamma globulin (immune substance), cholesterol, estrogen, and other hormones.

■ Blood Regulation

Storing extra blood and glycogen to be released on demand.

Regulating blood sugar. When the blood sugar is low, a healthy liver can convert glycogen into glucose to bring the blood sugar back to normal. When the blood sugar is elevated, the liver can remove the excess and convert it into stored glycogen or fat.

Creating a substance called Glucose Tolerance Factor from chromium, niacin, and other nutrients. Glucose Tolerance Factor works with the hormone insulin to regulate blood sugar levels. When the blood sugar isn't regulated properly, symptoms such as fatigue and anxiety are common.

THE IMPORTANCE OF BILE

The liver manufactures *bile*, which is a fluid that aids in the digestion of fats. When the liver is overburdened, fat metabolism is compromised. Bile is the major route for the excretion of cholesterol. In the clinic, patients have often lowered their cholesterol by cleansing their liver. It can be a much safer approach than treatment with drugs.

Bile is a major player in the detoxification process. It is a carrier of many of the toxins broken down by the liver, which are sent on to the intestines to be absorbed by fiber and excreted. Diets low in fiber inhibit this process, and toxins are often not eliminated.

THE LIVER & IMMUNITY

When we think of the immune system, we usually don't picture the liver. However, the liver is where 50% of all macrophages (white blood cells crucial for optimal immunity) are located. Remember the "Kupffer cells" (a type of macrophage located in the liver) discussed in the Chapter 5? They work in conjunction with resident liver cells called hepatocytes to clear bacteria entering this organ in the portal blood.

Kupffer cells are quite fast and have the ability to engulf bacteria within a fraction of a second after contact. When optimally functioning, they are able to clear 99% of the undesirable bacteria and toxins before blood is channeled back into the body. Rather than making antibodies like other white blood cells, the Kupffer cells take in and destroy their targets. Substances not handled by the Kupffer cells are moved along by the hepatoctyes to the bile.

PHASE I/PHASE II
DETOXIFICATION IN THE LIVER

In addition to the detoxification role of the Kupffer cells as explained above, the liver has extensive talent in using enzymes to transform toxic chemicals into substances that are easily excreted in the urine or bile. It does this with a Phase I-Phase II approach to detoxification, as introduced in Chapter 5.

Here's how the two-phase process works in the liver:

Phase I: Toxins such as environmental chemicals, drugs, and metabolic by-products enter the body and activate a group of enzymes called *cytochrome P450 mixed-function oxidases*. (Yes, the name is a mouthful, but it's what they're called!) In this phase, the toxins are transformed into an intermediate state that can be further broken down in Phase II.

Phase II: In this step, the body adds specific nutrients to transform the toxin into a water-soluble compound for a safe exit via urination or bowel movements.

THE 21ST CENTURY LIVER

In an optimally healthy person, the liver's detoxification system performs at its peak. Unfortunately, in most people, the reality of the increase of toxins in our environment has given the liver more than it can handle, or for that matter, was ever designed to handle. In addition to the toxins being an extra burden, nutrients needed to support the detoxification enzyme system are often deficient in the diet.

Since 1976, the EPA has been conducting the National Human Adipose Tissue Survey (NHATS). NHATS collects a nationwide sample of human fat tissue specimens and analyzes them for their toxic compounds. Adipose (fat) is chosen because toxins tend to store there in high concentrations. In 1982, the study expanded its list to examine environmental compounds. The results were astounding. Some of the most dangerous chemicals, such as dioxin, xylene, and ethylphenol, were found in 100% of the samples.[1] And DDE, which is a chemical that represents the breakdown of DDT in the system, showed up in 93% of the samples.[2] (Remember, DDT is a highly toxic pesticide that was banned from use in the United States but enters our country in produce from nations where it is still in use.) The increasingly alarming results of NHATS are demonstrative that most people's livers obviously aren't able to efficiently eliminate all unwanted chemicals. Thus, most people would benefit from practicing healthy habits to support better liver function.

SYMPTOMS OF A SLUGGISH LIVER

Symptoms of an overworked liver are not necessarily signs of actual liver disease. However, compromised liver function is so common that its symptoms seem almost normal. These include:

- Fatigue
- Tiredness after meals
- Depression
- Mood swings
- Anger/irritability
- PMS and other hormonal imbalances
- Digestion/elimination problems
- High cholesterol
- Pain in the muscles and/or joints
- Allergies
- Acne, psoriasis, and other skin disorders
- Blood sugar imbalances
- Fibromyalgia
- Headaches

- High blood pressure
- Brain fog
- Indigestion/acid reflux
- Constipation
- Diarrhea
- Nausea
- Bloating
- Difficulty losing or gaining weight

Other signs of a compromised liver can be observed as lines on the face between the eyebrows, a bitter taste in the mouth, dark circles under the eyes, body odor, bad breath, a coated tongue, and age or "liver" spots.

A liver that is sluggish isn't filtering the poisons out of the bloodstream adequately. The skin, being an elimination organ itself, becomes overwhelmed and must release poisons at the surface. Acne, rashes, psoriasis, and itchy skin can often be the result of a sluggish liver.

Optimal liver health is essential for mood stabilization. Thus symptoms of depression, anxiety, and irritability can often be signs of a challenged liver. In Traditional Chinese Medicine (TCM), a tendency to get easily angered, to have a "short fuse," is often associated with a sluggish liver. In South America, when people get angry, they are called "livery" and given some herbal tea to soothe their liver and calm their emotions.

When the liver is challenged, fat metabolism is often compromised. Effects of this will include difficulty in achieving and maintaining ideal weight, high cholesterol and triglycerides levels, an accumulation of cellulite, and poor fat digestion.

Poor blood sugar management is another common result of an overworked liver. Mismanagement can lead to hypoglycemia, diabetes, and a tendency to store carbohydrates as fat.

As mentioned earlier, hormonal imbalances are also frequently tied to a sluggish liver. Symptoms such as PMS, breast diseases, and menopausal symptoms are traditionally treated in TCM and other forms of natural medicine by supporting optimal liver function. At this time, Western medicine does not appear to be addressing this key causative factor.

Lastly, as the liver is a key player in immunity, its compromised function will often result in repeated colds, flus, sinus and other infections; asthma; allergies; chronic fatigue; and chemical sensitivity.

THE LIVER &
THE COMMON PROBLEM OF AN
UNDERACTIVE THYROID

Currently, thyroid imbalances are commonplace, practically an epidemic. This can be troublesome as the thyroid, a hormone producer, controls metabolism and thus affects every cell in your body. The liver regulates this butterfly-shaped endocrine gland by converting the thyroid hormone *thyroxine (T4)* into the more *active tri-iodothyronine (T3)*. A compromised liver can limit this conversion process.

Thyroid imbalances can result in difficulty losing or gaining weight (sluggish metabolism), hair falling out, blood sugar swings, a tendency to feel chilly, poor memory, mood swings, lethargy, menstrual problems, water retention, headaches, and trouble swallowing. These symptoms and others have driven thyroid hormone prescriptions to an all-time high. According to the *L.A. Times*, Synthroid, a synthetic hormone, is prescribed for underactive thyroid to the tune of 36.2 million prescriptions annually. It is the second highest-selling drug in America.

Despite the prevalence of drug therapy, many patients with sluggish thyroids have had success with detoxification protocols. Since environmental chemicals have been reported to cause a reduction of both T4 and T3,[3] reducing the toxic load allows the thyroid function to improve significantly.

A severely compromised immune system may manifest itself in more serious health challenges such as cancer and heart disease. It's interesting to note that almost all of the most renowned cancer treatment centers whose focus is on natural healing have liver detoxification as a key therapy.

It may seem strange and overwhelming to think that so many symptoms could be related to the liver. As stated earlier, in our culture, we tend to think of the liver only in cases of alcoholism, cirrhosis of the liver, hepatitis, and liver cancer. The symptoms above related to the liver are classically recognized in traditional medical systems in addition to

TCM (a system that dates back at least 5,000 years), such as naturo-pathic medicine, Ayurvedic (a classic system from India) medicine, and most forms of traditional herbal medicine.

THE LIVER & IDEAL WEIGHT

When liver health is compromised, the entire metabolism is sluggish. Many patients who come into the clinic have tried every diet that has come down the pike, but they still struggle with their weight. Diet pills temporarily speed up the metabolism, exhausting it so it becomes sluggish in the long run. Removing toxins from the body, especially the liver, allows the body to improve its overall metabolic functioning. This often results in the healthy attainment of ideal weight.

THE LIVER & EMOTIONAL HEALTH

In many traditional medical systems, the health of the liver is considered directly related to emotional stability. In Traditional Chinese Medicine, for example, conditions such as depression, anxiety, and panic disorders have sophisticated treatments prescribed that address various aspects of liver imbalance. I have had the pleasure of witnessing numerous cases of improved emotional health corresponding with improved liver health. The ancient Greeks treated emotional health by treating the liver. The term melancholy comes from the Greek for "black bile"—indicating the sluggish nature of the bile in the liver.

Stress chemicals and hormones, such as adrenaline and cortisol, must be processed by the liver for neutralization or elimination. Sometimes these chemicals are stored in the liver when the amount released into the bloodstream is too much for the liver to clear efficiently. This can contribute to emotional imbalances such as depression and anger, as well as stress-related illnesses, such as cancer and heart disease.

FACTORS CONTRIBUTING TO A COMPROMISED LIVER

The liver is one of the organs that is most assaulted by our habits and actions. Each year, 40,000 Americans die from liver diseases, such as hepatitis, cirrhosis, or jaundice. As has been noted, many of us are suffering from suboptimal liver function, resulting from a combination of factors. The following are the major elements that impact the health of our liver.

- History of mono, hepatitis, alcoholism, drug abuse
- Exposure to chemicals (pesticides, herbicides, industrial chemicals, etc.)
- Pharmaceutical drugs
- Toxic bowel
- Candida, parasites, fungus, viruses, bacteria
- Emotional stress/stored anger
- Hypothyroid
- Improper digestion
- Tobacco and marijuana smoking/recreational drug use

In today's world, most people could benefit by being aware of factors affecting their liver health. However anyone who lives in a heavily polluted area or works in a job that exposes them to paints, solvents, pesticides, herbicides, or industrial chemicals should take special note. If you regularly consume alcohol or take recreational drugs, you may also be putting your liver at risk.

It's not just recreational drugs that tax our liver. Steroids, oral contraceptives, chemotherapy, aspirin, antibiotics, and hormone replacement therapy all add to the liver's burden. In particular, Tylenol (acetaminophen) can deplete the body's stores of the antioxidant glutathione, and if consumed with alcohol, presents the risk of liver damage. In fact, in the mid-90s, a 39-year-old former special assistant to President Bush was awarded a multi-million settlement because of liver damage believed to be associated with the ingestion of Tylenol during a period when he regularly drank wine. The man required a liver transplant. It's thought that the regular consumption of wine may have reduced the ability of this man's liver to detoxify acetaminophen.

In Chapter 3, you learned that some toxic factors are under our control while others are not. This is true also for the elements that affect our liver health. For this very reason, it can be important to eliminate as many negative influences as possible. Let's look now at the dietary factors that may impair your liver function.

LIVER DIETARY DISASTERS

You now know the huge influence that the food you eat has on both your toxic load and your everyday health. Well, your diet can also either be supportive or detrimental to your liver too. It's not just the foods you eat but also your dietary habits that can stress this essential organ. The following items can translate into a dietary disaster for the liver:

- Overeating
- Excess of refined carbohydrates
- Excess of processed fats
- Excess of poorly assimilated protein
- Deficiency of essential fatty acids, vitamins, minerals
- Low vegetable intake
- Not enough fiber

- Alcohol
- Sugar
- Fried foods
- Pasteurized/homogenized dairy
- Eating while feeling stressed
- Eating in a rushed manner
- Excess of cooked and processed foods

Remember, a major task for the liver is to detoxify substances that come through your system. Diet is an area where you can make huge strides toward supporting your liver health. Note that not only are the original chemicals contained in food a factor, but also those that are produced inside the body as these compounds flow through. For instance, formaldehyde can result when Nutrasweet is detoxified by the body.

HOW TO SUPPORT
BETTER LIVER FUNCTION

By now, you understand how essential proper functioning of the liver is. Here are some of the basic things you can do to promote the health of this vital organ.

1. **Once again, drink plenty of pure water.** Consume an amount equaling at least half your body weight in ounces. For example, if you weight 140 pounds, drink 70 ounces. Add lemon whenever possible.

2. **Upon arising, drink a cup of hot water with lemon.** This can stimulate the release of bile and aid in cleansing the liver and bowels first thing in the morning. For those of you who drink coffee to stimulate bowel movements, you can replace the coffee with the hot lemon water for a healthier beverage.

3. **Increase green vegetables, especially the bitter lettuces.** Greens such as arugula, dandelion greens, mustard greens, endive, and dark salad greens are suggested. Make it a point to have a salad at least once a day that includes these vegetables. The bitterness of the greens supports the flow of bile, which aids in the detoxification processes of the liver. The greens themselves are power-packed with nutrients to support overall detoxification and rejuvenation. A dressing that includes olive oil and fresh lemon juice provides extra support for the liver.

4. **In addition to the greens, increase raw and steamed vegetables in your diet.** Beets, carrots, daikon radish, cabbage, broccoli, and Brussels sprouts contain phytonutrients that stimulate detoxification enzymes and have been well researched for their anti-cancer properties.

5. **Include enzyme-rich food in your diet and supplement when necessary.** The liver uses raw materials from completely digested food to construct thousands of essential nutrients. Also, eating enzyme-depleted food adds another burden to the liver in the digestive process.

6. **Use fresh herbs such as turmeric, rosemary, caraway, and dill as much as possible in your cooking.** These herbs have been researched to support optimal liver function.

7. **Add essential fatty acids to your diet.** At a minimum, take one tablespoon of fresh, unheated flax oil daily. Other oils to use could be borage, hemp, evening primrose, or a formulated blend.

8. **Limit sugar intake.** Try to include fresh, organic fruit when you have a sweet craving. The fruit contains vitamins and antioxidants which aid in liver function.

9. **Eat as organic as possible.** Avoid artificial food additives and pesticides. Toxic chemicals in food give extra work to an already busy liver.

10. **Avoid overeating.** All that food can stress your entire digestive tract, including the liver. The increased burden on the liver compromises its detoxification abilities. Also, don't rush through your meals.

11. **Partake in a regular enjoyable exercise program.** Whenever possible, try to fit in at least 20 to 30 minutes of exercise every day. This can be broken into two shorter sessions. Enhanced circulation improves overall liver function.
12. **Choose joy, compassion, peace, and love as much as possible.** Reject the indulgence of anger, blame, fear, or worry. In addition to improving the quality of your emotional outlook, these choices reduce the amount of stress chemicals that the liver would have to process.
13. **Make sure your breath patterns are full and even.** If you notice that you breathe in a shallow or uneven manner, consider training in breath work, yoga, stress reduction, or meditation.
14. **Supplement your diet with herbal formulas.** There are wonderful herbs clinically proven to improve liver function. Chapter 11 provides extensive detail regarding botanical liver support.
15. **Stimulate the liver by gently massaging the area just under your right rib once each day.** This can help keep your liver from becoming congested.

ASSESSING LIVER FUNCTION WITH LAB TESTS

If you are experiencing any symptoms of a compromised liver, you may wonder why your doctor has never detected that your liver needs support. Remember, what we're talking about here is not liver disease, but any variance in the high level of functioning of the liver that is essential for optimal health. While your liver might not actually be diseased (with hepatitis or cirrhosis, for example), it could be compromised. Such suboptimal functioning of the liver can contribute to cancer, PMS, heart disease, migraines, hormone imbalances, allergies, fatigue, immune dysfunction, and chronic pain.

On a standard blood test, two liver enzymes *SGPT* and *SGOT* are measured. If they are elevated, your doctor might suspect *hepatitis or an infection.* This is the basic test run by most physicians. It does *not* measure the toxic load your liver is handling, nor its detoxification efficiency.

There are other tests available to evaluate more specific functions of the liver, especially its ability to effectively clear toxins. See Chapter 15 for more information.

LIVER CLEANSE DRINK

A liver flush has been used traditionally to support detoxification. This cleansing drink increases bile flow, encouraging the elimination of wastes.

Many patients have used this recipe over the years with wonderful results.

Put the following in a blender:

- One cup of citrus: use orange, grapefruit, tangerine, lemon, and /or lime. Make the combination as sour as possible. You can dilute this mixture with purified water.

- One to two cloves of garlic

- One small piece of fresh ginger

- One tablespoon of organic olive oil

- Blend the above ingredients and drink immediately.

Follow with two cups of a cleansing tea, such as Jason Winters or dandelion tea.

It is preferable to do the liver flush drink in the morning on an empty stomach, and then wait an hour before eating.

It is suggested to do the liver flush four times a year (as the seasons change) or whenever you feel you need a boost. Five days in a row each time is recommended.

CARING FOR YOUR LIVER

The liver is so forgiving. Remember, it can regenerate itself, assuming the abuse—such as toxicity—stops and the support is there. The liver is happy to respond to proper care.

You may have a lifetime of accumulation in your liver, so don't expect it to be completely clean in only a month. This is a common misconception. I have asked many patients the question, "Have you ever done a liver cleansing program?" The answer is either "No," or "Yes, I cleaned out my liver years ago with a three-day fast."

The good news is that liver support, cleansing, and regeneration is very easy, as many things are when you have the right information. Earlier you were provided with steps that you could take to support optimal liver functioning. Another important element can be an efficient liver cleanse with herbs as presented in Chapter 11.

Throughout history, liver cleansing has been practiced by cultures throughout the world. In many traditions, liver cleansing was done seasonally, often in the spring. It is quite ironic that now that we have more toxins than ever before, this time-tested ritual seems to have fallen by the wayside in mainstream medicine. Fortunately, however, more progressive practitioners often include liver support in their treatments.

WHAT'S AHEAD

We can't separate the organs and truly address them in isolation, nor should we attempt to do so and expect positive results. Actions you take to support one area will benefit others too. However, by focusing on colon and liver health, you will be way ahead of the game. The whole body and all other systems will automatically improve with a boost in digestion and elimination.

It is still important, however, to understand, evaluate, and maximize the health of other body systems involved in detoxification and energy production. Thus additional systems—respiratory, lymphatic, urinary, and dermal—are described in the next chapter.

E I G H T

All Systems Go:
Other Players in the Detox Process

The kidneys are so beautifully organized; they do their
work of regulation with such a miraculous—it's hard to
find another word—such a positively divine precision,
such knowledge and wisdom, that there is no reason
why our archetypal man, whoever he is, or anyone
else, for that matter, should be ashamed to own a pair.

I know all about love already.
I know precious little about kidneys.

—Aldous Huxley, in *Antic Hay*

We have already explored two primary sites of detoxification in depth—the intestinal tract and the liver. It is now time to increase your awareness of the other systems in the body that also facilitate the detoxification process. As indicated in Chapter 5, there is much more involved! In this chapter, we will explore four important systems:

The **Respiratory System** (lungs, nose, throat, and trachea)
The **Lymphatic System** (lymph glands, nodes, and vessels)
The **Dermal System** (skin, sweat, sebaceous [oil] glands, and tears)
The **Urinary System** (kidneys, bladder, ureters, and urethra)

THE RESPIRATORY SYSTEM

■ Functions
The oxygen inhaled in the breath is a nutrient essential to every

metabolic process in the human body. Oxygen is considered the most essential nutrient of all. You can live for up to 40 days without food, up to a week without water, but couldn't survive more than a few minutes without oxygen.

With every breath, the respiratory system assists in preventing us from taking in unwanted toxins. The hairs in our nose trap dust, bacteria, and other pollutants. Mucus coating the inside of the lungs attracts particulate matter and keeps it from entering further into the chamber. Foreign substances may be exhaled through coughing.

Toxins that do travel in deeper face possible attack by immune cells. The lungs are also able to transform invading toxins into water-soluble chemicals, which can be excreted by the kidneys. However, some persistent toxins are retained in the lungs and can cause pathological changes. Others that evade an assault from the respiratory system may be deposited in different organs or tissues.

An important detoxification aspect of the lungs that we experience every moment is the expelling of the metabolic by-product carbon dioxide. This carbon dioxide is delivered to the lungs in the blood through small sacs called the alveoli. Some toxins, such as volatile organic compounds, are also released when you exhale.

Note: It's important to remember to breathe fully, all the way into your abdomen, rather than simply into your chest. This increases your intake of oxygen, which will help to revitalize your cells. Fuller breathing will also optimize the release of toxins that you exhale. Relaxed full breathing brings psychological detox benefits too as it modifies the functioning of your nervous system. Finally, abdominal breathing more effectively stimulates the circulation of cleansing lymphatic fluid. As published in the journal *Lymphology*, deep, diaphragmatic breathing creates a vacuum effect that increases the rate of toxic elimination through the lymph as much as 15 times the normal rate.[1]

▪ How the Respiratory System Gets Challenged

Most people are aware of some of the toxins they might breathe in (such as cigarette smoke in restaurants) and try to avoid them. However, if you are in a toxic environment frequently, your body can get desensitized even as toxins continue to accumulate in your system. Some examples of this would be people who get "used" to smog in a polluted city or to toxic air where they work (at a print shop, gas station, oil refinery, etc.). Even office workers in their "sterile" environments can have daily exposure to toxic outgassing from carpet, paint, air conditioning, printing, etc. Some inhaled toxins are deceptive, as they have no odor, such as carbon monoxide.

Toxins taken in from the air (a topic covered extensively in Chapter 3) usually affect the lungs most directly, though they can be passed along to other parts of the body. Also, toxins taken in through other systems can circulate and affect the lungs as well as the whole body.

The concept of systemic toxicity is displayed in fascinating data from the American Cancer Society. In a recent study involving 781,351 people, researchers found that cigarette smokers are 40% more likely to die of colon cancer than are non-smokers.[2]

The link between smoking and lung disease is known by most people. However, when smokers decide to quit, they usually don't think of the toxic reside that is left behind. Toxins may be retained in the lungs long after they have been inhaled. For example, why do you think people who haven't smoked for 20 years can still develop lung cancer? The detoxification of their lungs wasn't efficient. All ex-smokers should undergo at least a basic detoxification plan. Also, chest x-rays of people who live in polluted cities often reveal similar lung damage to that of smokers.

Conditions Associated with Lung Toxicity or Impaired Function

- Congestion
- Shallow breathing
- Fatigue
- Sighing
- Wheezing
- Chronic coughs
- Asthma

- Bronchitis
- Emphysema
- Allergies
- Recurrent colds/flus
- Lung cancer
- Emphysema

Respiratory System Stressors

- Smoking cigarettes and/or marijuana
- Environmental pollutants
- Lack of fresh air

- Excessive sadness
- Congesting foods: Pasteurized dairy, wheat, refined sugar and flour

Habits for Healthy Lungs

- Optimal water intake
- Generous intake of vegetables
- Yoga

- Aerobic exercise in a clean air environment
- Deep breathing exercises
- Steam inhalation

THE LYMPHATIC SYSTEM

▪ Functions

The lymphatic system is crucial to cleansing of the body. It is similar to the circulatory (blood vessel) system in that it has a network of vessels all over the body. In addition, there are numerous organs, glands, and nodes in this system including the tonsils, adenoids, appendix, spleen, thymus, and the Peyer's patches in the small intestine. However, when most people think of their lymph system in action, they usually just recall a gland being swollen such as under the arm.

The truth is that you have more lymph fluid than you do blood! The vessels of the lymphatic system contain approximately 15 liters of lymph fluid, *three times the amount of blood in the body.* The entire system derives its name from the clear, colorless appearance of lymphatic fluid (*lympha* means water).

The lymphatic system works like a trash collector. It has over 600 collection sites called "nodes" that are scattered throughout the body. One of its many duties is to collect and carry away waste products from your body's cells. Its vessels and nodes house white blood cells such as lymphocytes and macrophages (the T-cells and B-cells of the immune system); these defenders engulf and destroy harmful bacteria, viruses, fungi, and other toxic materials.

While the circulatory system has a heart to pump the blood, there is no similar forceful organ for the lymph. Still lymph flow occurs despite the fact that most of the movement is against gravity. Instead of a pump, the lymphatic system relies on the body's daily exercise routine and breathing in order to function optimally. During exercise, for instance, the rate of flow may increase as much as 10 to 15 times!

▪ How the Lymphatic System Gets Challenged

The lymph shows signs of compromised function when it is overloaded with toxins. When this occurs, the results can be fatigue, lowered immune response, and localized swelling. I remember as a little girl having numerous tonsil infections that prompted prescriptions of antibiotics. Other kids were getting their tonsils out and eating ice cream in the hospital. Once the doctor looked in my throat and said, "One more infection, and we will have to take your tonsils out." Mind over matter—I never had an infection again! We had plenty of ice cream in our freezer at home.

That was back in the days when they thought there was no purpose to the tonsils, the appendix, etc. When I see children or adults with infections and swelling in the glands, it is clear that their lymphatic system needs some support. During an infection, the glands closest to the affected area swell. This is indicating that the lymph system is working hard to eliminate the infection, *not that there is something inherently wrong with the actual gland*—tonsils, appendix, etc.

Conditions Associated with Impaired Lymphatic Function

- Swollen/tender lymph nodes
- Cellulite
- Fatigue
- Repeated infections
- Appendicitis
- Cancer
- HIV/AIDS

Lymphatic System Stressors

- Pasteurized dairy
- Caffeine
- Fried foods
- Refined/processed foods
- Sugars
- Alcohol
- Excessive cooked protein
- Emotional stress

Lymphatic System Supporters

- Optimal water intake
- Optimal nutrition (as detailed in Chapter 9), with an emphasis on lemon water and greens
- Massage

- Exercise, especially walking, dancing, swimming, and rebounding
- Dry skin brushing
- Healthy emotional expression

THE DERMAL SYSTEM (SKIN)

■ Functions

The skin is the largest organ of elimination, and it cleanses over one pound of toxins a day. Still most people think of the skin just as a protective covering. Toxins are removed by our skin through normal perspiration. Saunas and steam baths can accelerate this process. Sweat is an important detoxification fluid, similar chemically to urine. It carries toxins to the skin's surface for discharge.

It is interesting to note that when someone starts a detoxification program, many times he or she will experience skin eruptions. This is sometimes referred to as a "cleansing reaction." Toxins that were lodged deep in the tissues are now circulating through the bloodstream looking for a quick exit. Many skin disorders, such as acne and psoriasis, are not a result of the skin itself having a problem, but usually an outer manifestation of internal toxicity. When skin problems are attributed to a hormonal imbalance, once again, it may be an issue of internal toxicity. The liver can become so overloaded that it cannot process hormones efficiently.

Many dermatologists don't address the detoxification issue when treating skin disorders. I have consulted with many patients for skin problems, and some of these people had seen numerous dermatologists previously without results. Most were amazed at how their skin not only cleared up through a detoxification and rejuvenation regimen, but also acquired a healthier, youthful glow.

Another aspect of the skin of which people are often unaware is that it "breathes," like our lungs. Our skin gives off carbon dioxide and takes in oxygen—in fact, this makes up one-seventh of the body's total respiration!

There are many other interesting detox duties assigned to the dermal system. For instance, did you know that friendly bacteria live on the surface of the skin and prevent entry of microorganisms such as viruses, bacteria, fungi, and parasites? Also, the skin has the ability to convert certain toxins into a water-soluble form that can be excreted by the kidneys.

▪ How the Dermal System (Skin) Gets Challenged

The skin encounters toxins directly from the environment, as well as those generated from within the body. Free radicals from sun exposure and other environmental factors cause damage to the skin. Skin cancer, acne, and wrinkles are some examples of this damage.

Just like the rest of the body, the skin can also suffer from nutritional deficiencies. When the diet is lacking in vitamins, mineral, enzymes, protein, and essential fatty acids, the cells of the skin suffer. Of course, a nutritional lack simultaneously affects every cell in the body; it is just *noticeable* on the skin, as other organ cells are shielded from our view.

Conditions Associated with Compromised Dermal (Skin) Function

- Acne
- Excessively oily and/or dry skin
- Rashes
- Allergic reactions
- Cellulite
- Eczema
- Skin cancer
- Wrinkles
- Rosacea
- Premature signs of aging

Dermal (Skin) System Stressors

- Overexposure to sun
- Lack of water
- Excess processed fats
- Poorly digested protein
- Lack of fruits and vegetables
- Excess refined sugar and flour
- Caffeine
- Alcohol
- Fried foods
- Synthetic cosmetics
- Showering with unpurified water

Dermal System Supporters

- Optimal water intake
- Good quality protein
- Oily fish (salmon, sardines, etc.)
- Fresh raw nuts and seeds
- Generous fruits and vegetables
- 1 tbsp. fresh flax oil daily
- Skin brushing
- Sauna/steam
- Aerobic exercise
- Natural cosmetics
- Using sunscreen during any sun exposure

THE URINARY SYSTEM

▪ Functions

Center stage in this system are your two bean-shaped kidneys. Located to either side of the spine at the mid-lower back, each kidney is about the size of a fist. Blood flows into the kidneys at a rate of more than one quart per minute. As the kidneys filter over five hundred gallons of blood every 24 hours, they siphon toxins and fluids that are eventually excreted in the urine. The kidneys receive toxins that were broken down and transformed by the liver.

While the amount of water you drink varies from day to day, the kidneys function to maintain a steady balance of body water. By regulating retention and excretion of water, the kidneys support the proper concentration of minerals in the blood. Besides the urine, water is also lost from the body through the skin, in exhaled breath, and in the intestinal tract. The kidneys make sure that the total amount of water you lose in a day is about the same as what you've taken in. Depending on your needs, the kidneys adjust the concentration of the urine. This is accomplished through intricate exchanges of water and salt.

The kidneys are also responsible for eliminating the waste products created when protein is broken down into amino acids. These wastes include urea and ammonia. Specific mechanisms in the kidneys address the handling of these materials.

A proper balance of electrolytes are also overseen by the kidneys. Many of the compounds dissolved in body water are electrolytes including sodium, chloride, potassium, magnesium, and calcium. These electrolyte compounds must be present for proper cell functioning including the production of subtle electric current. At the kidneys, excess amounts of these substances are sent along to be excreted in urine.

A pair of 10-to-12-inch tubes called the left and right ureters transport urine from the kidneys to the bladder. The bladder serves as a temporary reservoir for urine, and it can hold about a pint at a time. From there, another tube called the urethra carries the urine during the final phase of its journey. Though sterile when it leaves the body, urine removes unwanted yeast, organic chemicals, and various toxins including medications when it leaves your body. A point of trivia: The yellow color of urine comes from compounds in bile from the liver.

▪ How the Urinary System Gets Challenged

All of the toxins explored ultimately affect the kidneys, as everything that is circulating through the bloodstream eventually is filtered through the kidneys.

Toxins that can put an extra burden on the kidney's detox ability include prescription drugs (especially painkillers), certain metals such as lead and mercury (including those found in dental fillings), and many environmental chemicals. When the kidneys are overloaded, many symptoms can manifest such as water retention and swelling, hypertension, hypotension, toxemia during pregnancy, sexual dysfunction, low back pain, low energy and a susceptibility to infection.

Conditions Associated with
Compromised Kidney Function

- Water retention
- Swelling (ex. fingers and ankles)
- Kidney stones
- Back pain (esp. low back pain)
- Puffiness around eyes
- High blood pressure
- Dark-colored urine
- Blood in urine
- Frequent unexplained chills, fever, nausea
- Difficult/painful/irritated urination
- Congestive heart failure
- Kidney and bladder cancer

Urinary System Stressors

- Inadequate water intake
- Caffeine
- Alcohol
- Excessive protein
- Food additives, such as artificial sweeteners and other synthetic substances

- Pesticides
- Refined table salt
- Excessive fear
- Prescription drugs
- Heavy metals (i.e., mercury fillings)

Urinary System Supporters

- Organic whole foods diet

  With emphasis on:

  Water
  Greens/all vegetables
  Vegetable juices

  Asparagus
  Beets
  Dandelion greens
  Watermelon
  Cucumbers
  Lemon/lime in water

That concludes the tour through the main systems involved in the detoxification of the body. Of course, you cannot really separate organs and systems, but they were categorized here for information. Every habit, beneficial or toxic, will affect the whole body, not just an individual organ or system.

As mentioned in Chapter 5 and throughout *The Detox Solution*, every system in the body is important in the detox process of the body. As you improve the functioning of your digestive, respiratory, lymphatic, dermal, and urinary systems, you will naturally be improving the functioning of other systems such as the endocrine, reproductive, and sensory.

WHAT'S AHEAD

As you now know, your body's detox mechanisms are very complex and intricate. One way to support their optimal functioning is to eat a clean, nutritious diet. In the next chapter, "The Nutrition/Detox Connection," we'll explore how to do just that along with other important issues concerning the foods you eat. This will not simply be a rehash of what you've read in the past. Ready to learn some important new information about how to eat for optimal health? Let's move on to Chapter 9.

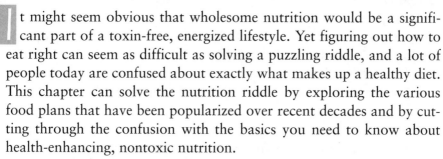

NINE

The Nutrition/Detox Connection:
Cutting Through the Confusion

Let thy food by thy medicine
and thy medicine be thy food.

—Hippocrates

It might seem obvious that wholesome nutrition would be a significant part of a toxin-free, energized lifestyle. Yet figuring out how to eat right can seem as difficult as solving a puzzling riddle, and a lot of people today are confused about exactly what makes up a healthy diet. This chapter can solve the nutrition riddle by exploring the various food plans that have been popularized over recent decades and by cutting through the confusion with the basics you need to know about health-enhancing, nontoxic nutrition.

As you consider making shifts in your diet, it's important to remember some key points. First, this book is mainly about creating routines that will boost your quality of life. After all, isn't the point to produce a high quality of living rather than to simply exist in survival mode? Eating right is one of those essential life-enhancing routines. Secondly, although this chapter will present foods as well as eating habits that negatively affect our health, it is not my intention that these be your focus. It is preferable to place most of your energy at this point into considering what beneficial foods and habits you can *add* to your life.

When patients come to the clinic to discuss their health concerns, one of the first evaluations that is performed is a thorough assessment of their diet—before any cleansing protocols are considered. They are instructed on how to make simple changes, if necessary, that can greatly enhance their health. What I find very exciting and rewarding is that many patients are able to create a lifestyle that incorporates healthy, enjoyable eating—without feeling confused or deprived. Though they often arrive at the clinic with misconceptions about proper nutrition as well as personal food issues that need to be addressed, they succeed in improving their diet. This is because they are supplied with some basic principles that are often overlooked in today's eating plans. Because core elements of nutrition are often missed or are misrepresented today, some of what you learn in this chapter may surprise you.

HEALTHY EATING & DETOXIFICATION

Optimal nutrition is essential to support the body's ongoing detoxification process. Remember, *our bodies are constantly detoxifying.* It is important to cultivate eating habits that will assist detoxification throughout your life, rather than thinking of the nutritional aspect of detoxification as an occasional two-day juice fast or a one-week radical detox diet. As you feed yourself foods that support this continual detox process and supply your system with the nutrients needed for optimal health, you'll naturally lose cravings for foods that don't serve you. You'll find yourself drawn to smarter, health-promoting eating choices.

There are many misconceptions today about healthy eating and detoxification. Many cleansing books and products support the illusions. As profits are often generated by hype and quick fixes (which consumers buy into), many people think of a "detox diet" as a temporary near-starvation way of eating—a fasting regimen or extreme short-term eating plan. The cultivation of a lifetime of healthy eating choices is overlooked, and instead consumers adopt the false belief that a few days of a juice fast or brown rice regimen can clean up toxins built up over a lifetime. When I ask a new patient with significant health challenges whether he or she has ever done any cleansing, I will often hear a proud response such as: "Oh, yes! About five years ago, I spent a weekend on nothing but juices and broth." Something occasional and extreme is not usually an effective or a safe way to detox.

At a birthday party recently, I ran into a former patient. Brenda is a corporate CEO who travels frequently. On the road or off, Brenda's expense account covers ample rich food and alcohol—all free of charge to her. Sadly, Brenda has become significantly overweight and a heavy drinker. During this party, I learned that Brenda was on the second day of a five-day juice fast. When she saw me, Brenda proudly explained her regimen. She was hungry and weak, but was convinced that the juice fast was a healthy idea. Brenda said she did this occasionally and felt she was "cleaning out her system." However, whether she was "cleansing" or indulging in her typical poor eating habits, Brenda never felt well and actually looked quite a bit older than her actual age. Unfortunately, the idea of cultivating a lifetime of healthy eating choices wasn't something that had ever sunk in with Brenda.

The way that diet programs are marketed also contributes to the "on again, off again" extreme way of eating. These programs often play with the idea of the quick fix. However, whatever aspect of good health you are considering, remember that it is not a state that occurs overnight. It is the *cultivation of healthy choices* that will have the biggest impact on our well-being.

Cultivation. In our fast-paced society, cultivation is not something that we hear about very often. Since it seems as if everything we want is just a mouse click away, it is easy to forget that optimal health does not develop instantly. If we buy into advertising and other media hype, we can begin to believe that looking and feeling good can be acquired simply with the right pills or latest plastic surgery breakthrough. However, deep down, we know that is not true. Regularly consuming high-quality nutrition is essential to creating the radiant health that is your birthright. Enhancing detoxification will also be among the benefits.

THE DECISION TO MAKE CHANGES IS YOURS

Some patients come into the clinic rather sheepishly and say they delayed their initial visit because they believed that they would "have to" give up foods they love. The truth is that many times the foods people claim they love are actually things they're addicted to and feel guilty about—*which is anything but love*. What I tell them is that I will not force them to do anything. Instead we will work *together* to balance their body chemistry, reduce cravings, and increase their energy and health. That's when I notice their body language expressing a loud "Whew!" and see that they're getting excited about exploring a new approach to eating.

This partnership helps patients realize their own truth, in a gentle way. They come to understand that they will *feel a lot better* if they gradually change their eating habits to ones that serve them. When they truly grasp this insight, they are usually ready to start making some improvements. By following the suggestions in this chapter, you can go through the same process.

Aren't you bigger than your habits? If you make the commitment to healthier eating, it will be so satisfying to look back later and see all the improvements you've made. And it would be equally frustrating to continue on your present path with ups and downs in eating habits. You can learn to make modifications in your food choices that *you* can feel good about. *The Detox Solution* is about feeling good about yourself, and *not* feeling deprived.

The decision to make better food selections comes naturally when you *truly* understand why you're making them. Supplying you with that information is what this chapter is all about.

CUTTING THROUGH THE CONFUSION ABOUT POPULAR DIET PLANS

During my fifteen years of counseling people on nutrition for healing and wellness, I have seen many food trends—Atkins, Scarsdale, Pritikin, wheatgrass, raw foods, fasting, macrobiotics, the Zone, Sugar Busters, Protein Power, etc. There are actually only a few real categories of these popular diets; they just get repackaged year after year.

Most of the nutrition/diet books out recently have been emphasizing the importance of the proper protein/carbohydrate/fat balance. The main difference in these books is the ratio of protein, carbohydrates, and fat suggested. Because nutritional needs vary, many have been helped by the different plans. By trying out so many plans, a consumer eventually finds one that fits his or her needs. In contrast to the trial and error approach, this chapter will cover the nutrition basics (which are often overlooked in search of a more "boutique" approach) that apply to everyone.

Before we explore those basics, let's review the characteristics, benefits, and concerns related to the popular eating programs. In general, the upside of these diet books is they prompt you to think about nutrition, and usually the plans don't include much junk food. The downside is that most present a relatively restricted program.

Atkins – This is essentially a high-protein, low carbohydrate diet. Robert Atkins, M.D., first came out with the approach in the '60s, and then he reintroduced it periodically. For instance, in 1989, Atkins published *Dr. Atkins' Diet Revolution,* and 10 years later, he put out another updated version. By the year 2000, an estimated 10 million books by Atkins had been sold worldwide. Other current popular diets with a similar focus are *Protein Power, Sugar Busters,* and the *Carbohydrate Addict's Eating Plan.*

Since many people today are eating too many carbohydrates and too little protein, Atkins and similar programs have helped bring this issue to light. Increasing protein in a diet that has been too high in carbohydrates can have many health benefits in addition to weight loss. A downside is that these programs can contain too much protein for many people and can be high in trans fatty acids. Some users report food cravings and/or constipation due to the increased protein and decreased fiber.

Macrobiotics – This is primarily a vegetarian diet that highlights whole grains. Some have found it useful on a short-term basis as a therapeutic regimen, as the program introduces the follower to health-generating whole foods and eliminates depleted processed ones.

The term "macrobiotics" was coined by Japanese philosopher-writer George Ohsawa during the 1920s. Michio Kushi of Boston was one of the leaders who popularized Ohsawa's ideas in the U.S. The macrobiotic system evaluates foods according to their yin and yang properties; ancient Chinese philosophies say these two complementary forces should be kept in balance to achieve good health and to promote longevity.

The macrobiotic diet has made an important contribution in increasing awareness of the importance of whole, organic food. However, as this diet recommends eating 50 to 60% whole grains and no meat, eggs, or dairy, some people find they need more protein than it provides. (The allotment for protein comes mainly from small amounts of fish, along with soy products and grain/legume combinations.) The diet is also low in raw foods. Water consumption is undervalued.

Raw Foods/Juicing – This plan is based on eating 75 to 100% raw foods, which provides the precious enzymes, vitamins, minerals, and phytonutrients that are usually deficient in the Standard American Diet (S.A.D.). Raw foodists eat fruits, vegetables, freshly made juices, grains, sprouts, nuts, seeds, and other organic unprocessed foods. The emphasis is on including a high proportion of foods that have not been cooked. On the Internet, you will find sites hosted by raw foods advocates, *www.rawfood.com* and *www.living-foods.com*. These sites feature impressive menu plans.

Some raw fooders run into trouble from overdoing fruits and sweets, which can result in poor blood sugar management. Also, note that an exclusive raw foods diet isn't recommended during colder months.

Although eating completely raw is not for everyone, increasing raw foods in the diet is beneficial for most, as the beneficial enzymes and nutrients are in their peak state. This is the only time in history that humankind has attempted to thrive on a diet so high in cooked foods. Enzyme experts have linked the increase in consumption of cooked foods to an increase in degenerative disease.

Low Fat – In this diet, the main theme is cutting back on all types of fats. Meals are centered on carbohydrates (whole grains/fresh produce) and lean protein. A benefit is that toxic sources of fat may be cut. What's dangerous is that good fats may also be avoided.

Nathan Pritikin engineered the low-fat diet in the '70s as part of a program to help those with heart disease. Another proponent of low-fat eating is Dean Ornish, M.D., author of *Eat More, Weigh Less*. Ornish also runs a rehabilitation program for those recovering from heart conditions.

Problems resulting from consuming too little fat include a deficiency in essential fatty acids (see section on fats later in the chapter) as well as in vitamins A, E, folic acid, calcium, iron, and zinc. Also, often people replace their fat calories with even more refined carbohydrate calories; these excess carbohydrates are rapidly processed into fat in the body. This is one reason we're seeing weight gain among those on low-fat regimens. An additional concern is that high-carbo-hydrate eating can contribute to degenerative conditions; research has shown that, for some, it may even raise their risk of heart disease and cancer—the very ailments the diet was designed to prevent.

While the low-fat diet increased awareness of the importance of eliminating sources of toxic, nutrient-poor fat, it is important to remember to include beneficial sources of fat in your diet every day.

Fasting – For centuries, fasting has been a practice observed by a broad range of cultures. During a fast, solid foods are cut from the diet and replaced with juice, broth, tea, and/or water. The fast is seen as a time when the body can take a break from most of its digestive duties in order to focus on healing and cleansing. While fasting can eliminate the digestive distress that comes from overeating and consuming the wrong foods, the practice can also trigger a rapid release of toxins that is too much for the body to handle all at once.

Fasting can be particularly challenging for those with health condi-tions such as diabetes, hypoglycemia, eating disorders, kidney disease, epilepsy, and ulcerative colitis. It is best to have professional guidance if you are interested in fasting. As mentioned earlier, regular healthy eating habits that support your body's ongoing detoxification are rec-ommended as opposed to extreme dietary changes like a fast.

Blood Type – The basic premise of this plan is that your blood type should be considered among the factors affecting your dietary needs. In this plan, each blood type—A, B, AB, and O—is given a particular food regimen. The blood type diet theory was presented in Peter D'Adamo's book *Eat Right for Your Type*. The author and his father, James, are both naturopathic physicians who have been researching the impact of blood type on diet and disease for many years.

In the book, Type Os (believed to be the first blood type to emerge on Earth) are said to require a diet with a high meat content. Type As (the next blood type to evolve) are steered to an "adaptive vegetarian" regimen that adds occasional servings of fish, chicken, and turkey to the veggie fare. For Type Bs (a type which appeared about 10,000 years ago), dairy, animal products, and carbohydrates are recommended. Lastly, Type AB (a rare type) is said to be likely to fall either toward the Type A or B protocol. This program is further explained in *Your Body Knows Best* by Ann Louise Gittleman.

The Zone – This program, designed by Barry Sears, Ph.D., calls

THE PENDULUM SWING
OF DIET TRENDS

During the earlier part of this century into the '70s, most nutrition books were geared towards weight loss. The emphasis was on caloric intake and tabloid-type promises. Then, in the '70s, Nathan Pritikin made international news with his low-fat plan. Some benefits were realized, as many Americans were eating too much of the wrong types of fat. Also, Pritikin's diet was centered on fresh fruits and vegetables, lean protein, plus whole grains. The missing link was that his original plan didn't include enough essential fatty acids.

Pritikin's plan seemed to spur the trend in believing that eating whole grains (high carbohydrate diets) was the way to go. This was a natural pendulum swing since most Americans were consuming an excess of refined carbohydrates (still a common concern). As the whole grains supplied much-needed nutrients and fiber, some people reported improvements from this particular focus.

Of course, any time something is in excess, we're going to see a deficiency in something else. Many health and diet-conscious Americans started playing up whole grains and then wondered why they weren't losing weight. In fact, the excess carbohydrates were actually making them fatter. Next came books to clarify the problem and save the day. Atkins was back, and people began to "enter the Zone." Now Americans are on a low-carb kick.

While the proportion of protein, fat, and carbohydrates is definitely an individual need, an excess of one type of macronutrient never seems to be the answer. Instead it is wise to educate yourself about the whole range of nutrition basics so you can come to understand your own unique needs.

basically for 40% carbohydrates, 30% protein, and 30% fat, and is sometimes referred to as simply "40/30/30." The ratio was selected based on the hormonal responses our bodies have to food, particularly with the goal in mind of keeping insulin at a desirable level.

As you can see, Sears recommends that your diet be balanced between the three macronutrients (carbohydrates, proteins, fats). The emphasis on *balance* is a desperately needed message today. Sears also brings into awareness the unhealthy aspects of excess carbohydrates commonly recommended in diets thought to be healthy. Limitations are that the Zone does not emphasize whole and organic foods. Also, not everyone needs exactly 40/30/30, and determining individual protein needs has been confusing for some people.

When considering diet plans, it is important to realize that while we all share some basic nutritional requirements, each of us also has unique needs. This breakthrough concept, known as "biochemical individuality," was developed by Roger Williams, a renowned biochemist. In 1956, Williams published a landmark nutrition book that featured the term as its title. Within the pages of *Biochemical Individuality*, Williams presented scientific research to back the notion of individual dietary requirements. Specific differences explain why a friend might work well with one diet plan while you benefit more from another.

If you want to learn more about the specific nutritional factors that may apply to you, as well as understand further details about the pros and cons of the popular diets, I strongly recommend Gittleman's book *Your Body Knows Best*. This book describes how your ancestral background, genetic heritage, metabolism, and blood type influence your nutritional needs. *Your Body Knows Best* is one of the most practical and accurate nutrition books I've ever seen. It can be very helpful in determining which food choices will be best for you.

DIETARY DOS & DON'TS FOR EVERY BODY

Cutting through the confusion of the plethora of nutrition information available first requires an education in some of the dietary fundamentals that apply to everyone. I'd like to introduce you to some simple principles that I share with clients every day in the clinic. Underlying these principles is the idea that the goal of any diet (I prefer to use the term "eating plan") should first and foremost be *reaching optimal health*. A person in a high state of health is not too fat or too thin, has plenty of energy, sleeps well, digests foods comfortably and efficiently, is served by a healthy immune system, and exhibits a general zest for life. While each person has individual needs, here are points that are important for *everyone* to keep in mind regarding eating for optimal health:

Each of us needs . . .

- to avoid toxic foods
- to consume clean, whole foods and pure water
- to get in touch with real hunger
- to understand our own body's requirements
- to eat foods that digest easily and avoid ones that are digestive stressors
- to eat a wide variety of foods

- to avoid overeating
- to limit intake of caffeine and stimulants
- to choose foods that support balanced blood sugar
- to practice healthy moderation
- to incorporate nutrient-dense foods into our diet, to get the most mileage from what is eaten.

At the same time that you apply these general principles, keep two categories in mind: (1) foods you want to cut from your diet, and (2) those you would like to add. As you progress, this second list will become your main focus. To get you started, here are lists of the basic categories.

Toxic items to cut from your diet include....

- highly processed foods such as table sugar, white bread, luncheon meats, and TV dinners
- commercial oils, including hydrogenated ones
- fruits and vegetables that have been irradiated, sprayed, waxed, or dyed
- deep fried or barbecued foods
- food additives, including MSG, artificial sweeteners, and chemical preservatives, flavorings, and dyes

- canned fruits and vegetables
- commercial eggs, due to antibiotic and hormone content
- refined salt
- sodas, whether made with sugar or artificial sweeteners
- commercial milk and milk products
- commercial meat that has residues of hormones, pesticides, and antibiotics
- genetically modified foods
- empty-calorie, non-nutritious foods

Nontoxic items to include in your diet are . . .

- pure, clean water
- herb teas
- fresh, organic produce
- unrefined oils, including flax, olive, and coconut
- whole grains
- raw, cultured organic dairy products
- fish and seafood from deep water areas
- organically raised meat and poultry
- natural sea salt
- organic herbs and spices
- free-range eggs without residues from hormones and antibiotics
- unprocessed foods in their natural state

Chapter 3 on external toxins and this chapter go into more detail about toxic and nontoxic food choices. The main point here is to do the best you can to feed yourself supportive nutrition. If some of your favorite foods are on the avoidance list, at least make sure you enjoy them in moderation.

GOOD NUTRITION IN A NUTSHELL

At some point in your life, it is likely that a physician or friend has commented that all you really need to do is *eat a balanced diet.* This concise advice would have been enough to say on its own during almost any time in the known history of humankind except within the past hundred years. In earlier periods, the foods that now rob our nourishment—packaged foods, table sugar, processed oils, etc.—simply didn't exist. *In other words, most food was health food.* And it was certainly organic. A sign of the times is that we are the first group that has ever had to live with pesticide residues.

My general advice is that you *eat in a simple, pure way that is similar to your ancestors' diets.* The truth is that modern processing techniques and available food selections are a radical departure from the way humankind has been nourished for millions of years. Our species has a long history of being hunter-gatherers. As hunter-gatherers, we selected unadulterated foods that are far from what we can grab off most shelves of today's supermarkets. With our current reliance on processed and refined foods, we have seen increases in both degenerative diseases—heart conditions, cancer, diabetes—and obesity.

In contrast to the common modern diet, the main focus of the eating plan suggested in *The Detox Solution* is on *whole foods*. What is a "whole food"? some of you may wonder. A whole food is one that either has not been processed or was only minimally processed. Examples include organic fruits and vegetables, whole grain breads, and range-raised organic meats. As the basic categories of foods are covered in this chapter, whole food examples will be presented for each group.

Today, because of processing, most of what Americans eat are *not* whole foods. Our grains are bleached and stripped of fiber, vitamins, minerals, and essential fatty acids. Most of the sugar available to us is so highly processed that virtually none of the nutrients found in the original source (i.e., sugar cane or beets) remains. In these times, it is crucial to be both informed about and committed to finding foods that are straight from Nature.

ACHIEVING AND MAINTAINING YOUR IDEAL WEIGHT WITH EASE

I have never "put" a patient on a weight loss diet. Why? What I have observed is someone whose body is in health and balance doesn't crave foods that are not good for their body. Many people are overweight from eating the wrong foods and holding onto toxins that contribute to cravings.

Remember the original underlying principle? If you give the body what it needs and remove what is not beneficial, it will thrive. A healthy body is not an overweight body. If you focus on health and eating healthy, the body will normalize its weight. If you focus on weight loss, your life will be centered on deprivation.

You do not need to invest in a diet scale. Join the thousands of people who have learned how to create their ideal weight. A comprehensive detoxification program coupled with the development of healthy eating and exercise habits results in natural weight loss and maintenance of ideal weight.

To recap, the best food choices include whole fresh foods. Preferably *organic*. This approach to eating applies to everyone—unlike the extreme diet books, which can be only be beneficial to some.

The more whole food nutrients you consume, the more your cells will be provided with what they need. They will be detoxifying efficiently and producing energy—and you will, as a result, feel *energized*!! That—in a nutshell—is good, efficient nutrition at its best!

ORGANIC FOODS—LOSE THE PESTICIDE RESIDUES, GAIN THE NUTRIENTS!

As you've read in earlier chapters, the amount of pesticides currently utilized in crop production is mind-boggling. Ironically, while pesticide use has risen tenfold since it began in the 1940s, crop losses from insects have not declined. Instead they've doubled from about a 7% loss to around 13%![1] And while opponents of organic farming say they need pesticides to produce vegetables and fruits at reasonable prices, a Cornell University researcher who studied hundreds of farms formed a different conclusion. He found that pesticide use could be cut by half with no impact on crop yields and only a 1% increase in costs.[2]

Meanwhile residues from these pesticides are reaching our plates. The EPA has identified more than 55 pesticides that could leave carcinogens behind in food. During just one meal, you might take in as many as a dozen of them! These toxic chemicals build up in our fat tissue over time. The National Academy of Sciences estimates that the risk from a lifetime exposure to the 28 pesticides most commonly eaten can result in 6 cases of cancer per 1,000 people. This translates into 1.46 million cases of cancer over the average life span.[3]

Obviously an important step in improving your diet can be buying organic foods to reduce the pesticide residues you're taking in. However, there's an aspect of organic food that you may not be aware of that provides further benefits. Studies are showing that *organic produce actually is higher in its vitamin and mineral content!* In addition, *it is also lower in other toxic elements besides pesticides.*

A two-year-long study published in the *Journal of Applied Nutrition* found the nutritional value of organic produce to be about twice that of the commercial crops that were reviewed.[4] Among the foods purchased were apples, pears, potatoes, and wheat. Different

specimens taken over a two-year period produced similar results.
Here's what the researchers found:

Apples
Nutrients: 40% more of both calcium and magnesium, 60% more
boron, 10% more chromium, 30% more iron
Toxins: 90% less mercury, 34% less aluminum

Pears
Nutrients: 40% more calcium, 220% more chromium, 30% more
magnesium, 240% more iron, 180% more manganese, 110% more
potassium, 40% more selenium, 100% more zinc
Toxins: 80% less lead, 55% less aluminum, 40% less mercury

Potatoes
Nutrients: 50% more calcium, 220% more selenium, 60% more
zinc, 30% more potassium, 50% more magnesium
Toxins: 40% less aluminum

Wheat
Nutrients: 120% more calcium, 430% more magnesium, 360%
more potassium, 80% more zinc, 1300% more selenium
Toxins: 20% less aluminum, 65% less lead, 40% less mercury

As you can see, the nutritional differences were dramatic! The benefits of including organic foods are so much more than just to *avoid*
pesticides—the increased nutrient value is priceless.

Over the last two decades, we've seen the availability of organic produce increase with consumer demand. I remember the days when organic produce was hard to find, terribly expensive, and looked awful. Prices
still tend to be a little higher, but can only drop if more and more consumers prove their preference for organic produce by buying it. Two
ways to find the freshest and most reasonably priced organic fruits and
vegetables are to attend your local farmers markets or join a food co-op.

Of course, it follows that wholesome prepared meals made with
organic produce will also be more nutritious. And other organic foods
such as meat and dairy also deliver fewer toxins, such as pesticides,
animal medications, hormones, etc. To support your optimal health,

include as much organic food on your grocery list as possible—from produce, to meat, to dairy, to oil, to wine, to eggs, etc.

THE MOST BASIC (AND OFTEN OVERLOOKED) NUTRIENT: WATER

Water is essential for life. While we could survive for a month without food, we would last but a few days without water. Yet water does not receive its fair share of the marketing and advertising that's directed toward the American public, and far too many people don't drink the amount of water that their body requires. On average, the requirement is about nine 8-ounce glasses a day.

Remember that your body's requirements are just that—*essential nonnegotiable requirements!* This is something your body truly needs to function properly. To allow this idea to register, consider an analogy. Imagine you received a bill for $100, but you decided you only wanted to pay $75. Your creditor would call and ask why you only sent three-fourths of the bill. If you responded, "Well, it's close," that would not satisfy your creditor. In a similar way, if you do not take in the full amount of water that your body needs on a daily basis, you will build up a deficit and become dehydrated. Chronic dehydration can lead to a variety of physical problems. Conversely, consistent water intake is health promoting.

Looking at water's many functions in the body brings home its significance. Water's duties include:

- Transporting nutrients, hormones, and chemical messengers to appropriate sites within your system
- Diluting toxins and waste products and escorting them out of the body
- Acting as a solvent, ridding the bloodstream of excess fat
- Protecting the internal surfaces of your digestive tract and other systems
- Maintaining the body's operating temperature
- Keeping your joints "oiled" with water-based solutions
- Surrounding the brain and spinal cord with fluid to shield them from impact.

INITIAL CHANGES FOR HEALTHIER EATING

Although a lot of information was included in Chapter 3 about eliminating the sources of toxins in your diet, the current chapter offers the opportunity for you to tie all the aspects of good nutrition together into a plan that works best for you. If you have been reading all of the chapters, you've probably taken some of the following steps already. In any case, here are the initial changes you'll want to incorporate into your healthy eating plan.

1. **Boost your water intake.** According to a study of more than 34,000 people, drinking at least five glasses of water a day is associated with an approximately 50% decreased risk of heart attack and stroke compared to consumption of only two glasses of water daily.[5] This is just one of the many benefits you can gain by raising your daily water consumption to sufficient levels. Below, in the next section titled "The Most Basic (and Often Overlooked) Nutrient: Water," a formula is provided to determine daily water needs. On average, it is about nine 8-ounce glasses.

2. **Eat more vegetables.** Yes, grandma was right. You should eat your vegetables. New research comes out practically every day demonstrating how crucial consuming vegetables is to preventing cancer and other diseases. Many people report an increase in energy directly proportionate to their increase of vegetables.

3. **Increase the amount of raw foods you consume.** Heating food over 118° F destroys enzymes that assist in the digestion and assimilation of nutrients. Therefore you also want to include some enzyme-providing raw foods—such as raw fruits, vegetables, sprouts, nuts, and seeds—in your diet. Also lost during cooking or food processing are vital vitamins and minerals. An easy way to add nourishment to what you take in is to enjoy raw foods in the forms of salads, freshly made juices, and snacks of raw nuts or seeds.

4. **Try to have some protein at every meal.** Many Americans tend to indulge in refined carbohydrates at the expense of good quality protein. This results in mood swings and uneven energy levels.

It also negatively affects glucose metabolism, an outcome that has been linked to many diseases including cancer, heart disease, and diabetes. The majority of patients I have seen who thought they ate relatively healthy were actually consuming too many carbohydrates and too little protein. Many were surprised at how quickly the simple addition of protein at every meal (and at snack time too, when possible) made a tremendous difference in their energy, moods, and food cravings.

5. **Reduce the refined flours and sugars in your diet.** These foods are low in nutrients and high in empty calories. The body is hungry for a complete package of nutrient-loaded calories. When the diet is rich in empty calories, the body uses a lot of its resources to process this dead food. This results in nutritional deficiencies contributing to food cravings, low energy, obesity, and degenerative diseases such as cancer and heart disease.

6. **Go organic whenever possible.** Once more, let me remind you of the importance of moving to organic versions of all types of foods whenever you can! Since people in this century are the first to consume foods laden with pesticide residues, we do not fully know what the health consequences will be. However, it doesn't take a genius to realize that these chemicals are foreign and taxing to our systems. Buy organic produce, meat, dairy, etc., etc., etc.!

Actually, just about every function in the body is pegged in some way to the flow of water. The next time you sip a glass of this life-sustaining fluid, take a moment to reflect on its many vital contributions! In addition to health maintenance, water consumption also can prevent and heal disease. F. Batmanghelidj, author of *Your Body's Many Cries for Water* (*www.watercure.com*), has made it his life's work to investigate the link between chronic dehydration and disease. He has learned that our thirst mechanism begins to malfunction when we do not consume enough water. So we can easily be unaware of our need for more water. Fortunately this function kicks back in when adequate water drinking resumes. Among Batmanghelidj's findings on ill health is the discovery that increased water intake can contribute to the healing of peptic ulcers. In his research, he has also made connections between dehydration and heartburn, arthritis, back pain, high blood pressure, migraines, colitis, and asthma. I have observed clinically incredible improvements in health from the addition of *adequate* water consumption.

At a conference, I once had a friendly conversation with a nurse who had been in practice for over 30 years. She "coincidentally" volunteered her belief (not knowing my professional background or interest in health) that most of the illness she sees are the result of toxicity and dehydration. Her eyes lit up when I told her I was writing a book covering this. *Don't expect any results from this plan unless you get serious about drinking adequate amounts of water.* I've overseen many cases where this single factor played an important part in a patient's improvement.

A simple way to calculate your specific needs for water is to divide your weight by two. That number is the minimum amount of ounces you need each day. For example, a woman weighing 130 pounds would require 65 ounces of water daily. A man at 180 pounds would need 90 ounces. Next, divide the total ounces by 8 to determine the number of glasses of water that you'll want to consume.

■　Other Beverages

Along with water, there are other fluids that are hydrating and beneficial to your body. In addition to setting a daily water goal, consider including some of these added sources of refreshment to your diet.

- **Herbal teas, iced or hot.** For iced tea, try Celestial Seasonings' Iced Delight, decaffeinated green tea, or other natural herbal caffeine-free tea mixes. These can be brewed right in the refrigerator. For a hot drink, consider mint or chamomile. When shopping, read labels carefully as some packages look like they contain an herbal product but actually offer a black tea and herbal mix. Also most bottled herbal teas contain a substantial amount of sugar. A wonderful line of low-sugar herbal teas is called Honest Tea (*www.honesttea.com*).

- **Homemade lemonade.** It's easy to make delicious lemonade at home without pouring in massive amounts of sugar. Here's how.

Start with an 8-ounce glass of pure spring water. To this, add 2 tablespoons of organic lemon juice (Santa Cruz is a good brand to use) or the juice of one organic lemon. Add drops of the natural sweetener stevia to taste.

▪ **Vegetable juices.** Buy organic, fresh vegetable juices at the health food store or be creative with your own juicer. One great blend to try is an organic carrot, celery, and parsley combination.

▪ **Apple Cider Refresher.** This detoxifying drink may be an acquired taste, however I've found that most people enjoy it. Add 1 tablespoon of raw apple cider vinegar to an 8-ounce glass of purified water. Sweeten with drops of stevia to taste. The flavor of the Apple Cider Refresher is much like apple juice, however this drink does not contain the sugar or the calories.

▪ **Fresh Coconut Juice.** Where do you find this? Drain it straight out of a coconut, of course. Coconut juice is an extremely nutritious, naturally-detoxifying drink.

▪ **Vegetable broths.** There are several brands of healthy instant vegetable broth powders available. They are usually found at health food stores. Vegetable broth can be a nice pick-me-up in the middle of the afternoon, and the powders are easy to prepare—just add hot water. Read the labels carefully, avoiding products with MSG and artificial additives.

▪ **Fruit-flavored drinks sweetened with stevia.** Most fruit-flavored drinks and drink mixes on the market are sweetened with sugar or toxic artificial sweeteners and loaded with artificial colors, flavors, and preservatives. An alternative is a product called Stevita (*www.stevitastevia.com*), a fruit-flavored drink that comes in cherry, grape, lemon, and orange flavors. These drinks are free of calories, sugar, and artificial ingredients.

Remember that most commercial beverages—such as bottled iced teas, commercial juice, or prepared lemonade—are made with a lot of sugar. And even if it is a "natural" sugar, usually there's too much of it. If you want something sweet, it's better to eat a piece of fruit than drink the fruit juice. The fruit sugar will enter your bloodstream a lot slower than the sugar in juice, due to the fiber content and the fact that the fruit takes longer to eat. Slower delivery of simple sugars is much less stressful to your system. If you must have fruit juice, try diluting it with sparking water; at least, add as much water as juice. Note: A glass of regular orange juice contains as much sugar as a candy bar!

Overall, what beverages should you avoid or limit to low levels? *Beverages with questionable health value include caffeinated coffee and teas, sodas (both those sweetened with sugar or artificial ingredients), undiluted fruit juices, other processed drinks, and alcohol.* Of this group, one particular source of concern is soda consumption. Far too many people today reach for a can of soda to quench their thirst. Some even drink it at breakfast! In fact, Americans presently drink an average of 60 gallons of soda per person per year;[6] this is nearly double the amount consumed in 1970.[7]

What's wrong with sodas? A lot. First, they are either overloaded with sugar (the average 12-ounce can contains ten teaspoons of sugar!) or spiked with toxic artificial sweeteners. In addition, when you drink soda, you also get empty calories, bone-weakening phosphoric acid, blood-sugar-altering caffeine, and other toxic artificial ingredients such as flavorings, colorings, and preservatives. Not exactly the image you get in those dazzling ads featuring people whose lives seem to be transformed by their choice of soft drink!

■ Caffeine

Beverages can be a significant source of caffeine in our diets. Just think of the surge of coffee houses we have seen established over the past 10 years! The extensive variety in coffee drinks, from espresso to café latte to cappuccino and more, is quite a phenomenon. Despite these trends, it's best to avoid caffeine-laden drinks as much as possible. This includes coffees, teas, and sodas. Caffeine has a disastrous effect on the immune system due to its overstimulation of the adrenal glands. Over time, chronic caffeine consumption weakens the adrenals. This can lead to a vicious fatigue cycle in which you are drawn to drink even more caffeine-containing drinks to stay alert or even wake. Also, caffeine can cause blood sugar mechanisms to over-react, resulting in low blood sugar. In addition, the diuretic aspect of caffeine leads to a loss of bodily fluid and nutrients.

Another problem with most of the coffees and teas is pesticide contamination. If you drink tea or coffee occasionally, seek organic sources.

For information on tapering off a caffeine habit, see the section "Dietary Addictions: Why They Occur & How to Recover" later in this chapter.

THE MACRONUTRIENTS: PROTEIN, CARBOHYDRATES & FAT

The three main components of food are known as macronutrients: *protein, carbohydrates, and fat.* Along with an increased awareness that the ratio of these nutrients is essential for optimal health, it is important to be familiar with the purpose of each nutrient and the best choices available in each category.

■ Protein

The term *protein* comes from Greek term *proteos*, which means "to come first." It makes sense to select protein as the first macronutrient to discuss, as this is a primary ingredient in each of your cells. Protein makes up about three-fourths of the solid structure of the body.

During digestion, protein from food is further broken down into smaller units called *amino acids.* There are 20 different types that are present in the body at significant amounts. Amino acids are used to make and repair skin, hair, nails, organs, tissues, hormones, enzymes, DNA, RNA, antibodies, and more. Sometimes referred to as the building blocks of protein, amino acids are crucially needed to support detoxification enzyme systems.

Sources of protein are classified as being either *complete* or *incomplete.* Animal proteins are considered complete because they supply all nine of the amino acids that we must get from the foods we eat. These nine are called the *essential amino acids.* Except for soybeans, plant proteins lack one or more essential amino acids, and are thus categorized as incomplete proteins. A diet blending both complete and incomplete sources can insure that your protein requirements are met for optimal health. The following chart highlights the major sources of complete and incomplete protein.

Since many people have been overindulging in carbohydrates for some time, symptoms of a protein imbalance often occur from taking in too little protein. Symptoms of protein malnourishment include anemia, hair loss, lack of mental clarity, poor memory, immune compromise,

COMPLETE PROTEINS

Eggs – A serving is two whole eggs or three whites. One large whole egg provides 6.3 grams of protein; the white alone, 3.5 grams. Despite common belief, recent studies are indicating that, for most people, eggs have no detrimental effects on blood cholesterol.[8] Be sure to select organic, free range, or fertile eggs only. Avoid nonorganic eggs, as they are high in pesticide residues and synthetic hormones.

Fish – A serving contains 4 ounces of cooked fish (15 to 25 grams of protein). Fish is a good source of health-promoting omega 3 fatty acids, which are discussed in greater detail in the section on fats below. Shark and swordfish are two fish that are best to avoid because of possible heavy metal contamination. Flounder, halibut, and sea bass, are usually safe; such deep-water fish tend to be wiser choices. (See Chapter 3 for longer lists of fish to buy and avoid.) Note: Conveniently packaged "burgers" made of fish such as salmon or tuna are available as an alternative to the filleted version.

Chicken, turkey, or other poultry – A serving contains 4 ounces of cooked poultry, with a protein content range of 20 to 25 grams. Choose free-range and hormone-free poultry; it contains as much as five times more essential fatty acids and significantly less cholesterol. Healthy brands of chicken include Shelton (*www.sheltons.com*) and Petuluma (*http://www.healthychicken choices.com*).

Beef, buffalo, lamb, and other meat – Here, again, a serving is 4 ounces, with the protein content ranging from 20 to 30 grams. Choose lean organic beef, such as Coleman's (*www. colemannatural.com*), to cut back on saturated fats and avoid toxic residues. Buffalo is lower in fat, cholesterol, and calories than commercial beef. It can be found in some restaurants and specialty markets. A lean cut of lamb to look for is foreshank; avoid fatty ground lamb. All of these meats are good sources of iron as well as protein. Buy organic brands whenever possible.

Tofu & tempeh (soy protein) – A serving is 3 ounces of tofu (13 grams of protein) or 4 ounces of tempeh (16 grams of protein). Soybeans are the only plant protein that provides all the essential amino acids. Benefits of eating soy protein include decreased menopausal symptoms, lowered cholesterol, enhanced immunity, and increased free radical protection. It is important to select fermented soy products (such as tofu or tempeh) rather than unfermented ones (such as soy milk). Unfermented soy products contain an enzyme inhibitor that can contribute to problems in protein assimilation and digestion. Soy protein powders are discussed on the next page.

Seitan (wheat gluten) – Another vegetarian source of protein, seitan (say-than) is derived from the protein portion of wheat. A 4-ounce serving contains 24 grams of protein. The easiest way to incorporate seitan into your diet is with prepared products made by such companies as White Wave or Lightlife Foods. These are sold in tubs or vacuum packs. You can also buy seitan powder, such as Arrowhead Mills Quick Seitan Mix, and make your own. Seitan has a meat-like texture, and it can be used as a meat substitute in recipes.

Dairy products (milk, yogurt, cottage cheese) – Serving sizes vary for these foods; a serving is 8 ounces for milk (8 grams of protein), 1 cup for yogurt (12 grams), and half a cup for cottage cheese (14 grams). Along with protein, these dairy products also provide calcium. Buy high-quality organic products that do not contain synthetic hormones and antibiotics. Consider goat's milk as an alternative to cow's milk. Raw milk products are preferred over the pasteurized and homogenized versions. (Other cheeses have not been listed as many do not contain significant protein.)

Veggie burgers – These patties can be made of a mixture of grains, soy products, vegetables, and/or dairy. Popular brands include Amy's, Boca Burger, and Garden Burger. Protein contents vary from about 6 to 18 grams per serving.

Vegetarian meat substitutes – There is an ever-increasing array of vegetarian sources of protein. Veggie dogs, lunchmeats, sausages, and frozen entrees provide an easy-to-prepare alternative to animal protein. Check the labels for organic ingredients.

Protein powders – These powders are a convenient choice for adding protein to a meal or drink. Sources of protein include whey, rice, soy, and pea. Many protein powders have added sugars that boost the carbohydrate content. It is best to avoid this and use powders that are mostly protein. Protein contents vary from 18 to 24 grams per serving. If using a soy protein powder, be sure it has been fermented to assure optimal digestibility. Look for organic products.

INCOMPLETE PROTEINS

Legumes – These are the best plant sources of protein, containing about 22% protein on average by dry weight. A serving of cooked legumes measures about one-half cup and delivers 7 to 8 grams of protein. Along with protein, legumes provide B vitamins, zinc, potassium, magnesium, calcium, and iron. In your diet, include beans such as kidney, lima, navy, pinto, and black as well as split peas and lentils.

Whole grains – A serving of whole-grain pasta or cereal equals half a cup and contains 2-3 grams of protein. A serving of whole-grain bread is one slice and delivers the same amount. A whole grain consists of all the edible parts. It is higher in fiber, Vitamin E, some B vitamins, and trace minerals. Whole grain products to look for include rice, corn, oats, barley, and whole wheat.

Raw nuts – Eat in small amounts (about 1 ounce, providing 1 to 7 grams of protein) as a snack or consume nuts as an accent ingredient in dishes or salads. Most *raw nuts* are permissible, especially almonds, walnuts, cashews, and pecans. Nuts are a nutrient-dense food, also rich in essential fatty acids. Skip peanuts (which can contain the mold aflatoxin) or any type of roasted and/or salted nuts. It's best to soak nuts overnight in purified water to improve digestibility by breaking down enzyme inhibitors.

Seeds – Consume seeds in a similar way to nuts, in small amounts (about 1 ounce; 7 grams of protein) as snacks or sprinkled on salads and casseroles. Good choices are sunflower and sesame. Seeds are also nutrient-dense, supplying iron, potassium, and phosphorus. Buy fresh seeds rather than those that have been dry roasted or salted.

Nut and Seed Butters – A great way to get the benefits of raw nuts and seeds is to partake of nut and seed butter. Yes, there's so much more to life than peanut butter! Nut and seed butters include almond, cashew, macadamia, pistachio, hemp seed, sunflower seed, pumpkin seed, and sesame seed. Nut and seed butters are loaded with quality protein, essential fatty acids, vitamins, and minerals. Maranatha and Rejuvenative Foods are two brands that offer superior nut and seed butters. A great website that further details the health benefits of raw organic nut and seed butters is *www.rejuvenative.com*.

fatigue, loss of muscle mass, cardiovascular disease, depression, anxiety, and metabolic imbalances. Often there is an accompanying fatty acid deficiency.

Protein requirements vary from individual to individual. The Recommended Daily Allowance (RDA) for protein is averaged at 50 grams for women and 63 for men, but can differ based on body weight and activity level. The website *www.zoneperfect.com* provides a simple online method to calculate your protein requirements based on the Zone's 40-30-30 plan, taking into account body fat and individual characteristics.

While it is virtually impossible to calculate your exact protein needs on a daily basis, try to include a serving of high-quality, easily digested protein at every meal. Many people also benefit from including protein with each snack. How do you gauge a serving, without bringing out the food scale? There's an easy way to determine a complete serving of meat, poultry, or fish protein. It's right in the palm of your hand! A serving tends to be about the size of your palm—this amount is about three to four ounces (21 to 28 grams).

When shopping for protein, seek out organic sources. According to the EPA, 90 to 95% of all pesticide residues are found at the top of the food chain in meat, fish, eggs, and dairy products. Also, most animals raised commercially are constantly exposed to artificial light, hormones, steroids, and antibiotics. In addition, avoid farm-raised fish, which tends to contain more toxins (for further information, see "Trouble on the Fish Farm" on page 77).

A last concern regarding protein is that many people tend not to be digesting it well. As a result, they are not receiving all the benefits of the amino acids it contains. Also, partially-digested protein can turn into carcinogenic material in the body. This is one of the causes of colon cancer. To enhance the digestion of cooked protein, include the use of a digestive enzyme with any meal that contains it.

A NOTE ON VEGETARIANISM

Over the years, I have observed that many people who are vegetarians are not actually eating healthfully. It's easy to start out making healthy choices as a vegetarian. However, with the demands of our modern, fast-paced lifestyle, many vegetarians find it challenging to provide themselves with a nutrient-dense diet. Instead they frequently fall into the trap of eating an excess of carbohydrates (often refined) with the basic rule of vegetarianism in mind—"eat anything but animal products."

A healthy vegetarian diet consists of an abundance of fresh organic vegetables, fruits, whole grains, beans, tofu, tempeh, nuts, seeds, and vegetarian meat substitutes. Some vegetarians include milk, cheese, yogurt, and eggs for extra protein. Some people eat a primarily vegetarian diet, but occasionally include fish or poultry when vegetarian protein sources aren't readily available—a situation common when traveling in unfamiliar areas.

There are times when you might be traveling when it seems that the only vegetarian foods available are doughnuts or junk food. If you are committed to vegetarianism, it is wise to be as committed to making healthy choices. Plan ahead if you are unsure of foods available when eating out or traveling.

Some vegetarian items that travel well include protein bars, nuts, seeds, vegetarian cheese substitutes, dried veggie "jerky," dehydrated vegetables and fruits, and trail mix.

▪ The "Got Milk?" Debate

Celebrity after celebrity has signed up to be part of the "Got Milk?" promotion campaign. But behind all the glitz and glamour lies an often-ignored fact: *We are the only species on earth that consumes another animal's milk after we are weaned.* Experts feel this unnatural habit can be detrimental to our health. Food products made from cow's milk are often hard for the human body to digest. They also cause stress to our immune system, as the undigested particles irritate the immune cells in the intestinal lining.

Some people's bodies are more intolerant of dairy than others. Their systems don't make enough *lactase*—the enzyme that's needed to digest the lactose (milk sugar) in dairy—so they have allergic reactions. However, raw, fresh milk usually provides enough lactase for smooth digestion of this dairy product. Buy certified raw milk, if possible, not pasteurized. If raw milk is not available in your area, at least purchase an organic product. Non-organic milk—and other dairy products made with it—contain bovine growth hormone and antibiotics—substances you want to avoid. You can also find cheese made with raw milk too, which is preferred over the pasteurized variety.

Other dairy options are products made with goat's milk. The protein structure of goat's milk is closer in chemical composition to that of human milk than is milk from a cow. This results in better digestibility and fewer allergies. When compared to cow's milk, goat's milk has 25% more vitamin B6, 13% more calcium, 47% more vitamin A, 134% more potassium, 27% more selenium, and 350% more niacin.[9] In the clinic, I have seen goat's milk be particularly helpful as a healthier alternative to formula for infants who are not being breast-fed.

You can also consider fermented dairy products. Fermenting (a practice common in many traditional cattle-herding circles) breaks down lactose. The resulting dairy products are more easily digested by those who are intolerant of regular milk products. Fermented products usually include beneficial bacteria that have immune-enhancing properties and other health benefits. Fermented dairy products include yogurt, cottage cheese, kefir, clabber, and others.

It was suggested earlier that a digestive enzyme be taken with meals containing protein. If you are using a full spectrum enzyme, it will also include lactase—the dairy-digesting enzyme. Supplementing your diet with a digestive enzyme can also be helpful in digesting dairy comfortably.

For those who absolutely cannot tolerate dairy, or who want a healthy alternative, try homemade almond or sesame milk. Soak one cup of almonds or sesame seeds overnight. Drain and blend in 2 cups purified water. Dates, vanilla extract, or carob powder can be added for flavor. Pour through a fine strainer. This milk will stay fresh in the refrigerator for two to three days.

If you do partake in dairy, do so in limited amounts. Think of it as a condiment or side dish, not as the staple of the meal. For example, adding milk to hot beverages is preferred over consuming glass after glass of milk. Adding some feta cheese to a Greek salad is preferred over a triple-cheese pizza. Including yogurt in a protein drink is preferred over a bowl of ice cream. (Okay, enjoy an occasional ice cream.)

▪ Carbohydrates

Carbohydrates are the principal source of fuel for the body. Items in the carbohydrate category can easily be used by the body for cellular energy or stored for future needs. It is essential to be judicious about how you consume carbohydrates, for they can be stored in almost unlimited amounts in the form of body fat. In addition to grain products and starchy foods, this macronutrient classification is also comprised of sugars as well as fruits and vegetables. The three general categories for carbohydrates are: (1) Simple Carbohydrates, (2) Complex carbohydrates, and (3) Fiber.

Simple Carbohydrates

These foods require less digestive processing than complex carbohydrates, and thus are quick sources of energy. Simple carbohydrates include fruits such as apricots, bananas, berries, cherries, coconut, dates, figs, grapefruit, grapes, guava, lemons, limes, mangoes, melons, nectarines, oranges, papaya, peaches, pears, pineapple, plums, prunes, raisins, and tangerines. This macronutrient category also contains sweeteners such as honey, molasses, cane sugar, beet sugar, etc. To avoid wide energy fluctuations, it's best to limit the intake of all concentrated sweeteners, and if possible, completely avoid refined white (cane and/or beet) sugar, which supplies a too explosive source of energy. Foods that also supply simple carbohydrate energy too quickly include many desserts—such as cakes, pies, cookies, ice cream—as well as most breakfast cereals!

THE GLYCEMIC INDEX

One way to assess whether a carbohydrate offers long-term energy or just a quick spurt is to refer to the *glycemic index*. This index evaluates the rate at which a carbohydrate will be broken down into glucose, a type of sugar that is then released into the bloodstream. Foods that are processed more rapidly will create a spike in your blood sugar level, resulting in a subsequent crash and fatigue. What you want is a more steady and slower source of energy.

Some foods that release glucose quickly and therefore have a high glycemic index rate are rice cakes (133), white bread (100), breakfast cereal (100), Russet potatoes (98), parsnips (97), carrots (92), honey (87), and bananas (82). Foods low on the index include apples (39), chick-peas (36), pears (34), lentils (29), peaches (29), and cherries (23). A detailed chart including the glycemic indices of hundreds of foods can be found at *www.mendosa.com/gilists.htm*.

Eating a high-glycemic-index carbohydrate with a more slowly digested food such as protein helps to slow the release of glucose. It is beneficial for most people to limit foods high on the glycemic index in order to minimize blood sugar fluctuations.

You want to include some fresh fruit in your diet, but don't overdo it. Choose fruit over juice, and dilute the juice with sparkling water if you do drink it occasionally. Avoid nonorganic fruit products, especially those that have been imported from Mexico or other foreign countries. DDT and some of the other most harmful pesticides are still legal in many nations. *These dangerous pesticide residues are imported along with the fruit!*

Did you know? Sugar is often a hidden ingredient in the foods we eat. Or if it is not hidden, we may not be aware of the large amount of sugar the food contains. For instance, there are twelve spoonfuls of sugar in a 16-ounce cola. This is as much sugar as you'd eat in a 5-ounce serving of pecan pie!!

Refined Sugar
One type of simple carbohydrate that calls for specific discussion

is refined sugar. The average American is consuming *150 to 170 pounds of sugar each year!* Where is all this sugar coming from in their diet? Well, people add it to their coffee or tea, sip it in their sodas, and ingest it when they eat processed foods—in everything from salad dressings to boxed cereal to spaghetti sauce to bread. One form of refined sugar—corn syrup—seems to be used as a sweetener in just about every type of prepared food these days; this development was encouraged by the low-fat craze. To create low-fat products, fat was taken out of food, and corn syrup and other sugars were added to enhance the flavor. U.S. Department of Agriculture (USDA) statistics show that consumption of added sugars—cane, beet, corn, and other sugars—has increased 30% since 1983. Some other names that disguise refined sugar's presence in foods include brown sugar, turbinado sugar, and evaporated cane juice.

If you find yourself craving sugar, it's usually not because your body needs it. The craving comes because the sugar content of your blood is low, and the healthiest response is actually to eat a combination of protein and carbohydrates. For example, you might snack on cottage cheese and fruit or some chicken breast on whole multigrain bread. If you just eat the sugar, you'll get a quick fix, but then you are just setting yourself up for another decline in energy a short time later.

Sugar has a profound effect on the immune system. An immunosuppressant, sugar decreases the activity of infection-fighting white blood cells for up to five hours after you eat it.[10] One study showed that sucrose, fructose, honey, and orange juice all decreased the capability of infection-fighting blood cells to kill harmful, disease-producing bacteria. Excess sugar consumption has been linked to countless other health concerns including various cancers, heart disease, elevated cholesterol, fatigue, kidney stones, arthritis, depression, asthma, allergies, obesity, PMS, eating disorders, tooth decay, hormonal imbalances, diabetes, and hypoglycemia.

One reason that refined sugar plays havoc with our systems is that it has been stripped of its vital nutrients. These nutrients—including B vitamins, magnesium, and chromium—help to maintain healthy blood sugar when *unrefined sugars* are consumed. So when you eat *refined sugar,* your body gets a feeling of quick energy, yet it is denied the natural combination of nutrients that would keep the body in balance. In order to compensate, the body has to dip into its own reserves. So instead of supplying nourishment, refined sugar actually leaves us more depleted.

As alternatives to white table sugar, healthier choices include *organic raw honey, date sugar,* and *maple syrup*—used in moderation. These natural sweeteners contain significant amounts of vitamins and minerals. *Stevia* may be used more liberally as it seems to have the least effect on blood sugar levels. This natural, noncaloric sweetener, derived from a South American plant from the daisy family, has been consumed by certain Indian tribes in the southern hemisphere for hundreds of years. Stevia is now one of the predominant products used in Japan, both as a tabletop sweetener and as a sweet substance used in prepared foods. About 40% of the low-calorie soft drinks in Japan are sweetened with it. See "Stevia: A Sweet Alternative" below. Another natural, noncaloric sweetener, derived from the lo han fruit, is called HerbaSweet, and can be found in health food stores.

STEVIA: A SWEET ALTERNATIVE

While not yet replacing table sugar on the kitchen tables in most American homes, the word is spreading about a natural sweetener called stevia. It's derived from a plant (*stevia rebaudiana*) originally found in northeastern Paraguay near the Brazilian border. South Americans have used it for centuries to sweeten a tea-like beverage called yerba maté. An Italian botanist discovered the plant while exploring Paraguay in 1887. Today stevia is grown and used in Japan, Thailand, China, and Korea, as well as Paraguay and Brazil.

In the United States, you'll find stevia on the shelves of your local health food store, where it is sold as a dietary supplement. (It has not yet been approved as a sweetener in this country.) When using it, remember not to add too much, as 1 teaspoon of stevia powder equals about a cup of sugar. Stevia also comes in a liquid form made from the powder; about two to four drops equal a teaspoon of sugar. Because stevia is from 100 to 300 times sweeter than sugar, liquid forms are easier to use in hot drinks—you won't be adding much! When you first start cooking with stevia, you may wish to combine it with honey or maple syrup—until you adapt to its use.

It is crucial to avoid artificial sweeteners, especially Nutrasweet (aspartame) and saccharin. Not only are they toxic and addictive, but studies have also shown that people who use these additives often gain weight rather than lose it. Aspartame has been linked to headaches, behavioral problems, tumors, and neurological disorders.

Complex Carbohydrates

This subdivision of carbohydrates includes foods that have a more complex structure than the simple variety. They require several steps in digestion before the glucose they contain can be released for cellular energy. Complex carbohydrates include potatoes, whole grain foods, most vegetables, and legumes. The best sources of complex carbohydrates are unrefined and organic; avoid refined products as they release energy too quickly into your system.

Consider expanding the variety of the complex carbohydrates that you eat—most people consume the same sources frequently (such as wheat products rather than other grains), virtually ignoring the hundreds of other choices.

Breads/Cereals: Choose whole grains, preferably brown rice, millet, spelt, kamut, barley, amaranth, quinoa, buckwheat (kashi), corn, and soy. Limit or avoid wheat, as many people are allergic to it. Select organic grains whenever possible. Choose whole grain cereals low in sugar. Pasta should be whole grain, and wheat-free if available (semolina is wheat). Breads should be yeast-free if possible. Avoid white, refined bread, pasta, and flour products.

Vegetables: Consume all organic vegetables including leafy greens, yellow vegetables, root varieties, and starchy vegetables. Fresh veggies are always the first choice; frozen is OK, if absolutely necessary. Eat as many vegetables as possible! Include sprouts and benefit from their uniquely high enzyme, vitamin, and mineral content. Vegetables can be consumed raw, slightly steamed, or baked. Choices include alfalfa sprouts, artichokes, bean sprouts, beans, beets, cabbage, carrots, cauliflower, celery, corn, cucumber, eggplant, kale, legumes, lettuce (avoid iceberg, the darker green the better), olives, onions, peas, peppers, potatoes, pumpkin, radish, spinach, squash, sweet potatoes, Swiss chard, tomatoes, turnips, water chestnuts, and yams. Pass on canned or otherwise processed vegetables. Nonorganic products run the risk of pesticide residues. Avoid fried vegetables.

ARE YOU CARBOHYDRATE-ADDICTED?

Over the past few years, there has been an increased awareness of the carbohydrate overindulgence that occurs from an addiction to this macronutrient. When people are carbohydrate-addicted, they have strong frequent cravings for carbohydrates, such as sweets, breads, pastas, crackers, pretzels, chips, fruit, fruit juice, or popcorn. If you suspect that you may have been taking in too many carbohydrates, be extra attentive to including protein at each meal.

One of the problems with consuming excessive carbohydrates is the resulting inflated insulin level in your blood. When insulin levels are high, food is easily converted into body fat. Eating a high carbohydrate diet also leaves you less satiated, so you crave more and more food. Our supermarkets today are filled with refined carbohydrates—breads, pasta, cereal, and other processed foods. These foods are very addictive as well as stressful to your body. Hypoglycemic tendencies are very common among carbohydrate addicts (and symptoms become even worse if meals are delayed or missed). Symptoms pointing to compromised blood sugar management include fatigue, headaches, depression, mood swings, anxiety, poor memory, lack of concentration, sugar cravings, caffeine dependence, and allergies.

To support healthy blood sugar management, decrease your consumption of simple sugars, alcohol, refined flours, and caffeine. Eat three meals, and two to three snacks. Each meal should include a significant amount of protein. It's wise to also increase vegetable consumption. Use digestive enzymes with all meals and snacks to help you get the most nourishment from the foods you eat. Supplementing your diet with 200 mcg. of chromium and 1,500 mg. of L-glutamine (500 mg. three times a day is usually suggested) daily will help ease your cravings for carbohydrates. Lastly, learn how to manage stress. The excess cortisol and adrenaline that is secreted when you are under constant stress contributes to poor blood sugar management.

If your symptoms don't improve, consult with a health professional. Carbohydrate addiction is one of the most common complaints seen in the clinic, and natural medicine has a lot to offer. You do not have to suffer needlessly.

Refined Grains (White Flour, White Pasta, Etc.)

While choosing healthy complex carbohydrates, it's important to replace refined white flour products with whole grain versions. This includes breads, pastas, and pastries. Refined flour has most of the vital nutrients and fiber stripped from it. This refinement process was not developed for the sake of your health, but to provide a longer shelf life to benefit the manufacturers. Whole grains have more vitamins, minerals, fiber, phytonutrients, and essential fatty acids than their refined counterparts.

Another downside to refined grains—excess amounts are easily transformed into body fat. If we are what we eat, and most Americans are eating too many refined grains, no wonder many people in the U.S. look like doughboys and doughgirls. Eating too much of these foods produces a bloated, puffy, doughy look.

Fiber

Fiber refers to portions of complex carbohydrates (always plant foods) that cannot be broken down by human enzymes or digestive juices. Therefore, instead of being used for energy, fiber—also called "roughage"—passes through the body undigested.

While not a source of nutrients, fiber plays important health roles. Its part in intestinal health was covered extensively in the colon chapter. A key point made there was that bulk in the intestines created by fiber increases bowel transit time and reduces your exposure to toxins in foods. In addition to colon benefits, fiber is also helpful in lowering cholesterol and triglyceride levels. It slows the absorption of sugars and fats too. Finally, research has shown that high-fiber diets are associated with lower incidences of colon and rectal cancer, heart disease, diabetes, diverticulitis, hemorrhoids, colitis, and constipation.

On average, most people eat only 11 grams of fiber a day. For optimal health benefits, 20 to 35 grams are needed. One reason for avoiding refined grains is that they have been stripped of their fiber. The use of processed packaged foods has also reduced the amount of fiber Americans are getting in their diet.

Let's turn now to the two categories of fiber: (1) insoluble and (2) soluble.

Insoluble fiber: This type of fiber increases the weight, bulk, and softness of the stool. Eating insoluble fiber has been linked to lower colon cancer risk, due to increased bowel transit time. In other words, when you consume more insoluble fiber, you will have more frequent bowel movements. Insoluble fiber binds bile salts, enhancing the excretion (rather than the absorption) of cholesterol by the body. Sources of insoluble fiber include wheat bran, fruit, whole grains, and dehydrated cereal grasses including wheat, oats, barley, and rye (more on cereal grasses in the next chapter).

Soluble fiber: These fibers don't add bulk, but instead dissolve in water to become gummy or viscous. They tend to slow the rate at which sugar is absorbed, and therefore help balance blood sugar levels. Adding soluble fiber to the diet can be useful in managing diabetes. Consuming soluble fiber has also been linked to healthy blood cholesterol levels. Sources of soluble fiber include oat bran, rice bran, legumes, fruits, vegetables, apple pectin, beans, and some seeds.

If you are considering "bulking up" (adding more fiber to your diet), do so gradually. Your body will need time to adjust. Making this change too fast can result in cramping, bloating, and gas. Also, optimal water is essential. Without enough water, the extra fiber can result in constipation, instead of the increased bowel transit time you're actually looking for.

It's not difficult to get your daily requirement of fiber if your diet includes whole, fresh foods and excludes refined versions. To learn more about the fiber content of foods, visit *www.slrhc.org/healthinfo /dietaryfiber*. Sponsored by Continuum Health Partners, this site lists everything you could ever need to know about fiber, including the most extensive fiber chart I have ever seen.

If adding enough fiber to your diet isn't something you can easily see yourself doing sometime soon, there are commercial formulas available made from natural food fibers. Possible ingredients include flaxseed, apple pectin, beet fiber, prune fiber, rice bran, citrus pulp/peel, and cellulose. A typical serving of a fiber formula will contain about 6 to 8 grams of dietary fiber.

▪ Fat

For years, fats received a bad rap. Consumers were told to greatly restrict their fat intake. However, the real problem was, and still is, people tend to eat the *wrong kinds* of fats—that is, those that are highly refined and processed. For optimal health, we really do need to include the *right kinds* of fats in our diet—in general, these are organic and minimally or unprocessed oils. No-fat diets can actually be dangerous to our well-being.

Why are fats so important? Well, this is a workhorse macronutrient with lots of duties in our bodies. For instance, some vitamins dissolve in fat. Without fat, vitamins A, D, E, and K could not be absorbed into our bloodstream to nourish the body. Fats are used for energy, and can be stored for later use in times of deprivation. The membrane of every one of our cells is made of fat. This macronutrient slows the movement of carbohydrates into the bloodstream, preventing wide blood sugar swings and excess insulin secretion. In addition, fats enhance immune function, protect us against cardiovascular disease, and support hormonal balance. For fat, it is all in a day's work, and that's just part of the list!

Recently we've been hearing more and more about another one of fat's important roles. And that is in supplying the two *essential fatty acids (EFAs)* that are not produced by our bodies—*Omega 3 EFA* and *Omega 6 EFA*. These two EFAs are vital to normal cell formation and body function. We need to eat them in about equal amounts, but Americans tend to get more Omega 6s in their diet. An essential fatty acid deficiency is very common in this country because most of the fat Americans consume has been refined and adulterated. Commercial refinement strips fats of their essential fatty acids or alters them into toxic compounds. At this time, there is simply not enough EFA-rich oil being included in the American diet because of mass refinement.

It is estimated that as many as 80% of Americans suffer from an essential fatty acid deficiency. Symptoms of this deficiency include depression; cardiovascular disease; high blood pressure; skin conditions such as eczema, psoriasis, dry skin, and acne; slow metabolism; difficulty losing weight; PMS; cancer; joint pain; chronic fatigue; autoimmune disorders; and decreased immune response. To make sure you're receiving your daily EFA requirements, it is wise to supplement your diet with a tablespoon or two a day of a prepared oil blend. Typical ingredients include flax, hemp, evening primrose, and borage oils. You'll find these blends at the health food store. Most people need between 20 to 40 grams of EFAs a day, which is roughly two to five tablespoons of oil a day.

An EFA deficiency is common among those with a diet that is also high in dangerous *trans fatty acids*. Trans fats are found in processed foods made with hydrogenated or partially hydrogenated oils like margarine, vegetable shortening, and soybean oil. The functions of the Omega 3 and 6 fatty acids you do take in are altered by the presence of trans fatty acids. Trans fats have been linked with cancer, heart disease, immune system breakdowns, depression, fatigue, and hormonal imbalances. Foods highest in trans fats include commercially made breads, crackers, rolls, cookies, pies, and doughnuts.

Be aware that trans fats often show up in commercial products that are marketed as being "cholesterol-free." The trans fats come from the partially hydrogenated oils that these foods contain. Remember, no plant-based oil will ever have cholesterol (only animal fats do). And just because there's no cholesterol does not mean that an oil is good for you. Partially hydrogenated vegetable oils are used more and more by fast foods restaurants because of the concerns about cholesterol. However, even though greasy French fries may not have cholesterol, they are a dietary disaster due to the toxicity of the fried fat. It is loaded with trans fats.

Basic rules of thumb in choosing oils are to always purchase those that are organic, cold-pressed, and/or minimally processed or unprocessed. Here's a rundown of the common oils, their best uses, and status as a smart or undesirable choice:

Extra virgin olive oil: This antioxidant-rich oil is great to use for cooking. Olive is one of the safest oils you can choose. However, like any other cooking oil, use it sparingly.

Flax oil: Flax is a terrific source of omega 3 fatty acids. Never heat flax oil, as high temperatures destroy the precious EFAs. The daily suggested amount is a tablespoon or two every day. Your daily intake of flax oil can also be consumed in a salad or over pasta. Keep flax oil refrigerated to keep it from going rancid. Research shows that flax oil has anti-cancer, anti-viral, anti-bacterial, and anti-fungal properties. Its anti-estrogenic effects can be helpful in preventing breast cancer. Ingestion of flax oil helps curb sugar cravings; improves the condition of skin, nails, and the internal organs; increases fat burning; and lowers cholesterol and blood pressure (therefore reducing heart attack risk). As an anti-inflammatory, flax can reduce the symptoms of arthritis. Flax is also helpful in the management of diabetes, and it reduces the risk of stroke. It's no wonder that Mahatma Gandhi said,

"Whenever flax becomes a regular food among the people, there will be better health."

Hemp, evening primrose, and borage oils: These oils are used along with flax oil in prepared oil blends supplying the essential fatty acids (Omega 3 and 6). Look for product sold in protective opaque containers. The oils should not be heated, since high temperatures destroy the EFAs.

Coconut oil: Use for sauté cooking, stir frying, baking, or on breads or pasta. Select an organic, unrefined product. Omega's Coconut Butter contains no trans fatty acids and is not hydrogenated. Coconut oil is a good source of lauric acid, an infection fighter. Although consumption of coconut oil has been criticized in the past, it appears that hydrogenation was the problem—not the oil itself.

Butter: Choose natural butter over synthetic margarine, selecting organic sources. Butter that is not organic can contain steroids, vaccines, pesticides, and antibiotics. Buy certified *raw* organic butter, if possible. The Alta Dena Dairy of California is one source of raw product. Butter has long been an important component in many traditional diets. It provides vitamins A, D, E, and K.

Ghee: This specially prepared fat can be made from organic butter. Advantages of using ghee are that no refrigeration is necessary after it has been made and that it stores for several months. Also, ghee does not smoke or burn like butter does at high temperatures. Prepared ghee can be purchased at Indian markets and health food stores. You can also make your own. Simply place 1 pound of butter in a saucepan over moderate heat. Bring it to a boil, and then cover and lower the heat as much as possible. Cook for about 45 minutes. The milk solids will go to the bottom, and the butter on top will gradually begin to appear transparent. Strain the clear ghee through cheesecloth to remove all the solids. Discard the solids. Store the ghee in a glass jar with a tight lid in a cool, dark place. Use for cooking.

Avocado: This tasty food, from the fruit category, is exceptionally high in essential fatty acids. It is strong in beta-carotene, and also supplies vitamin B6, potassium, magnesium, iron, and fiber. The fat found in avocados is similar to what's in olive oil. Use avocado liberally—perhaps adding slices to a salad or sandwich or mashing it into a guacamole dip. Ripen at room temperature before eating. Placing the avocado in a paper bag will speed the ripening process.

Salmon, tuna, and other cold-water fish: Some fish are good food sources of EPA and DHA fatty acids. These fatty acids are important for proper brain function, nerve response, and maintenance of the retinas, adrenal glands, and sex organs. Research shows they also inhibit the growth of tumors. Best sources are fresh salmon, sardines,

---

THE CHOLESTEROL CONTROVERSY

Few foods have generated the controversy that has surrounded dietary cholesterol. In recent years, researchers have learned that while removing cholesterol from the body is important to prevent heart disease, other factors are probably more central to the issue than the amount of cholesterol in our diet. It seems that there isn't a direct correlation between the amount of cholesterol we ingest and how much is in our system. Why? For 70% of people, the quantity of cholesterol in the blood is safely regulated regardless of how much cholesterol is ingested. Excess cholesterol is cleared efficiently, and more cholesterol is produced internally when dietary intake of it is too low. For the other 30% of people, whose bodies are unable to adjust for the cholesterol that is ingested, dietary cholesterol is cause for concern.

The body's regulation of cholesterol is affected by factors other than the cholesterol in the food we are eating. It is important to eat a high fiber diet so that cholesterol (in the form of bile acids and cholesterol molecules) can travel out of our bodies in our stools. Adding essential fatty acids in the form of flax or olive oil also helps in the metabolism of cholesterol. Be sure to limit the intake of high-glycemic foods, which inhibit cholesterol regulation.

It may be surprising to know that not enough cholesterol in the diet can actually be dangerous. A study by the National Cholesterol Education Program found that arbitrary elimination of cholesterol in the diet can lead to increases in death due to suicide and cancer. Suicide seems to increase because of a rise in aggression related to lower serotonin levels in the brain. A hike in cancer rates may be due to resulting reduced levels of oil-soluble antioxidants—including vitamins A, E and carotene. Consult with a health professional if you are unsure of your particular needs.

mackerel, trout, and eel. Eat raw as sushi or sashimi, or prepare by lightly boiling. Do not fry. Buy fish that lives in deep-sea areas, not farm-raised.

Peanut oil/sesame oil: Use occasionally for stir-frying. Frequent use is not suggested due to an excessive level of omega 6 fatty acids and a relative deficiency of omega 3 in these oils.

Canola oil: Use only in an organic, cold-pressed form. Store in the refrigerator as this oil goes rancid rapidly. Avoid eating canola oil in a hydrogenated form; it can often be found as such in prepared food products.

Safflower, corn, sunflower, soybean, and cottonseed: All of these oils are too high in omega 6 in proportion to their omega 3 content; they are also potentially high in pesticides. Use them sparingly, if at all.

Margarines, fake butters, and shortenings: Avoid these fats totally. Hydrogenation is used to make them. They are high in dangerous trans fatty acids. Margarine consumption has been linked with high blood cholesterol as well as cancer and heart disease.

Other hydrogenated or partially hydrogenated oils: Avoid completely. These are often found in prepared foods such as breads, crackers, rolls, cookies, pies, and doughnuts.

It is important to use care in selecting the fats that you include in your diet. While highly processed fats should be avoided, others are absolutely required to support the optimal functioning of our body. These healthy fats—olive oil, flax oil, butter, coconut oil, etc.—also play a role in preventing chronic illnesses, such as heart disease, cancer, and diabetes. Research has shown cholesterol in the diet should not be the main concern for the majority of people. (See "The Cholesterol Controversy" below.) It actually is the widely used processing techniques that are creating the fats that are the most detrimental to our health.

PUTTING IT ALL TOGETHER: BALANCING PROTEINS, CARBOHYDRATES & FATS

Over the years, one of the most important aspects of health information has been that of how to determine the proper balance of protein, carbohydrate, and fat in the diet. Research shows that the proper balance reduces food cravings, boosts immunity, supplies consistent energy, calms inflammation, prevents cancer and heart disease, and aids in achieving ideal weight.

A range that applies to many people is 40% carbohydrates, 30% protein, and 30% fats, plus or minus 10% in any one group depending on your individual requirements. Various books, including Barry Sears' *Enter the Zone,* are now calling for the 40-30-30 ratio. To discover what's right for you, get in touch with your body's individual needs. Reading Ann Louise Gittleman's book, *Your Body Knows Best,* will teach you ideas about some of the reasons for individual variation. These include your genetic and ancestral background. Some of our unique needs spring from regional differences.

Also, as you give your body more of what it needs founded on the nutrition basics covered in this chapter, you will be better able to get in touch with what works best for you and what doesn't. Part of the transition in diet will be eliminating toxic foods from what you're eating.

While recommended ratios of the macronutrients vary significantly in different popular plans, what we have noticed in recent years is that many people overdo carbohydrates. The typical American diet is overloaded with them: Breakfast, a donut, muffin, bagel or cereal and coffee; lunch, a sandwich with deli meat and cheese with chips and a cola; dinner, pasta with sauce, bread, a salad, and a cola. More of a balance needs to be achieved between protein, carbohydrates, and fats. Most people need to increase their protein intake and cut back on carbohydrates. Again, it is also crucial for abundant health to include beneficial fats.

No one ratio is appropriate for everyone. If it was, then the diet plan book that has that answer would probably outsell the Bible, which is the #1 best-selling book of all time.

FOOD ADDITIVES VS. HEALTHY
SEASONINGS & CONDIMENTS

As detailed in Chapter 3, manufacturers alter our foods with over 3,000 additives and preservatives. Many of these added ingredients are meant to enhance the flavorings of foods. Unfortunately, this often comes at the price of impacting our health with synthetic stressful substances. It is best to avoid food additives as much as possible. While

Eating Habits to Avoid

The nourishment we receive from foods is not only affected by the quality of the food, but also by the quality of our eating habits. Below are six eating habits to avoid:

1. Skipping meals, especially breakfast.
2. Rushing through meals in a chaotic environment.
3. Waiting until you feel starved before you eat, rather than noticing when hunger first calls.
4. Eating portions that are too large or too small.
5. Snacking late at night.
6. Having a meal or snack when you are stressed.

Eating Habits to Encourage

Some habits can create the optimal circumstances in which to eat. Here are half a dozen habits to incorporate into your routine.

1. Eating meals with people you love.
2. Creating a calm, relaxing atmosphere for your meals.
3. Chewing your food thoroughly, rather than gulping it down.
4. Savoring your food, instead of gobbling it up while distracted by television or other stimulus.
5. Taking the time to calm down before you eat if you are stressed.
6. Being grateful for the food before you.

certain ingredients have already been shown to be detrimental (such as aspartame and MSG), we are serving as human guinea pigs for many others. Don't wait for all the research to come through; use common sense and eliminate these foreign substances from your diet as much as you can. (For more information on MSG and its many disguises, see "The Name Game & Hidden MSG" in Chapter 3.)

When enhanced flavor is the goal, there are many natural alternatives to artificial ingredients to use. Today, in health food stores, you can find mustards, ketchups, and other condiments without synthetic additives. Many people are growing their own herbs (rosemary, basil, oregano, etc.), and non-irradiated versions of spices are now available in natural and specialty markets. Other ideas for healthy condiments include fresh natural salsas, garlic, lemon, raw apple cider vinegar, and Bragg's Liquid Aminos.

Over the years, there have been questions about adding one of the most basic seasonings—*salt*—to our food. Now we find the issues about salt are much like the problems with sugar—they have to do with its refinement. Most of the concerns in studies on salt stem from the consumption of *refined salt compounds* in combination with a sedentary lifestyle. Some sources of harmful refined salts include fast foods, packaged goods, spice mixes, cured meats, and table salt. Unlike refined products, natural sea salts—such as the Celtic Sea Salt brand—contain no synthetic additives (like aluminum compounds) and deliver more minerals.

A no-salt diet can actually be harmful, as we do need some healthy sources of it in our diet. Salt powerfully activates enzymes in our bodies. It is also important for its chloride content, a substance that contributes to the manufacturing of the hydrochloric acid used in digestion. A large study found dietary salt intake had no impact on blood pressure; in some cases, salt restriction caused blood pressure levels to *rise!*[11]

For more information on the health benefits of natural sea salts, visit the Celtic website at *www.celtic-seasalt.com.* Other brands include Lima (from Brittany, like Celtic), Muramoto and "Si" (from Mexico), and Maldon (from England).

DIETARY ADDICTIONS: WHY THEY OCCUR & HOW TO RECOVER

While reading the earlier sections about curbing your *sugar* and *caffeine* intake, you may have thought, "But wait, I'm addicted to both of them!" Usually we have addictions to fill needs. People consume both caffeine and sugar for energy, for stimulation, and to offset low moods. However, since both sugar and caffeine are addicting, you only want more.

When ridding yourself of a food addiction, the goal is to transform your desire for it—to not actually want it. Sound impossible? If you're thinking "mission impossible," it's probably because dieting is often based on a deprivation point of view. It's all about the things you want but can't have.

One of the benefits of the nutritional ideas in this book is that they can help you free yourself naturally from food addictions. You see, when your blood sugar remains balanced with a healthy diet and sufficient water, you'll begin to notice an increased consistency in your available energy—and less of a desire for both caffeine and sugar. Still some people will need to make a concentrated effort to rid themselves of sugar and/or caffeine cravings. Here are some tips for those who need some extra support.

In general, to motivate yourself to end a food addiction, it's important to understand why the substance isn't healthy. You'll find many reasons in this book for quitting caffeine and sugar as well as in other publications. In addition, plan to give yourself some time to withdrawal. Going cold turkey doesn't work for most people. Also, look for healthy habits that can replace the old toxic ones. Taking something away without a positive replacement invites a reemergence of the addictive substance in your diet. Lastly, set reasonable goals. Allow for a transitional period. Don't set yourself up for failure.

Keeping those points in mind, let's look at specific ideas for ending a caffeine or sugar habit.

Sugar: Many people can cut sugar from their diet without much difficulty. Having some protein at every meal and snack can help tremendously. As mentioned earlier, supplementing your diet daily with 1,500 mg. of L-glutamine (an amino acid) and 200 mcg. of chromium (a mineral) can help cut sugar cravings. Try to eliminate sweets from your diet as well as hidden sugars in packaged foods (corn syrup, etc.). Have a piece of fruit if you really want something sweet. Drink lots of water. If you have a serious sugar addiction, you may need to consult a health professional (see Chapter 15).

If *artificial sweeteners* are your issue, increase water intake. People who consume beverages that include these substances are often dehydrated. Taper off of the artificial sugar by choosing water and the healthy drinks that are discussed above in the "Other Beverages" section earlier in this chapter.

Caffeine: Allow two or three weeks to kick the caffeine habit. Withdrawing from caffeine will be easier with adrenal support. You can gain this support by taking buffered Vitamin C throughout the day for a total of several grams. Try sipping sparkling water with lemon or a hot herb tea when you normally would grab a glass of cola or a mug of java. If you feel you need a more gradual program, begin tapering off caffeinated drinks by mixing in decaffeinated versions. A black tea might also be a good replacement for coffee at first, since it contains less caffeine if not steeped too long. Baking soda or potassium bicarbonate tablets can be used to reduce withdrawal symptoms. Be careful not to begin to depend on sugar as a substitute stimulus for caffeine.

The exhaustion that prompts many people to consume caffeine often comes from poor nutritional intake, emotional stress, not enough sleep, etc. Examine your life and improve those areas that are depleting you. It is important to increase your water intake, as caffeine cravings can be a sign of dehydration.

Eventually you may decide to replace caffeinated coffee with decaf or one of the many coffee substitutes that are available. Tecchino and Cafix are two possibilities; check with your health food store or specialty market to find a coffee substitute that you like. Others may prefer to skip coffee and coffee-like drinks completely and to drink herbal teas instead.

Alcohol: A discussion of dietary addictions would not be complete without addressing alcohol. When there is significant abuse of alcohol, support is often needed in the form of a twelve-step program, acupuncture, psychological therapy, or spiritual counseling. During the time while you may be working on underlying issues related to alcohol use, nutritional support often makes the transition easier.

Since alcohol is dehydrating, you'll want to increase your water intake. It is important to upgrade your diet and supplemental regimen as discussed generally in other sections of this book. You may also wish to consult with a nutritionist to address the additional changes in diet and supplementation that you may require. Hypoglycemia and/or candida may also be an issue. These factors contribute to alcohol cravings.

Some general tips. Taking 1,500 mg. of the amino acid L-glutamine can reduce cravings. A daily dose of 30 mg. of zinc is also helpful. Avoid sugar as it can increase the desire for an alcoholic drink. Eat sufficient fiber to promote optimal bowel function.

To overcome addictions, support from a spiritual practice can be essential. Make time to cultivate a quiet inner space with yoga, prayer, meditation, Tai Chi, breath work, etc. Bringing in the light (beneficial activity) can help you transform the darkness (toxic behavior and addiction). Strengthening your spiritual life will also make it easier to "act as if" you are already a healthy eater. Remember that you are bigger than your addiction. With this empowering attitude, your body is more likely to respond in kind by allowing your unhealthy cravings to cease.

A final note: There are many food cravings that people experience beyond sugar, caffeine, and alcohol. Many of these cravings are actually a sign of food allergies! That's right; often people are drawn to the very foods to which they are allergic. Common foods that trigger allergic reactions include eggs, milk, cheese, wheat, and soy. See Chapter 15 to learn where allergy testing is available. A breakthough allergy testing and treatment protocol called NAET (*www.naet.com*) is an excellent system for evaluating and eliminating food allergies.

EATING WITH WISDOM

By now, you may be thinking that whoever wrote this book does not live in the real world, or she must be some kind of saint. Actually I am a recovered junk foodaholic as well as a former caffeine and sugar addict, and now I have more energy than I know what to do with. And as each year passes, my energy and state of wellness only increases. How many patients and I have moved forward was though a commitment to the process, not with a "get-fit-quick" scheme.

It is so important in this process to recognize and cultivate your body's innate wisdom. Allow your body to speak. Listen to its unique needs. So often we are too busy to slow down and pay attention to all the wisdom our body has to share with us.

When we are out of touch with our body's needs, our cravings tend to be for quick energy in the form of junk. Now that you are making smarter food choices, your cravings are certain to be changing for the better. Your body's innate wisdom is now coming forward. Isn't it interesting how this works? Another example of the body's inner wisdom is when pregnant women have strange cravings that seem to come out of nowhere. One theory is that the developing baby has specific nutrient needs and that the cravings are for foods that will supply that nourishment.

HEALTHY FOOD PREPARATION TECHNIQUES

Adopting healthy techniques for preparing food will support the smarter choices you're making in the selection of foods. At this point, you're buying the freshest, most wholesome foods available. What you want are methods that retain as much of the original nutrients in these foods as possible. At the same time, you want to avoid adding or creating any toxic substances in the foods.

The "Food Preparation" section of Chapter 3 presented practices that can foster the presence of toxins in food. Using one of the best materials for cookware, stainless steel—not aluminum or nonstick types—was encouraged. The reasons to avoid microwaving, frying, and barbecuing of foods were also covered. Lastly, it was pointed out that dishes and glassware manufactured in other countries may leach toxins into the foods you serve.

Let's look now at some specific techniques you can incorporate into your kitchen routine:

Raw Foods: Not every meal needs to be cooked! And some meals can contain mostly raw ingredients. You might make a salad with a wide range of vegetables, topped with broiled fish or chicken breast. Or you could cut up a tray of veggies and eat them with a satisfying healthy dip. Raw foods supply ample enzymes, nutrients, and fiber.

Steaming: When you steam foods, you cook them over—instead of in—gently boiling water. Make sure the water doesn't touch the food. This method retains more of the nutrients than boiling. Steaming requires some type of rack or barrier with holes that allow the steam to come through. You can steam vegetables, either just one or in combinations. You may also wish to steam fish. Do not overcook the food; vegetables should remain slightly crunchy. Inexpensive stainless steel steamer baskets are available at houseware stores.

Stir-frying: Here a food is placed in a hot pan with a little oil (olive, peanut, or sesame are good choices) and cooked briskly while being stirred. Because the food is sliced into small uniform pieces, cooking time is short. To avoid using too much oil, you may find it helpful to use a wok for stir-frying. Specially made for this purpose, a wok allows foods to cook in the smallest amount of oil. Use stir-frying for vegetables or veggie/meat combinations.

Broiling: Use this method for chicken sections, fish, or skewers of meat. Choose firm-fleshed fish, such as Pacific salmon, halibut, shrimp, or sea bass, so that it doesn't fall apart when turned over. Broiling allows the fat to drip away from the food to a pan underneath.

The techniques detailed above help to retain the natural flavors of the food. Meals will be so much *more enjoyable* as well as nutritious when they are made with wholesome ingredients and prepared in a way that allows their unique qualities to be experienced.

Here are some guidelines to use along with your own wisdom:

1. **Diversify your diet,** choosing from the wide range of whole foods that are available. If you are new to a natural foods diet, you can look forward to a culinary adventure. The Standard American Diet (SAD) tends to have a recurring theme—meat, potatoes, and overcooked vegetables. There is such a variety of fresh vegetables, fruits, whole grains, and other delicious items at the natural foods market just waiting for your discovery.

2. **Avoid refined foods.** What you want to avoid includes prefab packaged foods, fast foods, processed oils, chemically laden meats and dairy, irradiated or genetically engineered products, commercial sugar and salt, sodas, canned fruits and vegetables, artificial sugar substitutes, etc. These foods are a nutritional wasteland.

3. **Use nutritional supplements** to complement your food intake. Due to commercial farming methods, essential vitamins and minerals are often deficient in foods and must be supplemented. See Chapter 10 for more information.

4. **DO NOT DIET!!!** Diets don't work. Just the idea of deprivation (on which weight-loss diets are based) is already something that is working against us. There has been a tremendous increase in the amount of diet products and plans and a corresponding increase in obesity. Obviously, traditional dieting is not the answer. Focus on eating healthy and learning how to incorporate health-promoting habits into your daily life.

5. **Avoid eating late at night.** It is more difficult for your body to digest food as the late hours progress. As you sleep, your body's energy should go mainly toward maintenance and repair rather than digestion.

Follow the natural workings of your body, common sense, the wisdom of experts, and your own inner knowing. The goal is to be freed from eating habits that do not serve you. Supported by a working knowledge of the foods you require, you'll find it easier to live, love, and eat with satisfaction and fulfillment! Remember that the foods you eat are an integral part of maintaining or regaining health.

MENU IDEAS

There are many great cookbooks that are loaded with natural food recipes. See the Recommended Reading List for suggestions. Following are some menu ideas to get you started.

Power Breakfasts
Start each day with an energy-sustaining meal.

- Dr. Patricia's Power Potion (see page 242)
- Organic eggs (scrambled or soft boiled) with vegetables
- Whole grain pancakes with added protein powder
- Organic oatmeal with almonds and sunflower seeds
- Organic yogurt with trail mix
- Raw almond butter on manna bread
- Tofu scramble with veggie sausage
- Natural organic energy bars (*www.nutiva.com*)

Luscious Lunches and Delectable Dinners
These meal ideas can be enjoyed at lunch or dinner time.

Many of the ideas above are for the main course. Be sure to add a salad to at least one meal a day. A salad a day is essential for good health. Get in the habit even if you have to force yourself in the beginning. Soon you (yes, you!) will find yourself craving that daily salad—and healthier foods for that matter. Cravings for junk food subside when healthier foods are substituted.

- Steamed vegetables with protein (seafood, chicken, turkey, lean meat, tofu, beans)
- Sandwich on whole grain bread with lean protein and veggies
- Burrito (seafood, chicken, veggie) on whole grain tortilla
- Soft tacos (seafood, chicken, veggie) on corn tortillas
- Broiled turkey or veggie burgers on whole-wheat bun
- Bieler's broth
- Sushi
- Stir-fry with veggies, chicken, tofu, or shrimp
- Vegetarian chili
- Turkey with mashed potatoes, broccoli, and green salad
- Black bean soup with salad and corn bread
- Indian vegetable curry with brown rice and shrimp, chicken, or tofu
- Seafood enchiladas
- Fish chowder
- Seaweed salad with tofu
- Baked turkey or veggie loaf with string beans
- Broiled fish with rich pilaf and spinach
- Pizza with vegetables on whole grain crust with a green salad
- Spanish omelette
- Shrimp and veggie fajitas
- Vegetarian lasagna
- Risotto with brown rice and shrimp

Scrumptious Snacks

Many people tend to snack on high-carbohydrate, high-fat junk food. This is stressful to blood sugar management and contributes to the carbohydrate/sugar-craving pattern. It can be beneficial to snack on foods that have a substantial protein content in addition to healthy carbohydrates and fats. Look for snacks that emphasize whole foods, not refined and processed ingredients. Tip: Before snacking, drink a glass or two of purified water. You may notice that the desire to snack will diminish or disappear.

- Celery filled with nut or seed butter
- Half sandwich with protein on whole grain bread
- Dr. Patricia's Power Potion
- Protein drink or bar
- Raw nuts, such as almonds, walnuts, cashews
- Raw seeds, such as sunflower or pumpkin
- Baked corn chips and guacamole
- Organic string cheese
- Fruit and cottage cheese
- Plain yogurt sweetened with stevia
- Raw carrots and hummus
- Dates filled with raw goat cheese
- Trail mix

Bieler's Broth

This recipe comes from the famous medical doctor and nutritionist, Henry Bieler, M.D. Dr. Bieler was a pioneer in the field of nutritional medicine and had a huge following for over fifty years, which included celebrities such as Greta Garbo and Gloria Swanson.

Ingredients:
- 6-8 zucchini
- $^1/_2$ cup parsley
- 1lb. fresh or frozen string beans
- 2 celery stalks

Chop vegetables and place in steamer. Steam well in purified water, but do not overcook. Put the steamed vegetables and water in a blender and puree. Optional ingredients include garlic, onion, lemon, sea salt, cayenne pepper, and fresh herbs to taste.

Dr. Patricia's Power Potion

This recipe has been enjoyed by hundreds of patients, friends, relatives, and colleagues over the years. It can be used as a satisfying meal replacement or as an in-between pick-me-up. This smoothie provides sustained energy, is concentrated in nutrients, and tastes delicious.

Ingredients:

- 2 heaping tbsp. organic protein powder (rice, fermented soy, or whey)
- 1-2 tbsp. flax-borage oil
- 1-2 tbsp. superfood formula (see chapter 10)
- 1 tbsp. fiber formula or ground flax seeds (FiPro FLAX™)
- 1-2 tbsp. plain yogurt or kefir

- Fresh or frozen fruit
- 1 tbsp. organic bee pollen
- 1 tbsp. lecithin
- sprinkle of powdered ginger (optional for metabolic/circulatory/immune support)
- 1 tbsp. goat whey (optional for added mineral content)
- stevia (optional for added sweetness)

Blend with water (and ice, if desired) for desired consistency. Measurements can be adjusted for taste and texture. Experiment to see what ingredients and proportions work for you. Make a toast to optimum health and enjoy!

THE NEXT STEP IN THE NUTRITION/DETOX CONNECTION

As you begin to make healthier meal choices, you will notice increased energy and an improved sense of well-being. The next chapter will help you take the fundamentals of nutrition once step further. As you enter the world of the micronutrients, you will be able to fine-tune your plan by including powerful substances that can dramatically improve your health.

TEN

The Small Wonders:
Vitamins, Minerals
& Phytonutrients

Each one of the substances of a man's diet
acts upon his body and changes it in some way,
and upon these changes, his whole life depends,
whether he be in health, in sickness, or convalescent.

— Hippocrates

In the previous chapter, we delved into the basics of nutrition—
including the importance of whole foods—and considered the
macronutrients—water, protein, carbohydrates, and fats. In this chapter, we will explore the so-called micronutrients—vitamins, minerals, and phytonutrients, as well as special foods that are especially rich in these precious substances. Earlier we extensively covered the important subject of enzymes, so these key micronutrients will not be covered in this chapter. Keep in mind that as you follow Chapter 9's advice to eat organic whole foods regularly, you will be naturally increasing your intake of vitamins, minerals, phytonutrients, and enzymes. The current chapter will clarify the specific benefits that come from many of the small wonders that are hidden in whole foods.

Isn't it ironic that most vitamins were discovered in the early 20th Century, just around the same time that food was starting to be processed and stripped of these very nutrients? Throughout the history of humankind, foods have never been tampered with as much as we've seen over the last century or so. Yet most of the advancements in nutritional science—including the discovery of vitamins, minerals, phytonutrients, antioxidants, etc.—have occurred over the last hundred years. In Nature's wisdom, She made sure that those people who might overindulge in processed foods would have a way to counterbalance an otherwise deficient diet. Luckily supplementation allows us to make up for what's missing in the modern diet.

Yes, the first vitamin was discovered just before the turn of the 20th Century. Dutch physician Christiaan Eijkman detected thiamin (now known as vitamin B_1) in 1896, during a period when science was responding to Louis Pasteur's germ theory of disease. In this scientific environment, it was difficult to convince people that dietary factors could cause disease (that it wasn't always germs). Not until 30 years later, in 1929, did Eijkman receive the Nobel Prize for his breakthrough finding. Indeed, the term *vitamin* itself wasn't coined until 1912! So the actual field of nutritional science is relatively new. Its late arrival is partially due to the fact that virtually all food was whole and nutritious until the 20th Century. Another reason is that scientific advances have moved more rapidly during modern times.

You can benefit richly from this increase in knowledge. We now know that there are basic nutrients that are required *by all humans*. These substances have various functions, and while you may see certain ones marketed specifically for detox support, *they all assist in some way in the detoxification process.*

WHY SUPPLEMENTATION IS NECESSARY

Supplementation has long been a topic of controversy. One statement you may have heard in the debate is that supplements are not necessary if you eat a good diet. As I often tell my patients, I wish this were true! Unfortunately today, due to many factors, we cannot rely on our foods alone to support us nutritionally. It is wise to be taking a multivitamin/multimineral supplement every day, no matter how healthy you think you eat. Here are a few of the issues that make additional support essential.

A refined/unnatural diet: As you now know, our food fare today varies greatly from the nutrient- and enzyme-rich diet upon which the human body long relied. Processed foods fall way short of meeting our nutritional needs. Most studies conducted on the American diet have shown deficiencies or suboptimal intake of many nutrients.

Deficient soil: Even with many food choices available, daily requirements are not met. Because the soil is deficient, even fresh fruits and vegetables have become deficient in providing the essential nutrients. Reasons for depleted soil include chemical fertilizers, overuse, acid rain, and erosion of the topsoil. To compensate, we must take supplements to add to the support that we do get from food.

Heavy toxic load: In modern times, we encounter unprecedented levels of chemical toxins. On average, individuals are exposed to more than 500 chemicals at home and 700 in drinking water. These toxins have been shown to deplete nutrients. Fortunately, our intake of vitamins, minerals, phytonutrients, etc., can enhance our body's ability to detoxify.

Exposure to radiation: Radiation—coming from nuclear technology, x-rays, computer terminals, microwaves, etc.—builds up in the body over time. Again, supplements can help us fight back to protect our health. According to the *American Journal of Clinical Nutrition* and *Nutrition Review,* exposure to radiation, in combination with chemical toxins, destroys vitamins A, C, E, K, some of the Bs, and essential fatty acids.

One of the main points of this chapter is to help ensure that your basic nutritional requirements are covered. For all the reasons explained above, supplements are needed in addition to good food choices. Every day that goes by without meeting your fundamental nutritional needs is like not paying your credit card bills completely. You build up interest—in this case, the interest can be in the form of failing energy, increased susceptibility to disease, and accelerated aging. This chapter can greatly assist you in supplying yourself with the basics every day.

While we have many basic requirements that must be met to reach a level of optimal health, marketing of supplements often focuses on a particular supplement that is supposed to be a miracle cure. The truth is that since many people are so deficient in nutrients, they may see dramatic results just by adding one or two of the potentially deficient ten or twenty nutrients. Don't get caught up in the hype! It is important to satisfy all of your basic nutritional requirements for optimal health and disease prevention, not just to attempt to cure a symptom with a nutrient that you have read about in a supermarket magazine.

Note to Reader: While the importance of supplementation is emphasized in this chapter, keep in mind that it is meant to be *in addition to* a whole foods diet. Supplementation is not an excuse to skip meals or to overlook the significant role food has in supporting optimal health.

BENEFITS OF SUPPLEMENTATION

In recent years, we've learned that supplementation is more than just a means to make up for deficiencies in the diet. We've been seeing growing evidence that additional amounts of nutrients can protect against disease and ward off premature aging. In fact, every year, thousands of medical journal articles are published on the various gains that can be achieved from vitamins and minerals. In just one year, 500 to 600 articles were written on vitamin E alone, and about the same number focused on vitamin C. Throughout this chapter, you'll discover benefit after benefit that comes from the world of the micronutrient. But before we begin to look at specific groups of these substances, here's an overview of the many advantages to be gained through intelligent supplementation.

Day-to-Day Health Maintenance: Vitamins, minerals, and the other micronutrients help your body function at an optimal level on an ongoing basis. Along with the macronutrients (water, protein, carbohydrates, and fat), the micronutrients serve as building blocks that maintain the body and its biochemical operations. You need these substances to create energy, repair tissue, and make enzymes, hormones, and new cells. So meeting your basic needs for the micronutrients is like drinking water when you're thirsty. They are among your body's standard requirements.

Detoxification Support: The chemical reactions that take place when your body detoxifies require various vitamins and nutrients. In this chapter, you will read about the roles specific micronutrients play in detoxification. For instance, a deficiency in vitamin A reduces your body's resistance to pesticides. And vitamin C can increase the production of compounds in the liver that help detoxify chemical air pollutants.

Prevention of Illness: Many people are aware that high dosages of vitamin C along with zinc can lessen the severity and duration of a cold. Well, research shows that more serious afflictions may be avoided or mitigated through the use of supplements. For instance, we've learned that various micronutrients, such as beta-carotene and vitamins C and E, can help prevent such health concerns as heart disease, cancer, arthritis, and cataracts. A smart prevention program includes a whole foods diet, regular exercise, *and* supplementation.

Promotion of Longevity: A recent discovery is that specific vitamins, such as niacin (vitamin B$_3$), can block the formation of DNA breakdown products that cause cells to become damaged and die prematurely. This is just one way that supplementation can help us not only stay healthy, but also live longer.

Let's move on to the wonderful and magical world of the micronutrient.

VITAMINS

"Thanks to the new science of nutrition, you can today multiply the benefits of healthy habits by taking, every day, the optimum amounts of the essential vitamins."
— Linus Pauling, *Nobel-Prize-winning scientist, health advocate*

Since your body is not able to make many vitamins (and creates the others in insufficient amounts), they must come in either your food or supplements. Though vitamins are vital to your health, they are only needed in minute amounts. Currently there are thirteen substances commonly recognized as vitamins—*A, C, D, E, K* and *the eight Bs (known as the B complex)*. In addition, there are other compounds considered part of the B complex, such as *inositol, folic acid,* and *biotin*. Since various substances that were earlier identified as vitamins later turned out to be duplicates or actually belonged in different classifications, there are gaps in the vitamin lettering system.

One reason that proper vitamin intake is so important is that these micronutrients serve as cofactors to enzymes (your body's catalysts). What this means is they "flip the switch" that turns enzymes on to do their varied work in creating the chemical reactions necessary for life. While not every enzyme requires a cofactor, many do and are thus inactive without them.

▪ Vitamin A (Retinol)

Nutrient Properties: Good eyesight, particularly night vision, is associated with vitamin A. This micronutrient blends with a protein to create visual purple, which adds to our ability to see after dark. Proper intake also promotes elasticity and reparability of body tissues, and thus healthy skin. Retinol's antioxidant ability can protect against infection as well as cancer of the skin, lung, and prostate. This vitamin is converted from the phytonutrient *beta-carotene* by the liver and intestines. Stress depletes vitamin A.

Detoxification Properties: Retinol prevents penetration of toxins by strengthening the walls of the cells. Proper amounts increase the efficiency of the thymus gland, allowing for greater immune resistance to invading toxins. Vitamin A lessens the negative effects of chemical toxins such as medications and pesticides. A report in the *Journal of the National Cancer Institute* noted that vitamin A can counteract ionizing gamma radiation.[1]

Foods Sources: Eggs, liver and other organ meats, fish liver oils, seafood, milk fat. (Beta-carotene: Carrots, broccoli, and leafy green vegetables such as collards and kale.)

Recommended Daily Amounts: Vitamin A 5,000 IU; beta-carotene 15,000 to 25,000 IU.

▪ Vitamin B1 (Thiamin)

Nutrient Properties: Vitamin B_1 was the first water-soluble vitamin to be discovered. It fights fatigue by promoting the release of energy from carbohydrates. Thiamin is required for hydrochloric acid production in the stomach. Proper functioning of the heart, GI tract, and nervous system are all supported by vitamin B_1. Deficiencies are seen in alcoholics, schizophrenics, and people with Alzheimer's. A daily dose of just 100 mg for eight weeks was shown to prompt improvements in Alzheimer's patients.[2] Shortages can be caused by a diet high in refined grains, sodas, and junk food.

Detoxification Properties: A powerful antioxidant, B_1 counteracts the effects of free radicals. It also enhances the Phase-2 detox pathway in the liver.

Food Sources: Pork, liver, and other organ meats; poultry; fish; eggs; wheat germ; whole grains including cereals; nuts; seeds including sunflower; legumes such as peas, avocados; spinach.

Recommended Daily Amounts: 10 to 25 mg

▪ Vitamin B2 (Riboflavin)

Nutrient Properties: This vitamin is responsible for the bright yellow color of urine that follows use of a multivitamin or a B-complex supplement. You might call B_2 the "energy vitamin," as it plays important roles in metabolism and food processing. Riboflavin also contributes to the health of skin, hair, and nails. In addition, it is needed for the production of red blood cells which are responsible for carrying oxygen to body cells. Riboflavin activates the other B vitamins.

Detoxification Properties: B_2 protects against chemical toxins by activating the powerful antioxidant glutathione. It aids in the scavenging and neutralization of free radicals. Riboflavin is also helpful in the Phase I detoxification process.

Food Sources: Dark green leafy vegetables, milk, eggs, cottage cheese, yogurt, mushrooms, asparagus, broccoli, avocado, Brussels sprouts, tuna, oysters, salmon, liver, almonds.

Recommended Daily Amounts: 10 to 25 mg

▪ Vitamin B3 (Niacin)

Nutrient Properties: Niacin (short for nicotinic acid) is also important in energy production. It assists your body in using sugars and fatty acids. B_3 also helps enzymes function properly in the nervous system. This vitamin is necessary for the formation of sex hormones. Consuming excess amounts leads to flushing of the skin, liver damage, and ulcers. Therapeutic doses of niacin may lower blood cholesterol. Research at the University of Kentucky found niacin protective against cancer.

Detoxification Properties: Vitamin B_3 is essential for recycling the antioxidant glutathione. It is also helpful in the Phase II detoxification process.

Food Sources: Chicken breast, tuna, mackerel, liver, veal, halibut, turkey, dairy products, sunflower seeds, bran, peas, and other legumes.
Recommended Daily Amounts: 50 mg

■ Vitamin B6 (Pyridoxine)

Nutrient Properties: Vitamin B_6's many roles in primary body processes, including metabolism, makes it one of the most important micronutrients. Involved more so in the breakdown of protein into amino acids, it also helps metabolize fat and carbohydrate. (High protein diets call for higher supplementation of this micronutrient.) Pyridoxine is needed for proper mental functioning. Volunteers put on a B_6-deficient diet became irritable, depressed, and confused within only two to three weeks. Optimal immune response and healthy skin also require adequate B_6. Note that a yeast overgrowth will interfere with vitamin B_6 processing.

Detoxification Properties: Pyridoxine is needed to clear formaldehyde. B_6 along with folic acid and betaine can detoxify excess homocysteine from a high protein diet. (Homocysteine has been linked with an increased risk of cardiovascular disease.) Certain chemicals found in herbicides, medicines, and petroleum products are B_6 antagonists. This vitamin is also important in Phase I detoxification.

Food Sources: Brewer's yeast, whole grains, sunflower seeds, legumes, liver, fish, chicken, bananas, prunes, raisins, nuts.
Recommended Daily Amounts: 10 to 25 mg

■ Vitamin B12 (Cobalamin)

Nutrient Properties: This was the last vitamin to be discovered (the year was 1948), and new functions are still being found. We do know that B_{12} is present in every cell, as it is a part of many body chemicals. It is used to process fatty acids and some amino acids. Cobalamin and folic acid work together to form normal red blood cells. You need cobalamin to maintain healthy nervous tissue. It's also used in the manufacture of genetic material. Strict vegetarians are at risk of developing a vitamin B_{12} deficiency. Therapeutic doses of B_{12} are helpful in treating depression.

Detoxification Properties: Vitamin B_{12} aids in the detoxification of fat-soluble toxic chemicals. It is helpful in mitigating reactions to sulfites, preservatives used at salad bars and in wine. Cobalamin helps clear excess estrogen and enhances the flow of bile. According to the *American Journal of Clinical Nutrition,* vitamin B_{12} may protect against the development of lung cancer. This vitamin is needed for Phase I detoxification.

Food Sources: Red meat, sardines, salmon, crab, poultry, kidney, eggs, yogurt.

Recommended Daily Amounts: 50 to 100 mcg

▪ Vitamin C (Ascorbic acid)

Nutrient Properties: One of most well researched micronutrients, vitamin C was studied extensively by Nobel laureate Linus Pauling, Ph.D., who recommended large doses to fight colds and flu. Subsequent research has shown that megadoses can cut the length and severity of colds by at least 30%. The National Academy of Sciences now recognizes that vitamin C also plays a role in preventing cancer. Ascorbic acid supports the strength of your connective tissue by building collagen. It also reduces the impact of stress by supporting the adrenal glands.

Detoxification Properties: Since vitamin C boosts our immune system activity, it can be helpful in counteracting the effects of chemical toxins and radiation. Also, anemia is a common response to such exposures, and vitamin C helps by increasing the absorption of iron and subsequently the production of red blood cells. This micronutrient also serves as a powerful antioxidant, cleaning up free radicals. It activates other antioxidants as well. According to a study published in the *Journal of the American Medical Association,* vitamin C shows promise in reducing the levels of lead in the blood.[3] Vitamin C has been useful for detox by smokers and victims of carbon monoxide poisoning.

Food Sources: Citrus fruits such as lemons, limes, grapefruits, and oranges; green vegetables including Brussels sprouts, spinach, broccoli, and peppers; parsley, bean sprouts, melons, papaya, kiwi, berries, tomatoes.

Recommended Daily Amounts: 2,000 to 5,000 mg

▪ Vitamin E (Tocopherol)

Nutrient Properties: Vitamin E, an effective antioxidant, has also been researched extensively. It has been found to protect the walls of the blood vessels from oxidative damage from fat, reducing the likelihood of heart disease. Research indicates that it also may lessen the risk of developing cancers of the colon and prostate, as well as cataracts. Tocopherol is needed for effective immune response. It also supports the health and function of the nervous system.

Detoxification Properties: As part of its work as an antioxidant, vitamin E protects cell membranes and tissue (including the liver) from damage from free radicals produced by chemical toxins. A study at the National Cancer Institute found vitamin E to mitigate radiation damage. Research found it helpful against cesium-137, a type of radiation that comes from fallout and nuclear power leakage.[4] Vitamin E seems to guard against the effects of an array of toxins such as carbon monoxide, chlorine, cigarette smoke, mercury, nitrates, ozone, and various drug residues.

Food Sources: Fresh unprocessed vegetable oils, wheat germ, nuts such as almonds and walnuts, nut butters, seeds, organ meats, whole grains, green leafy vegetables.

Recommended Daily Amounts: 400 to 800 IU

▪ Biotin *(Part of the B-complex family)*

Nutrient Properties: This micronutrient is required for metabolism as well as the synthesis of carbohydrates, fatty acids, and amino acids. It also helps derive energy from glucose. Working with pantothenic acid, biotin assists in producing many body enzymes. Healthy skin, hair, and nails all require biotin. Some biotin is produced by bacteria in the digestive tract.

Detoxification Properties: Biotin is an important part of a detoxification program, for it is needed for Phase I detoxification.

Food Sources: Wheat germ; brewer's yeast; organ meats such as liver; oatmeal; cooked egg yolks; milk; whole grains including brown rice; cauliflower; mushrooms; legumes including split peas, lentils, and peas; tuna; sardines; molasses.

Recommended Daily Amounts: 200 mcg

▪ Choline *(Contained in Lecithin; part of the B-complex family)*

Nutrient Properties: This B-family relative is primarily known for its help in improving memory. Since it's a primary component of lecithin, studies have often looked at choline's effects in that form. Research has shown that lecithin supplementation enhances one's ability to remember names and locate misplaced items. In one study, the impact was greatest in the thirty-five to fifty age group, yet participants who were sixty-five to eighty also benefited. Researchers believe choline is lecithin's secret ingredient, as it is a substance that helps messages travel along nerve cells.

Detoxification Properties: Choline is also a potent antioxidant, and in that role, it aids detoxification. It also increases contractions of the intestine during digestion, which boosts the elimination of toxins. In the lecithin form, it has been shown to significantly thin the bile, making removal of toxins from the liver more efficient. Lecithin is protective against liver damage from alcohol.[5]

Food Sources: Apples, black currents, mangoes, papaya, citrus fruits, strawberries, cantaloupe, broccoli, Brussels sprouts, cabbage, cauliflower, green and red peppers, dark green vegetables, tomatoes, egg yolk, organ meats, wheat germ.

Recommended Daily Amounts: Choline, 500 to 1,000 mg; Lecithin, for memory enhancement, 2 tablespoons daily.

■ Folic Acid *(Also called Folacin or Folate; part of the B-complex family)*

Nutrient Properties: First found in green leafy vegetables, folic acid's name was derived from the word "foliage." This micronutrient is involved in many body processes including cell division and growth, and it also plays a role in the utilization of protein and amino acids. Folic acid and vitamin B_{12} are enlisted together in the production of red blood cells. Folate is also used to manufacture genetic material including DNA. Since deficiencies of folic acids are linked to neurological birth defects, women of childbearing age are especially encouraged to be aware of their intake. Elderly people may particularly suffer from insufficient supplies. Folic acid deficiencies also depress immune response and increase allergic reactions. Stress, physical injury, alcohol abuse, and the use of birth control pills deplete this micronutrient. Folic acid should be taken along with vitamin B_{12}.

Detoxification Properties: Folic acid is supportive of liver health. It has also been shown to reduce elevated homocysteine levels in the blood (an amino acid that contributes to cardiovascular disease). Folate plays a role in decreasing the risk of Alzheimer's and other neurodegenerative disorders. Adequate intake is thought to assist in preventing cancers of the colon and rectum; a study at the University of Alabama at Birmingham found shortages to be associated with cervical cancer. Together, folic acid and vitamin B_{12} stimulated the repair and replacement of red blood cells damaged by radiation in lab experiments.[6] Phase II detoxification requires folic acid.

Food Sources: Green leafy vegetables such as spinach, kale, Swiss chard, and beet greens; organ meats; wheat bran and whole grains; legumes including black eyed peas, lentils and lima beans; beets; avocado; broccoli; carrots; sunflower seeds; bananas.

Recommended Daily Amounts: 400 to 800 mcg

▪ Inositol *(Part of the B-complex family)*

Nutrient Properties: Inositol assists in metabolizing fat, turning it into fatty acids that contribute to healthier skin and body tissue. Since it is involved in nervous system function, deficiencies can result in anxiety, mood swings, and irritability. This micronutrient, along with choline, plays a role in converting estrogen to estriol, so it can be helpful in reducing PMS. Inositol is present in the cells of all animals and plants.

Detoxification Properties: Inositol protects cell membrane integrity. Its work in supporting fat metabolism is important for detoxification since toxins tend to be stored in body fat. Various studies show that inositol has strong anti-cancer properties.

Food Sources: Brewer's yeast; wheat germ; whole grains including barley, oats, and alfalfa; organ meats; seeds; nuts; legumes such as chick peas, green beans, and lentils; raisins; cantaloupe; oranges; grapefruit juice; milk; molasses.

Recommended Daily Amounts: 500 to 1,000 mg

MINERALS

If the term "minerals" summons mental images of huge mining operations, you're on the right track. These inorganic substances are basic elements of the earth's crust. Transported into soil, groundwater, and waterways, they are absorbed by plants and consumed by animals and humans. While there are over sixty minerals that can be found in the human body, only certain ones are of particular concern. We will look at six key minerals—*calcium, magnesium, manganese, potassium, selenium* and *zinc*. Of the six, only three (calcium, magnesium, and potassium) are needed in large quantities. While still crucial, manganese, selenium, and zinc are required only at trace amounts.

▪ Calcium

Nutrient Properties: Calcium is considered your chief mineral as it makes up the largest percentage of your body weight. This mineral's primary role is in building bone; 99% of the calcium in your body is found in either the bone or teeth. Meanwhile it's quite important for many other body processes. Calcium nourishes and relaxes the nervous system, helps muscles contract, and supports enzyme activity for healing and energy production. While calcium constructs bone, studies are indicating that it should be taken in a 2:1 magnesium-to-calcium combination. (See magnesium description below.)

Detoxification Properties: With lead toxicity, calcium plays both preventive and curative roles. It can protect against a buildup and also lower current lead levels. A study at the New Jersey Medical School in Newark found that a high-calcium diet was helpful in lowering blood lead levels in children. Calcium supports proper kidney function—an organ important for blood cleansing. This mineral can protect against toxicity caused by radiation and such heavy metals as cadmium, aluminum, fluoride, and mercury.[7]

Food Sources: Yogurt, cheese, milk, and additional dairy products; sardines and other small fish with edible bone; sesame seeds; dried figs and apricots; parsley; turnip greens; spinach; carrots; tofu; almonds; Brazil nuts.

Recommended Daily Amounts: 600 to 800 mg

▪ Magnesium

Nutrient Properties: Magnesium works in concert with calcium to build strong bone; extensive research by gynecologist Guy Abraham, M.D., indicates that it is best taken in a 2:1 magnesium-calcium ratio. Overuse of calcium (taken without sufficient magnesium) can lead to a buildup in the body that may contribute to clogging of the arteries. Americans are often deficient in magnesium. Yet it is needed for stress resistance, healthy nerve transmission, enzyme activity, muscle relaxation, athletic endurance, and the normal beating of your heart.

Detoxification Properties: Adequate magnesium intake is needed to support heavy metal and pesticide detoxification. In particular, it is helpful in counteracting a buildup of aluminum. While magnesium supports Phase I detox in the liver, it is used in just about every mechanism of detox in your body. Magnesium deficiencies are one of the most commonly seen in the chemically toxic. This mineral is depleted by coffee, alcohol, diuretics, and certain other drugs.

Food Sources: Beef, chicken, or fish broth; almonds and other nuts; sunflower seeds; green leafy vegetables including beet greens, kale, and collards; wheat germ and whole grains; bananas; apricots; avocados; dairy products such as milk and yogurt.

Daily Recommended Amounts: 500 to 800 mg

■ Manganese

Nutrient Properties: While abundant on earth, manganese is found only in minute amounts in the body. Still it makes critical contributions. It activates enzymes to unlock riches from the foods you eat. Manganese supports adrenal function, and is especially helpful in times of stress. It also helps maintain the integrity of your cells, nerves, skeletal structure, and connective tissues.

Detoxification Properties: As an antioxidant, manganese is an important body defender. It assists in the chelation of heavy metals, and can be helpful in offsetting an excess of iron. Manganese is an element of enzymes that detoxify sulfites, aldehydes, and aldehyde oxidase.

Food Sources: Nuts; pumpkin seeds; egg yolk; whole grain cereals; beets; leafy green vegetables such as spinach; blueberries; raisins; legumes including lima beans and lentils.

Recommended Daily Amounts: 5 to 10 mg

■ Potassium

Nutrient Properties: Your body's fluid and mineral balance are in part regulated by potassium. This micronutrient also helps to transmit nerve signals. It's needed for muscle contractions too, including the beating of your heart. Adequate intake assists in maintaining healthy blood pressure. A diet high in sodium, sugar, or refined carbohydrates causes a loss of potassium. While we should be eating about ten times as much potassium as sodium, the ratio is often reversed. Sluggishness and insomnia are early signs of a potassium deficiency.

Detoxification Properties: Potassium supports detoxification by the kidneys. It also helps the body cleanse itself of excess mercury. Deficiencies in potassium allow for greater absorption of certain radioactive elements, including cesium-137 from fallout.[8]

Food Sources: Yogurt; nuts; seeds; white potato; fruit such as banana, orange, or dried apricot; okra; winter squash; parsley; milk; turkey; haddock; baked sweet potato.

Recommended Daily Amounts: 500 mg

■ Selenium

Nutrient Properties: Needed in only trace amounts, selenium is yet a crucial nutrient. This active antioxidant joins forces with vitamin E to curb free radical damage to your cells. It is an important immune system supporter. Various studies indicate a role for selenium in fighting cancer. For example, rates of cancer have been found to be lower in areas where farmland is richer in selenium. Research also shows that groups with high blood selenium levels have less cancer. Selenium may also be protective against heart disease. This mineral is deficient in many disease conditions.

Detoxification Properties: Selenium is an essential part of glutathione peroxidase, an enzyme active in the liver. It is antagonistic to various heavy metals, including lead, mercury, aluminum, cadmium, and arsenic. This mineral binds with toxic metals so that they can be transported out of the body. Research indicates that selenium can detox peroxidized fats, lipids that can contribute to the growth of cancer tumors. It also neutralizes dangerous free radicals released during immune activity by lymphocytes.

Food Sources: Turkey, veal, organ meats such as liver and kidney, eggs, butter, Brewer's yeast, whole grain cereals, Brazil nuts, cashews, mushrooms, garlic, coconut, seafood, broccoli, and other vegetables grown in selenium-rich soil.

Recommended Daily Amounts: 200 to 400 mcg

■ Zinc

Nutrient Properties: This mineral is becoming known for its role in fighting the all-too-common "common cold." A study at Dartsmith College found zinc lozenges taken early to be helpful in curbing the seriousness and length of colds. This busy micronutrient is required for the functioning of more than three hundred enzymes. It is needed for white blood cell immune activity, the healing of wounds, proper operation of the thyroid, prostate health, and body development. Zinc helps fight aging and supports the absorption of other vitamins and minerals. Specifically it protects against age-related eye-deterioration. Deficiencies in zinc are common. There is a simple test to determine zinc status available through homeopathic pharmacies and holistic health professionals.

Detoxification Properties: Zinc increases production of metallothionein, providing protection to the kidney from arsenic, cadmium, and mercury. These heavy metals are often contributors to kidney damage. In a controlled trial published in *Lancet,* cirrhosis patients with enlarged livers showed improvement within eight days from zinc supplementation.[9]

Food Sources: Red meat, lamb chops, liver, herring, eggs, brewer's yeast, wheat germ, whole grains, oatmeal, legumes, pumpkin seeds, corn, ginger.

Recommended Daily Amounts: 15 to 50 mg

In addition to the six minerals detailed above, there are numerous minerals necessary for the detoxification process. Important ones to include are:

> Boron: 2 to 4 mg
> Chromium: 200 to 400 mcg
> Copper: 1.5 to 2 mg
> Iodine: 150 to 250 mcg
> Iron: 10 to 18 mg
> Molybdenum: 100 to 200 mcg
> Vanadium: 100 to 200 mcg

See the Resource section for suppliers of mineral products.

AMINO ACIDS

While protein is a macronutrient, it is made up of more than 20 different micronutrients—namely *amino acids*. Your own body can manufacture some of these to a degree, but others must always come in the form of food or supplements. When they are provided in food, the amino acids are released by digestive enzymes. They are then distributed throughout the body to meet certain needs. As you learned in the nutrition chapter, amino acids are used to repair parts of the body including your skin, organs, tissue, and DNA. They also help you resist disease. These micronutrients lend support to the detoxification process in various ways too. Let's look at work performed along your body's detoxification assembly line by four of the major amino acids.

Cysteine: Cysteine helps the body detoxify pesticides, plastics, hydrocarbons, and other chemical toxins. It assists in protecting the body against the adverse effects of alcohol, tobacco smoke, and air pollutants. This sulfur-containing amino acid is needed by the Phase II detox pathway. It is a component of the antioxidant glutathione, a substance that can be very helpful in heavy metal detoxification. Cysteine is used as a treatment for copper poisoning.

L-Glycine: One-third of the collagen in your body is made up of molecules of this amino acid. L-glycine is important in clearing wastes from the body. Along with cysteine and L-glutamine, it stimulates the production of the antioxidant glutathione. This amino acid is used in Phase II detoxification in the liver. It can be helpful in detoxifying benzoic acid (from coffee and other sources) and phenol (a central nervous system depressant).

L-Glutamine: This is a powerful detoxifier on a cellular level. In this work, it collaborates with vitamins A and E. L-glutamine is another building block of glutathione. It is required for Phase II detoxification. L-glutamine is helpful with chemical detoxification.

Taurine: Since this sulfur-containing amino acid was originally discovered in the bile of an ox, it was named after Taurus, the bull. Our body makes much of the taurine we use as a component of human bile from the gall bladder. Its main responsibility is in keeping the electrical system of our body in balance. For detox, taurine is used in Phase II. It aids in the chemical detoxification of chlorine, petroleum products, petrole, ammonia, and medicine residues.

To ensure that you take in enough amino acids to support detoxification, you might consider taking an amino acid detox blend. A good product may include a variety of amino acids along with the vitamins choline and inositol and the phytochemical quercetin. See the Resource section.

ANTIOXIDANTS

As you've learned in this chapter, various micronutrients (including vitamins and minerals) act as antioxidants in the body. Before we look at a particularly exciting antioxidant—Pycnogenol—which has been getting a lot of recent attention, let's review just why antioxidants are important.

In our bodies, oxygen is transported to the cells in the blood. Once the oxygen is delivered, the cells miraculously convert it into energy. Toxic by-products—free radicals—are created along with energy during this conversion process. These free radicals are highly reactive and destructive because they carry an unpaired electron. Harm is caused as the solitary electron attempts to couple with an electron from the area around it. Fortunately antioxidants can come to our defense. Sometimes they are able to destroy the free radical before damage occurs. Other times, they may supply the missing electron for the free radical as a stabilizer, or an antioxidant might combine with the free radical to create a safe substance.

So just what is this amazing antioxidant **Pycnogenol** (pronounced as "pick-nah-geh-nol.") that's creating all the buzz? This herbal product is a complex of over forty substances extracted from pine bark. Its origins have been traced back to native Indians of Canada. Among its active ingredients are flavonoids. Pycnogenol is thought to be fifty times more effective than vitamin E and twenty times more than vitamin C. This product also enhances the activity of the other antioxidants.

Pycnogenol is well absorbed because it is water-soluble. It works in the watery areas inside and around cells rather than in cell fat. Along with slowing aging, Pycnogenol is also said to fight arthritis, cancer, Alzheimer's, chronic fatigue syndrome, and heart disease. A 1996 study found it to be a strong immune enhancer. Researchers are suggesting that you take this supplement along with a broad spectrum of antioxidants from your diet to get the best results.

SPECIAL NUTRIENTS

There are so many unusual sounding supplements that are hyped today, that it all can become a little confusing. However there are some special nutrients that really are worth noting. These substances offer unique support for the body. Some should be, but are not found in our food. Here are what you might think of as the "Top 10" in the special nutrient category. For ease of use, they are listed alphabetically.

#1 Allicin: That old wives' tale that garlic is good for you is now being proven by science. Studies have found that an active ingredient in garlic—allicin—has both antibiotic and antifungal properties. Garlic is also rated high on the list of foods being investigated by the National Cancer Institute. Other large population studies have shown a correlation between garlic consumption and lower cancer rates. Two ways that allicin supports detox is that by enhancing the immune system with its antioxidant activity.

#2 Alpha Lipoic Acid (ALA): ALA is an exciting super antioxidant found in food in only minute amounts. For instance, it would take 7 pounds of spinach to produce just 1 mg of alpha lipoic acid. Therefore to reap its benefits, you must use supplements. Alpha lipoic acid has the ability to rapidly boost the body's supply of the crucial antioxidant glutathione. It can raise levels by as much as 30 to 70%. This trait makes it important for the prevention and treatment of many common diseases. ALA is an effective detoxifier of mercury, arsenic, and other heavy metals. It also protects the nerves from pesticide damage.

#3 Calcium D-Glucarate: This is the calcium salt of D-glucarate, a natural substance found in some fruits and vegetables. Some of the anti-cancer and detox properties of fruits and vegetable are said to come from D-glucarate. Calcium D-glucarate stimulates the liver's work in isolating carcinogens and eliminating them from the body. It is used in Phase II detoxification. Because calcium D-glucarate can be helpful in forcing fake estrogens (from pesticides, plastics, etc.) and other carcinogens out of the body, it looks promising in the prevention of breast cancer.[10]

#4 CoEnzyme Q10 (CoQ10): There is special interest in CoQ10 for its heart-protective properties. It is thought to lessen harm to heart tissue caused by free radicals. Studies have found that deficiencies of CoQ10 in the heart muscle are common among people with congestive heart failure. A ubiquitous substance, CoQ10 is found naturally in all body tissue. It is helpful as an antioxidant in protecting cell membranes. CoQ10 enhances the antioxidant efforts of vitamin E. This is another compound existing at such low levels in foods that supplementation is required to reap a benefit. One study found CoQ10 to be protective against occupational exposure to toxins in paint.

#5 Diindolyl-Methane (DIM): This substance is naturally created in the gastrointestinal tract by enzymes after consumption of cruciferous vegetables such as Brussels sprouts, cauliflower, or cabbage. It supports the Phase I removal of unwanted estrogens and promotes healthy estrogen metabolism. Supplementation is recommended to get this effect. Studies show that DIM intake may contribute to a decreased risk of breast and cervical cancer.[11]

#6 Glutathione: As you learned earlier, this key antioxidant contains cysteine, L-glycine, and L-glutamine—three amino acids that are important for detoxification. Glutathione itself has been identified as playing a crucial role in detoxifying harmful drug residues and environmental pollutants. It supports a strong immune system. Low levels of glutathione are a marker for disease and death. People with AIDS have low amounts in their systems. Environmental toxins (cigarette smoke, nitrates, etc.) and excessive alcohol intake are among the factors that deplete glutathione levels. This is one of the most important antioxidants for detox at a cellular level.

#7 N-Acety-L-Cysteine (NAC): This is an amino acid precursor to cysteine that increases antioxidant glutathione levels. It is a detoxification promoter, specifically helpful in eliminating internal toxins of the intestinal tract as well as foreign chemicals. In studies, NAC is being tied to extended life. Swiss researchers giving high doses of NAC to fruit flies found the insects lived 16% longer.

#8 Methyl Sulfonyl Methane (MSM): This is a natural form of organic sulfur found in humans and other animals. Though it is contained in vegetables, fruits, milk, fish, and grains, MSM is often depleted in food processing. This compound nourishes the immune system's defense mechanisms and helps form enzymes and hormones. Athletes use it to soothe sore muscles, tendons, and connective tissues. It can also offset other symptoms of stress. In detoxification, MSM supports the Phase II biotransformation pathways of the liver as they are often sulfur-deficient.

#9 Oligomeric Proanthocyanidins (OPCs): During Phase I detoxification particularly, foreign chemicals can cause free radical damage to the body. OPCs are powerful antioxidants that aid in clearing free radicals that are released during the detox process. OPCs join the antioxidant effort in the blood vessels, which serve as the route for the transportation of toxic chemicals from fat tissue to the liver and kidneys. Thus OPCs can prevent inflammation of these vessels.

#10 S-Adenosyl-L-Methionine (SAMe): Because of its long name, you'll usually just hear this compound referred to as SAMe (pronounced "Sammy"). This is a substance made by the body from the amino acid methionine. It's been getting recent attention for possible anti-aging effects. SAMe participates in perhaps hundreds of metabolic functions in the body. For instance, it helps to remove toxins and maintain healthy cell membranes. SAMe has been used for the treatment of depression, joint stiffness, fibromyalgia, and arthritis. It supports liver health and has been shown in studies to reverse the effects of liver damage.

PHYTONUTRIENTS – NATURE'S PHARMACY

"The medicine of the future will be found in foods."
—Oliver Wendell Holmes

Since the 1970s, science has been confirming what grandma told you all along—eating fruits and vegetables is good for you! Consistently research has shown that eating produce lowers the risk of most cancers. Now we're learning *why*. It seems that plant foods contain a variety of chemicals, dubbed phytonutrients, which improve overall health as well as prevent disease. In the plants themselves, these substances add color, work as chemical messengers, defend against threatening insects and plant diseases, block harmful ultraviolet rays, and attract critters for pollination. In the human body, they're active as well—blocking and carting away carcinogens, detoxifying environmental pollutants, boosting the immune system, and retarding various aging processes, among other duties. Twelve-thousand phytonutrients have been identified and many more are expected to be isolated.

In studying how phytonutrients work, scientists have found that many are antioxidants—destroyers of destructive and reactive molecules in our bodies. Others have different powers in fighting disease. These and other findings are exciting health and nutrition researchers, and the discoveries will have a major impact on the way we view food in the future. As part of their efforts, scientists have grouped phytonutrients into tongue-twisting categories based on their structure and content. Let's explore some of the main classifications.

▪ Carotenoids

Where Located: Carrot, yams, sweet potato, yellow squash, tomato, spinach, broccoli, parsley, apricot, mango, papaya, cantaloupe, peaches, mushrooms.

Benefits: With over 600 members, this group includes the well-known free radical scavenger, *Beta-carotene*—the most abundant carotenoid. Many others are also antioxidants. These compounds are anti-cancer agents and immune system boosters. The often brightly colored carotenoids can also reduce plaque in the arteries. Yellow-orange carotenoids have been linked with the prevention of breast, colorectal, lung, prostate, and uterine cancer.

Research Findings: A 19-year-long study in Western Europe showed a reduced incidence of lung cancer when a diet rich in carotenoids was consumed. Also, scientists observing people in northern Italy discovered that consumption of seven or more servings of raw tomatoes a week lead to a 60% less chance of developing colon, rectal, or stomach cancer compared to a diet with two or fewer servings. Tomatoes also contain *lycopene* (see description below). In yet another study, women who ate a carrot a day reduced their risk of stroke by 68%.

▪ Catechins

Where Located: Berries, black or green tea.

Benefits: This is another set of antioxidants. Green tea, specifically, is said to have one of the highest antioxidant values known. The catechins in super-powerful green tea support healthy digestion, neutralize harmful fats and oils, halt mechanisms that trigger cancer, attack bacteria and viruses, and lower the risk of stroke and ulcers.

Catechins are thought to be protective against stomach, kidney, and bladder cancer.

Research Findings: Several studies have shown that catechins can fight against viral infections. Research at Rutgers University found that green tea blocked stomach, skin, and lung cancers in mice. Additional studies have found oolong and black tea to also prevent cancers in animals.

▪ Flavonoids

Where Located: Citrus fruits, berries, apples, tea, carrot, peppers, cabbage, tomato, squash, eggplant, broccoli, yam, cucumber, onions, parsley, soybeans, soy products.

Benefits: Flavonoids prevent cancer-causing hormones from attaching to body cells by blocking the receptor sites. Thus they may offset the negative effects of excessive estrogen. These phytonutrients are also protective for the eyes and nerves. Symptoms of allergy, arthritis, and asthma have been seen to improve with consumption of flavonoids.

Research Findings: In lab experiments, bilberry extract has been shown to quench various free radicals. This action prevented cell damage. Based on such antioxidant activity, bilberry is thought to be helpful in improving eye health, vascular function, and wound healing, as well as in reducing inflammation. As reported in the *Lancet,* a Dutch study found a flavonoid-rich diet to reduce the risk for men of dying from coronary heart disease.

▪ Indoles

Where Located: Cabbage, cauliflower, broccoli, Brussels sprouts, kale, collard greens, kohlrabi, mustard greens.

Benefits: These compounds attach themselves to chemical carcinogens and stimulate the production of detox enzymes. They assist in neutralizing the fake estrogen found in many environmental chemical toxins. Indoles have a cell-protective capability against cancer. These phytonutrients are involved in Phase II detoxification.

Research Findings: Compounds in such cruciferous vegetables as broccoli, cabbage, and cauliflower have been found to increase the body's detoxification functions. Also, in the lab, a substance called indole-3-carbinol has been shown to break down harmful estrogens, the ones associated with reproductive cancers, into a benign form.[12]

▪ Isoflavone

Where Located: Legumes including lentils, kidney beans, and peas; soy products such as non-genetically-engineered tofu, miso, soy flour, tempeh, and soybeans.

Benefits: A reduced risk of breast cancer and other cancers is associated with consumption of the isoflavones found in soy foods. Soy isoflavones are converted into phytoestrogens in the body; these substances are thought to slow bone degeneration, alleviate hot flashes, and possibly reduce other symptoms of the menopausal years. Other legumes are also believed to generate the production of phytoestrogens when consumed.

Research Findings: In a study of five varieties of breast cancer cells, the isoflavone found in soy—genistein—was found to inhibit the growth of every type. Isoflavones have been found to be protective of the heart, thus the FDA now permits a soy protein claim for cardiovascular health benefits.

▪ Isothiocyanates

Where Located: Watercress, kale, mustard greens, Brussels sprouts, cabbage, turnip, horseradish, radishes, rutabaga, wasabi.

Benefits: Isothiocyanates are powerful stimulators of protective enzymes. Among these enzymes is a variety that guards against cell damage from potential carcinogens. DNA is defended by isothiocyanates.

Research Findings: Studies at Ohio State University show that this group has a role in inhibiting cancers of the esophagus and lung, among others.[13] Another study suggests watercress specifically can help in lung-cancer prevention. At the John Hopkins University School of Medicine, researchers have found that isothiocyanates curb Phase I cancer-promoting enzymes and stimulate Phase II cancer-battling enzymes.

▪ Lignans

Where Located: Berries, seeds (particularly flaxseed), whole grains, walnuts.

Benefits: Lignans are antioxidants and fibers that suppress cancer development, especially of the colon. They are also protective against heart disease. This group has anti-inflammatory properties. Lignans are believed to lower the risk of breast, uterine and cervical cancer by interfering with estrogen production.

Research Findings: Lignans reduced the growth of precancerous and cancerous cells in the breasts and colons of laboratory rats.

▪ Limonene

Where Located: Citrus fruit.

Benefits: These phytonutrients look promising for reducing cancers of the mouth, breast, and liver. They stimulate protective enzymes and appear to be part of the body's arsenal against harmful substances. Limonenes are involved in both Phase I and II detoxification.

Research Findings: In a six-month European study, patients with chronic bronchitis were given a supplement that contained the antioxidant limonene and two other substances. The frequency and intensity of their bronchitis flare-ups were reduced as well as their bouts of coughing.[14]

▪ Lutein

Where Located: Spinach, kale, mustard greens, orange pepper, broccoli, collard greens, zucchini, squash, kiwi, oranges, grapes, maize.

Benefits: This group appears to reduce the risk of macular degeneration and other diseases of the retina. Macular degeneration is a major cause of blindness in old age. These powerful antioxidant micronutrients also provide general protection against cell damage.

Research Findings: In the Beaver Dam Eye Study in Wisconsin, lutein surfaced as a major player in preventing macular degeneration related to aging.

▪ Luteolin

Where Located: Artichoke

Benefits: Artichokes are actually the buds of a Mediterranean thistle. These decorative vegetables have been shown to enhance detoxification and to protect the liver. They also promote healthy blood cholesterol levels and good digestion. This vegetable also offers protection from free radical damage.

Research Findings: Studies show that artichokes prevent oxidative stress and strongly inhibit tumor growth.

▪ Lycopene

Where Located: Tomato, red peppers, red grapefruit.

Benefit: An important subgroup of carotenoids, you might think of the bright-red pigment lycopenes as cousins of beta carotene. The antioxidant properties of these foods make them strong cell protectors. Lycopenes are associated with a lower risk of prostate cancer, the most common cancer affecting American men. They have also been linked with preventing the growth of breast, lung, gastrointestinal, cervical, bladder, and endometrial cancer cells.

Research Findings: A study at Harvard University found that a diet rich in tomatoes and tomato-based foods can result in a 21 to 43% reduced risk of prostate cancer. Research at the National Cancer Institute has confirmed that lycopenes can help reduce the risk of many cancers. Also, people in the Beaver Dam Eye Study with the lowest blood levels of lycopene were twice as susceptible to age-related macular degeneration. A university study in the Netherlands found lycopene to also lower the risk of clogged heart arteries.

▪ Monoterpenes

Where Located: Parsley, greens, broccoli, pepper, cabbage, eggplant, squash, carrot, yam, tomato, cucumber, parsnip, citrus fruit.

Benefits: These antioxidant phytonutrients are associated with the prevention of breast, liver, lung, and other cancers. Since monoterpenes can lower blood cholesterol, they are also linked to a lower risk of heart disease. Monoterpenes support protective enzyme activity. Parsley, in particular, can assist in detoxifying carcinogens, including neutralizing certain substances in cigarette smoke.

Research Findings: Research has shown monoterpenes to be helpful in the prevention of breast, liver, lung, and other cancers.[15]

▪ Organosulfur

Where Located: The onion family—garlic, onions, leeks, shallots; cruciferous vegetables—cabbage, broccoli, Brussels sprouts, bok choy, kale, and turnips.

Benefits: Garlic and onions have long been used for their healing properties. Rich sources of sulfur compounds, they offer natural antibiotic and antifungal properties.

Cooking can boost the protective powers of foods in the onion family.

Research Findings: In a Chinese study published in the *Journal of the National Cancer Institute,* consumption of vegetables in the onion family was found to protect against stomach cancer.

▪ Polyphenol

Where Located: Blueberries, raspberries, cranberries, red current, citrus fruits, apples, grapes, green tea, black tea, eggplant, purple bell peppers, red wine.

Benefits: In Greek, "poly" is the root for many. This group of "many" phenols are powerful antioxidants. They have been shown to prevent clots in the blood—a major cause of heart attack and stroke. Polyphenols also mitigate the effects of nitric oxide, a major type of free radical that can be harmful in excess amounts. These compounds can prevent LDL cholesterol from oxidizing (a factor in atherosclerosis and heart attack). They are associated with the prevention of heart disease and cancer.

Research Findings: At the University of California at Davis, tumor growth was reduced in animals given phenolic compounds found in wine.

▪ Quercetin

Where Located: Apple, citrus fruit, grape, onion, garlic, tea, legumes.

Benefits: A subgroup of the flavonoid family, these are among some of the most powerful members. In cancer, they suppress malignant changes and are thought to possibly alter hormone binding to curb the disease's development. Quercetin provides powerful protection against allergic reactions.

Research Findings: Studies have pinpointed quercetin as a weapon against macular degeneration and cataracts.

▪ Sulforaphane

Where Located: Cabbage, broccoli, cauliflower, Brussels sprouts, kale, green onions, horseradish, mustard.

Benefits: These compounds delay the onset of cancer, inhibiting the size and number of tumors. They enhance the effect of enzymes that impede carcinogens attempting to damage healthy cells. Sulforaphanes enhance Phase II detoxification.

Research Findings: Scientists at Johns Hopkins University investigating sulforaphanes believe they will become a leading substance used to fight cancer. The National Cancer Institute has found broccoli and cabbage to reduce the risk of bladder cancer in men.

▪ Sterols

Where Located: Pepper, eggplant, cucumber, soy, whole grains including cereals.

Benefits: These compounds are good for your heart, as they have been found to lower cholesterol. In cucumbers, they're primarily in the skin, so buy organic to avoid wax and pesticides.

Research Findings: Research suggests that plant sterols reduce cholesterol synthesis in the body.[16]

▪ Triterpenese

Where Located: Artichoke, licorice root, citrus fruits.

Benefits: Triterpeneses act as both cancer preventors and fighters. They appear to deactivate steroidal hormones that trigger tumor growth and to slow the division of unhealthy cells.

Research Findings: The National Cancer Institute and other researchers are very interested in licorice root in cancer prevention and treatment. Used in the Orient to heal ulcers and as a tonic for the heart and spleen, licorice is just starting to be looked into for its medicinal value in the U.S. American licorice candy is not usually made with licorice root, but rather with anise.

DAILY PHYTONUTRIENTS FOR HEALTH

A lot of the names of the phytonutrients themselves may seem confusing, but their sources are common plant foods, many of which you have eaten. With research mounting regularly proclaiming the wonderful health benefits of these gifts of Nature, it would be foolish not to indulge.

The best way to include more phytonutrients in your diet is to eat the vegetables in their freshest form. When that is not possible due to travel or time constraints, you do not have to skimp on your nutrition. The phytonutrients can often be found in a dehydrated, powdered form. Also, for those of you who are gradually incorporating more

A HEALING GARDEN OF CULINARY HERBS

While the cook (and his or her guests) may value culinary herbs for their flavor-enhancing abilities, did you know that these plants also have many medicinal properties? Although these remedies may have been common knowledge for our great-grandmothers, interest died down for a time. Now a resurgence of curiosity is taking place about using culinary herbs for their health benefits. In part, it's because people like to rely on Nature. Also, there's a movement toward taking actions every day to support your good health. If you think you might like to start your own healing garden, here are some of the culinary herbs to be sure to include:

Thyme: This herb comes from the *thymus* family, a species named after the Greek word for courage—"thymon." It was once used to give soldiers vigor and as a remedy for shyness. A powerful antiseptic, Thyme has traditionally been turned to fight a variety of bacterial, viral, and fungal infections. The herb inhibits helicobacter pylori, a bacteria believed to be associated with ulcers and stomach cancer.[17] It can be consumed as a tea for this purpose. Thyme tea also helps soothe congestion, sore throats, and coughs. Thyme is a detoxifying herb that helps cleanse and nourish the bloodstream.

Oregano: Growing wild and scenting the hillsides of Greece, this plant was dubbed "oros ganos"—joy of the mountains. Earlier, it had been utilized by the ancient Egyptians as a disinfectant. Today we know that Oregano has anti-cancer, antimicrobial, antiseptic and antioxidant properties. This spice can cleanse food of pathogens. It can be infused in a tea for coughs, stomach problems, headaches, irritability, and menstrual pain. Apply as an external poultice for muscle or joint soreness. Oregano contains flavonoids and provides valuable antioxidants.

Rosemary: The nickname for this herb is "dew of the sea." Once a symbol for fidelity, it was worn by brides as a wreath accented with many colored ribbons. Rosemary is known for its memory-enhancing abilities, and it's been helpful in the prevention of

Alzheimer's disease. It has exhibited anti-cancer properties in numerous studies. This herb can increase circulation and soothe pain where applied. It supports fat digestion. Try it as an anti-septic mouthwash or gargle. Rosemary stimulates Phase II detoxification, and its antioxidants reduce DNA damage from toxic chemicals.[18]

Sage: This healing plant is counted among the members of the *salvia officinalis* family. The name of this species comes from the Latin term "salvia"—meaning "to cure," "to save." Working best as a sole spice on foods, Sage aids fat digestion. As a digestive aid, it can also be consumed as a tea. Sage has antiseptic and antimicrobial properties, and can combat such bacteria as staphylococcus aureus.[19] A hot sage tea eases sore throat. Drink sage tea in small amounts, as overindulging can bring adverse effects.

Basil: India is the original home for this popular culinary herb. In that country where it is revered, Basil has been used to swear upon in court. Indians also rub the leaves on their skin as an insect repellent. There are many varieties of this tasty herb. In aromatherapy, Basil essential oil is used to relieve mental fatigue. The antioxidant phytonutrient monoterpene is found in Basil. It also contains many antiviral compounds.

Mint: In Rome, where Mint was considered a symbol of hospitality, it was once scattered in halls where feasts where to be held. There are over 600 varieties of this plant, including the well-known Peppermint and Spearmint. A Mint can be used alone or with other flavors in hot and cold teas. For instance, Peppermint tea is helpful in relieving indigestion and intestinal distress. Drops of essential Spearmint oil may be inhaled to soothe colds. Oils brewed with Mint leaves can later be massaged into areas to ease pain. Like Basil, Mint also contains the antioxidant phytonutrient monoterpene along with antiviral substances.

Since most culinary herbs take up relatively little space, you can grow a nice variety even if you've only got a small area to work with. Some other healing culinary herbs to consider are cumin, parsley, ginger, marjoram, chives, tarragon, bay leaf, saffron, cilantro, and tumeric.

vegetables into your diet, such a product may be helpful in the transition. This can be added to water, juice, or the protein smoothie described in the previous chapter. See Resource section for suggestions on phytonutrient powders.

SUPERFOODS FOR ENERGY

"I submit that scientists have not yet explored the hidden possibilities of the innumerable seeds, leaves, and fruits for giving the fullest possible nutrition to mankind."
— Mahatma Gandhi, *Nonviolent political activist of India*

There are certain foods that are very dense in vitamins, minerals, and phytonutrients, and they have been found to have unique properties that enhance the body's energy production and immune response. These foods have often been called "superfoods." They range from vegetables gathered from the sea, to bee pollen taken from a flowering field, to aloe vera harvested from the desert, among others.

Since diet is one area affecting our health over which we can exert control, it makes sense to include superfoods in our routine. Research has again and again shown that diet can improve the day-to-day state of our health as well as prevent many chronic conditions. The superfoods pack a lot of power to satisfy our body's needs.

Sea Vegetables (Seaweed): The only obvious exposure many Americans have to sea vegetables is in Asian foods. For instance, sushi is wrapped in a black-red algae called nori. However, as there are thousands of varieties, sea vegetables have also been put to other uses such as in emulsifiers for ice cream. It makes sense that basic sea vegetables are more of a staple in societies that are near the ocean.

Sea vegetables are a rich source of such minerals as potassium, calcium, magnesium, iron, and iodine. These minerals support healthy thyroid function. Also dense in phytonutrients, seaweeds have antioxidant, antiviral, and tumor-suppressing properties. It is thought that the high consumption of sea vegetables may contribute to the lower rate of breast cancer among Japanese women. Lab experiments have verified the ability of these plants to support a strong immune system and to fight colon cancer. They also help the body remove heavy metals, radioactive elements, and chemical pollutants.

You'll find sea vegetables in Asian markets and health food stores. Look for dulse, nori, kelp, kombu, hijiki, wakame, sea palm, arame, and agar-agar. The seaweeds come in various forms—sheets, flakes, powders, and granules. For information on cooking with sea vegetables, check out the book *Seaweed: A Cook's Guide* by Lesley Ellis.

Chlorophyll: The emerald pigment found in all plants, Chlorophyll converts light into energy through photosynthesis. This is the process by which the plant uses carbon dioxide, water, and light to make food. Chlorophyll can be considered the blood of plants—in fact, one molecule of Chlorophyll is virtually identical to a hemoglobin molecule from human blood. This resemblance enables this superfood to rejuvenate red blood cells and to raise the oxygen supply to tissue.

Rich sources of Chlorophyll include such cereal grasses such as barley, wheat, rye, kamut, and alfalfa. (Cereal grasses are the young green plants used to grow cereal grain.) In addition to supplying the powerful effects of Chlorophyll, cereal grasses are extremely high in nutrients including vitamins A, B_{12}, C, E, and K; the minerals potassium, selenium, zinc, calcium, and phosphorus; and over twenty amino acids. They are also great sources of enzymes and antioxidants. In cereal grasses, nutrients come in higher amounts than in their grain counterparts. Fiber and protein are two other important components of cereal grasses.

Chlorophyll has been found helpful in wound healing and detoxification. By boosting the oxygenation of the body, Chlorophyll-rich foods lessen the effects of pollutants. Consumption of cereal grasses has also been shown to heal scars inside the lungs from smog. Chlorophyll helps remove drug residues from the body, and it counters damage from BHT—a chemical preservative used in food. Research has found Chlorophyll effective in the treatment of both constipation and kidney stones.

Cereal grasses have anti-cancer, antibacterial, anti-ulcer and anti-inflammatory properties.

Using dehydrated organic cereal grasses as a daily nutritional supplement can be a convenient way to add more green foods to your diet. Unlike synthetic supplements, these are simply the dehydrated form of the original plants. Wheatgrass juice sold in health-food stores and at juice bars is another source.

All green plants contain Chlorophyll. Other sources include spirulina and chlorella from the sea, as well as common vegetables such as spinach, broccoli, and salad greens.

Sprouts: These small, tender shoots are produced when seeds from bean and grain plants are germinated. Various types of sprouts are now appearing in regular grocery stores as well as health food markets. There are sprouts made from radish seed, flax seed, alfalfa, soybeans, sunflower seed, mung beans, clover seed, chickpeas, and more. Sometimes a variety is offered in a mix.

These foods are good sources of protein, particularly for those on raw diets. They are also very high in enzymes and fiber. The vitamin content, especially of the B family, is greatly enhanced over that in the original seed. The supply of phytonutrients, such as carotene, is also concentrated in sprouts. Studies have found that they provide phytoestrogens (specifically alfalfa, soybean, clover sprouts) and antioxidants.

The consumption of sprouts has been traced back 5,000 years to ancient China, where they were used to treat various disorders. Two easy ways to add them to your diet today are as a garnish on a sandwich or an added ingredient in salads. Wash sprouts gently and refrigerate to store.

Bee Pollen: These microspores from flowers are the main food source for bees. This superfood was used extensively by Hippocrates, the great physician of ancient Greece, in treating his patients. It's no wonder that Bee Pollen is considered Nature's "perfect food;" it contains all the known vitamins, twenty-seven minerals, twenty-two amino acids, nineteen enzymes, and several hormone-like substances. Bee Pollen also delivers rutin, a bioflavonoid that supports cardiovascular health.

A natural antibiotic, Bee Pollen is effective against *E. coli*, *Salmonella*, and other pathogenic bacteria. It boosts immunity and can help fight cancer. In a Welsh study, pollen extract was effective in treating prostate cancer specifically. Because Bee Pollen raises oxygen in the blood, it increases energy and endurance. In a study of impotent men, 50% of participants taking this superfood experienced improvements in sexual performance. Since some individual have pollen allergies, it is generally recommended that you start with a small amount and increase your intake gradually. Bee Pollen is taken in capsules or tablets.

Royal Jelly: This thick, creamy fluid is the queen bee's sole food. Royal Jelly allows her to grow to maturity faster, be quite fertile, and live longer. Among the benefits for humans in consuming Royal Jelly is maintenance of healthy skin; it contains skin-protective fatty acids as well as collagen, lecithin, and vitamins A, C, D, and E. In studies, Royal Jelly has been found to lower cholesterol levels and slow the development of clogged arteries. Delivering the B-complex vitamins including a good supply of pantothenic acid, Royal Jelly has been used successfully in the treatment of stress, depression, and insomnia.

The immune system is bolstered by Royal Jelly in part because this superfood increases gamma globulin levels. Gamma globulin is a protein part of blood rich in antibodies. Royal Jelly also has antibacterial properties. In studies of mice, Royal Jelly was most effective in preventing tumor growth when given before any masses developed. To be effective, Royal Jelly must be freeze-dried within 24 hours after collection.

Aloe Vera: For years, people have been turning to a common household plant, Aloe Vera, to treat surface skin problems such as burns, sores, cuts, rashes, and abscesses. Now we are learning this succulent can also be helpful for internal disturbances along the gastrointestinal tract. Patient reports along with scientific research speak of Aloe's assistance in healing the lining of the stomach and intestine. It has been helpful in cases of ulcers, colitis, and Crohn's disease. Aloe promotes the growth of good bacteria in the digestive tract and inhibits the harmful types. As it assists in normalizing digestive functioning, Aloe Vera enhances immune function.

Aloe Vera has general antibacterial, antifungal and antiviral effects. It assists the body's detoxification processes by dilating the blood vessels and increasing blood and oxygen supply to the tissues. This substance also makes cells more permeable, allowing toxins to exit more easily. Aloe is believed to be a great immune supporter.

Historians have tracked the origins of Aloe Vera to the warm, dry climate of Africa. Explorers spread its use to other parts of the earth. Today it is utilized worldwide. Over $50 million worth of Aloe is imported each year into Japan alone for the treatment of ulcers and other digestive tract disorders. Aloe can be taken in juice form. Look for organic whole leaf aloe juice.

Flaxseed: One reason that Flaxseed is health-promoting is because it increases bulk and bowel transit time, transporting toxins through the body more quickly. It is also an effective remedy for constipation. To soothe digestive difficulties, mix one tablespoon of Flaxseed with 8 ounces of warm water. Drink after fifteen minutes when the mixture is gelatinous.

Flaxseeds contain lignans—phytonutrients with significant antioxidant effects. The seeds have increased estrogen activity in animals, showing promise in helping menopausal women who are deficient in this hormone. Flaxseed oil is an excellent source of Omega-6 fatty acids, and it contains more Omega-3s than other vegetable oils. Consumption of the oil has helped relieve eczema and also resulted in general improvements in the skin. In animal studies, Flaxseed oil has demonstrated an anti-tumor effect related to breast and colon cancer.

You can increase your consumption of Flaxseed oil by adding a tablespoon over your salads, vegetables, or cereal. The same amount of ground seed can be sprinkled on cereal, stews, or soups. Flaxseed oil can also be used in baking.

Taoist Mushrooms: Dubbed the "five Taoist mushrooms of immortality," the reishi, shiitake, maitake, cordyceps, and tremella varieties are said to have been selected for their ability to support the life force and enhance immunity. They are all being researched by the National Institutes of Health in the U.S. and Japan for their anti-cancer and immune-supportive properties. Taoist mushrooms have been used to treat chronic wasting diseases such as AIDS, cancer, hepatitis, and tuberculosis.

These superfoods contain phytonutrients that are forms of glucose—an important energy source. One of the phytonutrients—beta-glucans—has been shown in experiments to slow tumor growth. It is believed that the mushroom compound accomplishes this by both killing cancer cells and boosting immunity.

THE JOY OF JUICING

If juice brings to mind the large carton of sweet liquid you bought at the grocery store, think again! Fresh organic raw vegetable juices are a much better choice, providing an elixir of concentrated, vibrant nutrients. (Fruit juices tend to play havoc with your blood sugar.) Homemade vegetable juices provide the building blocks for optimal wellness, including many phytochemicals; vitamins A, C, and E; live enzymes; and potent antioxidants. They also are helping to support the recovery of people with cancer, liver disorders, ulcers, heart disease, and other ailments.

There are many tasty combinations to try. For instance:

- Carrot, beet, celery, and greens such as spinach, dandelion greens, parsley
- Cabbage, cucumber, parsley, asparagus, celery, and lemon
- Carrot and string beans
- Tomato, cucumber, cilantro, lime, and purple onion
- Beets, celery, dandelion greens, and watercress
- Carrot, spinach, cauliflower, and garlic

For specific recipes and other ideas, try *The Juicing Book* by Stephen Blauer, *Juicing for Life* by Cherie Calbom and Maureen Keene, and *Healing with Herbal Juices* by Siegfried Gursche. Or experiment with your own combinations!

To create these drinks at home, you'll need a strong juicer; look for one with at least a .4 horsepower motor. These machines will last longer and have more stamina during the juice creation process. A nice feature is the ejection of the vegetable pulp rather than the use of an inside basket. Pick an easy-to-clean machine with a large receptacle for the juice. An excellent website for information and purchasing of juicers is *www.living-foods.com/marketplace*. Also check out *www.vitamix.com/household* for a multi-purpose juicer and food processor.

Taoist mushrooms can be added to soups, stews, or pastas, as well as taken in supplement form.

Whey: This is the liquid part of milk that is separated out from the solids when cheese is made. It is rich in minerals. Whey derived from goat's milk is one of the best choices. One tablespoon of Whey taken in a small amount of water will promote good digestion by fostering the growth of healthy bacteria in the intestinal tract. This superfood is loaded with minerals in whole food form. Whey also keeps your joints, muscles, and ligaments flexible for movement. For stomach upsets, take one tablespoon of Whey three times a day.

SUPPLEMENTS—REINFORCING OUR OPTIMAL HEALTH

Of course, there's no magic bullet that can replace the cultivation of overall healthy lifelong habits to support our well-being. However I want to emphasize once more that it's important to make sure that your basic requirements are covered. The theme of this book has consistently been to give our body what it needs. Because there are vitamins and minerals that are essential, you'll want to take a daily multiple supplying both. Due to the modern refined diet, deficient soil, and our heavy toxic load, we are just not getting all the nutrients we need from our food today.

Taking the right multiple can support the optimal functioning of your body—not just allow you to get by. In addition, consider other micronutrients that will help you achieve higher levels of health. For optimal health, it is recommended to: (1) Increase your intake of phytonutrients and antioxidants by adding foods to your daily fare that provide a rich supply, (2) Incorporate the superfoods including a daily chlorophyll supplement, and (3) Learn to make nourishing, fresh vegetable juices for a rich source of vitamins, minerals, antioxidants, phytochemicals, live enzymes, etc.

Throughout the past century, there has been a revolutionary amount of new information available about the micronutrients that are now available to us. Why not put this cutting-edge knowledge to use in your life starting now? You'll be pleased with the results. Not only can you lower your risk for many of the major diseases, you are also likely to live out your days in a higher state of vibrant health!

WHAT'S AHEAD

Up to this point, *The Detox Solution* has provided information on what you can do on a regular basis to enhance your body's natural daily detox processes. The next chapter will explore how you can use herbs on a periodic basic to encourage the cleansing of the toxic residues that have built up over time.

E L E V E N

Wisdom of the Ages:
Herbal Cleansing & Rejuvenation

Balm brings you sympathy and Marjoram joy
Sage is long life . . . Sweet Woodruff augurs well
for health—A blessing richer far than wealth.
While Lavender means deep devotion,
Herb of sweet omen, Rosemary conveys
Affection and remembrance all your days.
May Heaven and Earth and Man combine
To keep those blessings ever thine.

— **Rachel Page Elliott**

This chapter will explore the use of herbs for cleansing the body internally, which is what comes to mind when most people think of detoxification. If you happened to skip ahead to this chapter to see what pills to pop, please make sure you have reviewed the previous sections before using the herbs. Ideas were provided earlier for lightening the body's load by removing toxins from your environment, diet, etc. Suggestions were also given to improve the functioning of your major detoxification systems with practical steps and smart eating habits. So if you haven't yet worked with the book, please go back and apply the ideas presented. If you have been implementing the plan, you're probably ready to "remove the residue" from years of toxic buildup. This cleanup will be accomplished through a series of herbal cleansing formulas.

Scan the following checklist to make sure you didn't overlook any of the major steps previously presented in *The Detox Solution:*

CLEANSING PREP CHECKLIST

Have you removed the obvious toxins from your environment and diet to the best of your ability? You want to be sure that you are minimizing toxins that may be entering your system before you cleanse to remove previous buildup.

Are you drinking plenty of water? Do not even think about starting the cleansing formulas unless you have been drinking at least half of your body weight in ounces for at least two weeks. For example, a man at 180 pounds would need to consume 90 ounces, or about eleven 8-ounce glasses. A woman who weighs 130 pounds would want to drink 65 ounces, or about eight 8-ounce glasses. This optimal water intake should continue throughout the cleanse and for the rest of your life.

Are you eating a diet rich in whole organic foods with adequate fiber? It is important to be eating a substantial amount of vegetables, preferably at least one salad daily.

Are you consuming essential fatty acids daily? Ingesting at least one tablespoon of organic flaxseed oil each day is a good idea.

Are you including plant-based digestive enzymes with any meal that has been cooked/processed? Since heating food over 118 degrees destroys all of the enzymes, supplementation is essential to enhance digestion and to prevent a toxic buildup. It would be foolish to start an herbal cleanse without using enzymes regularly—you could be adding toxins (via undigested food) at the same time you are attempting to remove them—not very efficient.

Are you taking probiotics (beneficial bacteria) daily? A supplement with the strains mentioned in Chapter 6 (*Lactobacillus acidolphilus, Bifidobacteria bifidum, Lactobacillus bulgaricus, Lactobacillus sporogenes, Lactobacillus salivarius, Lactobacillus plantarum*) is suggested to maintain optimal beneficial bacteria.

The above reminders are important as they emphasize what is key to enhancing the body's detoxification processes naturally—essentially adopting wise healthy habits. As emphasized throughout *The Detox Solution*, the "quick fix" approaches that are often glamorized, such as a "three-day fast" or a two-week diet of brown rice, are not efficient—or safe—detoxification methods.

Herbs are powerful aids to detoxification, and it is important to know that they can facilitate deeper cleansing. However, for optimal health, it is imperative to cultivate beneficial, nontoxic health habits. Think of the herbal aspect of detox described in this chapter as a way to "cleanse deeper," to remove toxic residue that has built up over many, many years. Herbal cleansing can be used periodically (I recommend at least twice a year, spring and fall) but not every day. Healthy, nontoxic habits, however, *are* for every day.

Herbal cleansing is like that periodic oil change that's performed for your car. Healthy daily habits are similar to selecting the right gasoline. The results from using bad gas can't be fixed by overdoing oil changes. Similarly, if your daily habits aren't supportive of the body's natural detox processes, your success with herbal cleansing is going to be limited.

Most individuals will benefit from the herbs suggested throughout the chapter. Those with chronic health conditions should seek the advice of a health care professional who is familiar with the use of herbs for detoxification. In all cases, proceed slowly. The herbs explored in this chapter have a long history of safety and effectiveness; however, each person has different needs and sensitivities.

WHY HERBS FOR CLEANSING?

The use of herbs for medicine is nothing new. Virtually every traditional health care system except Western medicine emphasizes cleansing, and herbs are a main component of various detoxification regimes around the globe. According to the World Health Organization, 80% of the world's population use herbs as their primary medicine, and a significant proportion of the use is for cleansing. In fact, every culture around the globe has a history of using plants for cleansing and healing.

In Western medicine, about 25% of today's prescription drugs are derived from plants, utilizing either a natural substance or a synthetic imitation—although cleansing and detoxification are not usually the emphasis.

Herbs in their pure state are rarely used by today's Western physicians. Training in herbal medicine is not usually part of the curriculum at medical schools in the States, although some universities have recently added a survey course to familiarize physicians with the herbs that

TO FAST OR NOT TO FAST?

Often when I mention to a patient that a detoxification program may help them, the first thought they have is that I want to put them on a fast. A fast is something I rarely endorse. Fasting seems to feed into the "all or nothing" mentality. What we want to develop is a toxin-free healthy lifestyle. I have found that a whole foods diet, coupled with cleansing herbs and lots of pure water, does a great job. Also, you won't experience a feeling of deprivation, like you can with a fast.

Fasting certainly has therapeutic benefits, and it's a practice with a lot of history behind it. However I usually caution against it for many people for the following reasons:

1. **The toxins that can be released through fasting are often a strain on detoxification organs.** These organs need additional herbal support to eliminate the toxins safely. This wasn't a problem until this toxin-laden century.
2. **Because of a diet of refined carbohydrates, many people today have imbalances that are contraindicated for fasting.** Conditions such as hypoglycemia, diabetes, and poor blood sugar management could be aggravated by a prolonged fast.

If you're really interested in fasting, please consult with a health practitioner who is knowledgeable about supervising such a process. In Chapter 15, "Working with a Health Professional," you'll find information about a scientifically proven liquid cleansing program called Ultra Clear. It's used by many alternative health practitioners as part of a fasting regimen.

many of their patients have elected to use. To locate a practitioner who has proper training in herbal medicine, refer to Chapter 15.

Some people have a funny feeling about herbs. However, medicinal herbs are basically just concentrated food from a plant source. They are richer in nutrients than a non-"herb" food. Many parts of plants are used to produce herbs; it might come from the leaf, root, flower, bark, fruit, or stem. Herbs used for cleansing have properties that enhance digestion; stimulate bowel movements; increase perspiration and urination; improve circulation; destroy unwanted bacteria, viruses, fungi, and parasites; and clear mucus from the intestinal tract and lungs.

It's important to use herbal products made with organically grown ingredients. Not only will they be free of toxic pesticides; these herbs are grown in better soil and will have more of the health-promoting properties you're seeking.

Some herbs—such as basil or thyme—are used for culinary purposes; others—including chamomile or peppermint—make a great tea. In this chapter, however, we will be presenting herbs that generally have cleansing actions. You may notice that some of the herbs included can also be used for culinary purposes or ingested in tea form.

All herbs presented in this chapter have a long history of safe use when taken properly. However it is always wise to proceed with caution whenever you try anything new. Start slowly; listen to your body and intuition. If you notice that you're having any unusual reactions, stop using the herbs and consult with a health practitioner familiar with natural medicine and detoxification techniques.

FIRST STOP: THE COLON (LARGE INTESTINE)

The first place to start with herbal cleansing is with the colon. Just like we clean our houses, outer bodies, etc., cleansing is just a process of "removing the dirt" periodically, and preventing a build-up to the best of your ability.

If you've never cleansed, you might compare your body to a house that needs regular cleaning as well as the previous build-up removed.

Why are we starting with the large intestine? The intestinal tract is a prime target for toxins that have not been properly eliminated. These toxins gradually accumulate in the colon. Many are the result of inefficient digestion. As you've learned, undigested proteins putrefy, carbohydrates ferment, and fats rancify.

Many people think their colons are clean until they actually attempt to cleanse. Embarking on a colon detoxification program is a wonderful way to prevent illness, increase your level of wellness and energy, as well as assess how much toxicity you have built up.

Caution: Do not begin a colon cleansing program if you are pregnant, or have any inflammatory bowel disease such as Crohn's disease, regional ileitis, or ulcerative colitis. See a health professional trained in detoxification for assistance.

COMMON QUESTIONS REGARDING COLON CLEANSING

Although cleansing the colon has been practiced for thousands of years, it is just now enjoying a renaissance in our culture. There has been some confusion and misunderstanding regarding this valuable therapy. Some of the most common questions can be found below:

"Doesn't the body cleanse itself naturally? Isn't that enough?" If we can rely on our natural detox mechanisms alone, then why are constipation, colon cancer, and various other health conditions related to slow bowel transit time and autointoxication so common? And why do people feel so much better after a cleansing program? Certain exterior cleansing practices, such as taking baths and showers and brushing our teeth, aren't usually questioned. The interior of our bodies also needs assistance in keeping clean. By this point in the book, you have seen the many factors that can have a negative effect on the body's natural detoxification processes. And many of you can recognize your body's many cries for assistance in cleansing.

"Is it true that colon cleansing causes the bowel to become weak?" In our modern world, many people's bowels are already weak, as evidenced by the high incidence of intestinal disorders. After following a proper cleansing program, most people notice increased intestinal health.

"Does the colon really retain toxicity that needs to be cleansed? The increase of colon and rectal cancers in "civilized" countries where the fiber content is low implies that retention of toxic materials needs to be addressed. Research presented in Chapter 6 details the toxic material found in the colon and the related health conditions that occur as a result of poorly digested food turning into poison.

When I suggest using colon cleansing to aid my patients' health challenges, 99% of the time the reaction is "that makes so much sense." Since many other organs "dump" into the colon, taking the initial step of emphasizing colon detoxification opens up the "exit" door.

Then when the time comes to cleanse the other organs, the effort is more efficient.

It is important to note that although we are emphasizing colon health and cleansing in this chapter, you are naturally cleansing the whole body to some degree when you take this step. Before using herbs for colon cleansing, it is important to review the "Guidelines for Optimal Colon Health" detailed in Chapter 6.

COLON CLEANSING WITH HERBS

There are various products on the market for colon cleansing. They usually fit into three basic categories.

A Cleansing Fiber Formula
A Bowel Stimulating Herbal Formula
A Chlorophyll Product

■ 1. Cleansing Fiber Formula
The Cleansing Fiber Formula will create bulk in the stool. It also assists with removing the toxic residue. Look for a formula that includes:

Psyllium Husk: This is an excellent source of indigestible fiber. It adds a lubricating soft bulk, scrubbing the bowel as it moves through and removes toxins and excess cholesterol. Psyllium increases bowel transit time. Studies show that it is protective against colon cancer and other digestive diseases, such as ulcerative colitis.[1]
Flaxseed: Another fiber source, Flaxseed also provides nutrition for beneficial intestinal bacteria. Flaxseed supplies omega-3 fatty acids and lignans, substances that guard against cancer.
Apple Pectin: This natural fiber not only absorbs cholesterol,[2] it also increases the excretion of heavy metals, including lead, mercury, manganese, and beryllium. Apple Pectin protects against lead poisoning when consumed near the time of exposure. It absorbs radiation as well. This is another food source for friendly bacteria. It prevents gallstones, assists blood sugar balancing, and reduces cancer risk.[3]
Guar Gum: Extracted from the seeds of an East Indian plant, Guar Gum is another natural fiber. It reduces cholesterol,[4] balances blood

sugar,[5] may protect against colon cancer,[6] and increases nutrient absorption. Guar Gum lends support to the detoxification process. If guar gum sounds familiar, this may be because it's a common thickening agent in foods.

Ginger: James Duke, an herb authority and author of *The Green Pharmacy*, has found that ginger furnishes eight liver-protecting compounds. Research shows that Ginger prevents nausea by clearing bile from the liver, settles the stomach, and reduces flatulence. It relieves pain and alleviates cramps. Ginger promotes cleansing through the bowels, kidneys, and skin.

Fennel: One of the oldest cultivated plants, Fennel can be used to calm the digestive system. It reduces gas and relieves constipation. Fennel has antibacterial properties, including effectiveness against Salmonella.[7] Research has shown that it helps fight cancer. This herb supports mental clarity. Its estrogenic effects promote healthy menstruation, increase libido, and relieve symptoms of "male menopause."[8]

Prune: Famous as a natural laxative, this high-fiber food adds bulk to the stool. One study found that twelve prunes a day substantially reduced LDL or "bad cholesterol."[9] The ability of prunes to reduce fecal acids may protect against colon cancer.

Alfalfa: High in essential enzymes, trace minerals, and vitamins A, K, and D, Alfalfa has long been turned to for its medicinal properties. Chinese and Indian physicians used it to treat digestive disorders and ulcers. Alfalfa is a liver supporter, detoxifier, and infection fighter.[10]

Slippery Elm: This herb is made from the bark of the slippery elm tree. It soothes tissues and draws impurities out of the mucous membranes, stomach, and bowel. The herb has been used to treat diverticulitis. Slippery Elm also reduces acidity in the stomach.

Citrus Peel: Traditional Chinese Medicine utilizes citrus peel as a digestive aid. The herb helps with abdominal pain and constipation. It is effective in dispelling gas and bloating, as well as clearing mucus.

Licorice Root: This is such an ancient remedy that a bundle of licorice was found in King Tut's tomb! This demulcent is soothing to digestive tract. It is also liver-protective. Licorice root has antimicrobial properties. It is immune-supportive and a blood purifier.

Triphala: This is an Ayurvedic remedy dating back thousands of years.

In India, Triphala is used commonly to increase bowel movements. It has detoxifying, antimicrobial,[11] and anti-cancer[12] properties. Triphala is liver protective.[13] This herb provides bioflavonoids, vitamin C, and linoleic oil.

Bentonite: This is a clay, also known as montmorillonite, has profound detoxification abilities.[14] The clay adsorbs toxins such as heavy metals, pesticides, and free radicals like a magnet and absorbs them like a sponge. Bentonite's ability to absorb pathogenic viruses, aflatoxin (a toxic mold), and pesticides (including Paraquat and Roundup) was reported in the *Canadian Journal of Microbiology*. The clay is eventually eliminated from the body with the toxins bound to its multiple surfaces. According to clay expert Ran Knishinsky, author of *The Clay Cure*, people eat or drink clay daily for its detoxifying benefits in over 200 cultures throughout the world. Sometimes you will see Bentonite sold separately in liquid form, or included in a fiber formula.

Activated Charcoal: Walnut and peach seeds or wood are processed to create Charcoal; the emphasis is on increasing the absorption of the final product. Acting like a sponge, Charcoal removes additives, pesticides, chemicals, radioactive waste, and other poisons from the gastrointestinal tract. It can also absorb harmful bacteria and viruses. Charcoal's actions protect the liver.[15] Charcoal is very helpful for flatulence, that often surprising and overpowering form of gas, which sometimes can temporarily increase during a cleanse. Charcoal will help you cleanse and avoid distancing your friends.

Whatever Cleansing Fiber Formula you purchase, be sure to follow the instructions on the package. Dosages suggested are generally one tablespoon mixed with 12 ounces of water one to three times a day. Start with one dose a day and build gradually, adding an extra dose every few days. Taking a formula like this more than three times a day is not usually suggested without professional supervision. As you increase the dosage, be sure to listen to your body—you only want to increase it if you are noticing increased *comfortable* bulkier bowel movements.

If you take too much of the fiber formula you may experience symptoms such as excess bloating, gas, abdominal distention, diarrhea, constipation, or mild cramping. If this is the case, be sure to drink more water, and either reduce the fiber formula or take a temporary break from it. When your symptoms subside, you can gradually resume the program. Be careful not to overdo this formula! Your body will need time to adjust to the additional fiber.

Note: With a Cleansing Fiber Formula, it is crucial to drink extra water. For each dose of the formula, drink 8 ounces more of water than your usual amount. (Just a reminder of how to determine your regular daily amount of water—drink one-half of body weight in ounces. For example, if you weigh 120 pounds, the minimum water amount would be 60 ounces.)

■ 2. Bowel Stimulating Herbal Formula

The Cleansing Fiber Formula detailed above includes ingredients that increase bulk in the stool and magnetize toxins to the colon for elimination. Now that we have all of these toxins "ready to exit," it is important to note that aid for increased peristaltic activity (bowel movements) is usually needed. Without these bowel stimulating herbs, the bulk created by the fiber could result in constipation. In other words—we need to keep things moving.

The following herbs, used in combination, will cause an increase in bowel movements, supporting the release of toxins absorbed in the Cleansing Fiber Formula.

Turkey Rhubarb: This root herb will promote bowel movements. It encourages the flow of bile. Used as a tonic, it is mildly stimulating to the liver.

Cascara Sagrada: A "sacred bark" from traditional Native American medicine, Cascara stimulates secretions throughout the digestive tract and increases the frequency of bowel movements. Cascara bark is known for its detoxification properties.

Aloe Vera: A traditional Chinese and Ayurvedic remedy, Aloe Vera has antibacterial and antifungal properties. It relieves constipation and assists healing of ulcers. Aloe helps restore intestinal health by thwarting the growth of Candida and reducing putrification.

Barberry: This ancient Egyptian herb, made from root bark, is a natural antibiotic. It supports the immune system by stimulating the action of white blood cells. Barberry improves bile flow, liver function, and digestion, and it increases bowel movements.

Ginger: Research shows that Ginger prevents nausea. This herb lowers cholesterol by clearing bile from the liver. Ginger settles the stomach, reduces flatulence, and is an effective pain reliever. It also promotes cleansing through the bowels, kidneys, and skin. This popular herb has antibacterial and anti-parasitic effects.

Sage: Both the Chinese and Romans valued this healing herb. Recent research shows it has antimicrobial abilities against *Staphylococcus aureus* bacteria.[16] Sage also contains a variety of antifungal compounds. This is a liver-supportive herb.

Black Walnut: Dating back to ancient Greece, this herb has traditionally been used for its remarkable ability to destroy worms and parasites. It is antifungal,[17] effective against candida and other related species. Black Walnut has demonstrated impressive antimicrobial effects.[18]

Slippery Elm: The bark of the slippery elm tree works well as a gentle laxative. Slippery Elm is soothing to the digestive tract. It absorbs toxins and helps heal tissue.

You will see Cleansing Fiber Formulas on the market with similar ingredients. The best formulas use organically grown herbs. Follow the instructions on the package. Be careful not to take too much or you could experience cramping and/or diarrhea.

Take the minimal amount of the Bowel Stimulating Formula needed to insure comfortable bowel movements, preferably at least three movements a day.

When you are taking a Cleansing Fiber Formula with a Bowel Stimulating Formula, you will most likely notice an increase in bowel movements. The stools should be bulky and on the soft side. They may be ropy or have strange colors. This is generally okay, unless you see blood. (Note: If you are eating beets, you may notice redness in the stool. This is nothing to be alarmed about.) Sometimes your stools could be runny or have small amounts of mucus. This is generally not a cause for concern unless an unusual pattern continues.

If you are experiencing cramping, cut down on both formulas. If your stools are dry, you may either be taking too much of the Cleansing Fiber Formula, or not be drinking enough water.

Caution: Herbs used to enhance bowel movements are to be used only during a cleanse or for occasional constipation. They are not to be

COLON HYDROTHERAPY (COLONICS)

Colon hydrotherapy is a safe, gentle way to enhance the removal of toxic waste material from the large intestine. Purified water is infused into the intestine, stimulating peristalsis.

Similar techniques date back to at least 1,500 B.C., when its use was recorded in the Egyptian medical document "Ebers Papyrus." Greek physicians Hippocrates and Galen also worked with this therapy extensively. Colon hydrotherapy was commonly practiced in hospitals and clinics in America until the 1940s, when natural healing methods began being replaced with treatment with pharmaceutical drugs.

"The irrigation or the washing of the colon is a procedure that has been practiced by humans in all civilizations in recorded history, and, no doubt, before," says Dr. Ann Wigmore, an internationally recognized detoxification expert. "With the new awakening that is presently occurring on Earth, colon hygiene once again is being recognized and practiced by an ever-growing number of individuals as a fundamental and essential aspect of health."

Colon hydrotherapy can be a valuable complement to an herbal cleansing program. Colon hydrotherapists are very familiar with detoxification, and in addition to the treatments, can often provide valuable advice on other types of cleansing.

Chapter 15 will give you referral information for practitioners who perform colon hydrotherapy.

used on a regular basis, for they can create a "lazy bowel" or a dependency. The "Guidelines for Optimal Colon Health" detailed in Chapter 6 should be followed to insure safe ways of ensuring healthy elimination without the use of herbs or laxatives.

■ 3. Chlorophyll

In Chapter 10, the importance of chlorophyll was detailed. To summarize: Chlorophyll acts as an antiseptic, strengthens tissues, and aids in detoxification. Pure chlorophyll comes from a variety of sources, such as alfalfa, barley grass, wheatgrass, etc. It is suggested to take chlorophyll during any cleansing program, as well as on a regular basis for enhanced nutrition.

Chlorophyll comes in two forms, liquid and powdered.

1. **Liquid:** DeSouza's is an excellent chlorophyll product, made from alfalfa. It is the only one on the market that I know of that is organic and doesn't have preservatives. It has a mild taste and is easy to mix. One to two tablespoons a day is usually suggested.

2. **Loose powder (to be mixed in water) or encapsulated powder:** The powder is basically a dehydrated version of the fresh product, specially formulated to be reconstituted with water. There are several powdered forms of chlorophyll available. I usually suggest organic barley grass juice. The taste is pleasant, and the texture easy to mix. The capsules might be more convenient for travel purposes. With powders or capsules, follow the instructions on the package. One to two teaspoons a day is usually suggested with the powder; if taking capsules, five twice a day is usually suggested. See the Resources section for product suggestions.

Unlike the other herbs and formulas mentioned in this chapter (which should only be utilized for periodic cleansing—not on a regular basis), chlorophyll can be used during the cleanse as well as on a daily basis for maintenance.

Even though chlorophyll is safe to take every day, remember that it does have cleansing properties. If you take too much, you may experience cleansing symptoms such as slight headaches, fatigue, skin breakout, etc. Adjust the dosage accordingly.

If the chlorophyll is used regularly for maintenance, it is suggested to vary between the different forms available: i.e., barley grass, alfalfa, wheat grass, etc.

THE LIVER CLEANSE

Cleansing the liver is a crucial part of any cleansing program. As detailed in Chapter 7, the liver is a main player in the body's detoxification processes. With the entry of numerous chemicals into our environment in the past century, the liver has an increased burden. Supporting and enhancing the liver's ability to detoxify is a wonderful way to give your overall health a significant upgrade. The liver can be compared to the oil filter in the body, and a liver cleanse is like an oil change.

TEMPORARY REACTIONS TO HERBAL CLEANSING

Most patients that I've seen over the years were able to incorporate herbal cleansing without any difficulty. When there are reactions, they are usually minor. The following is a list of possible reactions.

- Tongue coat
- Bad breath
- Nausea
- Brain fog
- Chilliness
- Headache/bodyache
- Weight loss
- Rashes
- Diarrhea/constipation
- Night sweats
- Fatigue

Most of these reactions happen because the body is cleansing quickly and the toxins are not being expelled (through the bowel movements, urine, sweat, etc.) efficiently. Symptoms can be reduced by increasing water, decreasing emotional stress, and insuring that the bowels are moving easily.

In other words, *"cleansing reactions"* occur because of dehydration, sluggish bowel movements, and/or a too rapid release of toxins. Another reason may be a history of chronic illness.

If you experience something severe (which is *extremely* rare), stop immediately and consult a health practitioner (see Chapter 15) who has experience in detoxification. If you are cleansing without professional supervision, it is wise not to overdo it. It is easy to get overly enthusiastic about cleansing.

It is generally suggested to do an herbal colon cleanse for one to three weeks before introducing herbs which are more specific for the liver. When you introduce the liver herbs, it is important to continue to take the colon herbal formulas in whatever amount ensures comfortable and frequent (at least three a day) bowel movements. If you take a liver cleansing formula, and your bowel is sluggish, you will probably not feel good. That is most likely because the toxins that are being released with the liver cleanse are not being "escorted out the door" with the colon cleansing formula, and the backup can definitely cause some problems. Keep it moving!

There is no hard and fast rule to know when to start the liver cleanse, but you want to make sure that you are not experiencing any discomfort (gas, bloating, cramping, fatigue, headaches, skin break-outs) from the colon cleanse. You should be experiencing at least three comfortable bowel movements a day.

Most liver cleansing herbal formulas suggest starting with a small dose and gradually recommend building up to a more potent one. The range suggested with most products is from a beginning dose of two or three capsules twice a day, building up to a maximum dose of between five and eight capsules twice a day. Most people benefit from taking the herbs for the liver for three to four weeks the first time they do an herbal liver cleanse.

Many individuals who have done a liver detox have found it help-ful to gradually increase the beginning dosage by one capsule every four or five days. You want to make sure that you don't experience any sig-nificant symptoms; a slight amount of passing fatigue, a mild headache, and/or a few pimples are nothing to worry about—they will subside. However, if you experience severe fatigue, viral symptoms (sore throat, achiness, fever, chills), or severe headaches, you will really have to pro-ceed slowly. Or better yet, seek guidance of a health care professional who has experience in detoxification.

These precautions are not meant to scare you. Most people are able to handle the increases of herbs easily and experience the remarkable benefits of detoxification.

Remember, you don't have to be "gung ho" and attempt to do an extreme detox. In fact, I caution against this. The purpose of this book is to remind you that our bodies are always detoxifying, and to guide you through gentle and effective detoxification support. It is better to take small doses of herbs for a longer period of time than to overwhelm your system.

Herbs that have been traditionally used to support liver detoxifica-tion are often found in various formulas and include:

Milk Thistle: This herb is one of the best-known liver protectors, and it has been used for this purpose for over 2,000 years. Milk Thistle reduces liver congestion, and prevents toxins from penetrating liver cells. It also promotes bile flow and healthy bowel movements. *Silymarin* is the bioflavanoid complex found in Milk Thistle. It has strong antioxidant properties. Silymarin protects the liver from incoming toxins and helps remove toxic buildup. It also supports liver cell regeneration. Silymarin is protective against common airborne pollutants and radiation (including that from x-rays). Milk thistle has also demonstrated remarkable anti-tumor properties.[19]

Turmeric: Also known as Curcumin, this is what gives curry its yellow tint. Turmeric protects the liver by increasing bile flow and preventing congestion. It enhances the production of the powerful antioxidant glutathione. This herb has antimicrobial effects. It also helps lower cholesterol. Turmeric has demonstrated anti-cancer properties.[20]

Artichoke Extract: The historical and folk uses of Artichoke are as a digestive aid and liver remedy. Studies have verified these applications. Artichoke aids the liver in detoxification by stimulating bile flow. It also helps to regenerate the liver. This herb protects LDL cholesterol from oxidation.[21]

Schisandra: Used in Traditional Chinese Medicine as a tonic, this antioxidant herb also helps to regenerate liver tissue.[22] It normalizes stomach acid as well. Schisandra restores a weak immune system. The herb increases mental focus as well as physical stamina and endurance.

Rosemary: This herb's medicinal history goes back to ancient Rome where it was used as a memory enhancer. It has high antioxidant properties. Rosemary increases anti-cancer enzymes by as much as 450%. The herb can block the carcinogenic effects of chemical toxins. Its ability to increase the liver detoxification function has been demonstrated.[23]

Bupleurum: An important herb in Traditional Chinese Medicine (TCM), this plant is used by TCM doctors to treat liver disturbances. Research shows that it is liver-enzyme supportive and inhibits damage to the organ. Bupleurum also strengthens the immune system.[24]

Boldo: This is an evergreen native to South America. The herb improves digestion by regulating gastric secretions. It supports the liver through increased bile flow. Boldo also appears to protect the liver against toxic chemicals by supporting enzyme levels.[25] Oxidation of blood fats are prevented by a chemical found in Boldo leaves and bark.[26]

Dandelion: Viewed by some as just a lawn weed, this is actually one of the best-known herbs to treat disorders of the liver. Dandelion is useful for treating liver and gall bladder inflammation as well as jaundiced states. Its bitterness increases bile flow and stimulates digestion. Dandelion is a rich source of vitamins A, C, D, and the B-complex. It is also abundant in the following minerals: iron, silicon, magnesium, zinc, manganese, and potassium.

Yellow Dock: This root herb is a bitter, a class of remedies traditionally used for stimulating appetite and improving digestion. Yellow Dock also promotes detoxification, and it was a Native American cleansing herb. This root has antifungal and antibacterial effects. It is rich in minerals, such as iron. Yellow Dock gently enhances elimination and also promotes bile secretion.

Gentian: Also a bitter, Gentian stimulates the production of saliva, stomach acid, and digestive juices. It also promotes the flow of bile and pancreatic juices. Gentian is protective of the liver, pancreas, spleen, and kidneys.

Eclipta: An Ayurvedic tonic, this herb guards the liver against damage from toxins.[27] It also has antifungal properties. Eclipta promotes bile flow.

Barberry: This root herb contains a natural antibiotic called berberine. It stimulates the immune system by increasing the activity of macrophages. Barberry boosts the flow of bile and enhances digestion. It has a strong curative effect on the liver, thus it is used for treating jaundice.

As you take the liver herbal formula, you can expect some changes. You may notice increased energy immediately, or you may notice some periods of fatigue interspersed with periods of increased energy. You may also experience some minor cleansing reactions, as described earlier in the chapter. Listen to your body. Make sure your water intake is optimal, that you are getting enough rest, and that you are not taking more herbs than your body can comfortably handle.

ADDRESSING OTHER DETOXIFICATION SYSTEMS WITH HERBS

The herbs detailed for the colon and liver cleanses have beneficial effects on the whole body, including other detoxification systems such as the respiratory, lymphatic, dermal, and urinary. However, there are additional herbs that have been used specifically for cleansing other organs such as the lungs, skin, and kidneys, as well as the lymph:

Nettle: Another prominent weed, this nutrient-rich herb provides vitamins A, C, D, and K as well as the minerals calcium, phosphorus, potassium, iron, and sulfur. Nettle has been used for centuries to clear the lungs, due to its antihistamine properties. A cleansing herb, it helpful for relieving fatigue and other effects of stress. Nettle curbs water retention. A Belgium study found it to inhibit HIV and cytomegalovirus.[28]

Red Root: This herb comes from a shrub named after its deep red roots. Red Root clears liver and lymph congestion. It is used for soreness and infections of the throat (including tonsillitis). An active component appears to be tannins.

Elecampagne: Also known as Wild Sunflower, Elecampagne is a common plant in North America. Its antiseptic expectorant action clears the lungs. Elecampagne is also thought to have antiamebic properties. It can improve weak digestion and clear the gut of mucus.

Cleavers: A common weed, Cleavers is an important herb for clearing lymph and liver congestion. It is used to reduce lymphatic swelling, as in tonsillitis, swollen glands, and lymphadema. Cleavers is also a kidney stimulant, detoxifier, and blood purifier. Its historical use is for the treatment of tumors.

Ligustrum: This herb comes from berries of a shrub grown in China and eastern Asia. It has been used traditionally for chronic toxicity. It appears to boost the immune system, clears phlegm, opens the lungs, and exhibits an anti-inflammatory effect.[29]

Scrofularia: Also known as figwort, this herb is used to clear skin disorders, such as acne, eczema, and psoriasis. Scrofularia stimulates bile flow, increases peristalsis, enhances lymph drainage, and acts as a diuretic.

Burdock: This herb also goes by the name Gobo Root. Burdock clears lymph and liver congestion. Its antimicrobial activity helps cleanse blood. Gobo Root promotes kidney function, a healthy immune system, and the balancing of blood sugar. It is known for healing skin conditions and ulcers. Burdock appears to slow the growth of tumors.[30]

Mullein: An expectorant used by the ancient Greeks, Mullein leaves or flowers have traditionally been used to soothe lung problems such as colds, bronchitis, or emphysema. This herb helps loosen and remove mucus. It also reduces the swelling of glands.

Goldenrod: Because of its diuretic and antiseptic properties, Goldenrod is used widely in Europe. It appears to be supportive of kidney and bladder health. Germans use it for yeast infections. Substances in Goldenrod combat fungus such as candida and parasites.

Chickweed: Traditional uses of the leaves of this plant are for relieving itching and healing skin problems. Chickweed can also soothe internal inflammation. It strengthens the stomach and intestines. This herb helps clear blood vessels and the body of fatty substances.

Horsetail: A flowerless weed, horsetail is known for its diuretic properties. Horsetail is used to treat various kidney and bladder ailments. It helps heal wounds and ulcers. The herb's astringent qualities assist in clearing toxins and preventing inflammation and infection.

Buchu: Originally from South Africa, Buchu (meaning "fragrant") was used there for treating mild stomach, intestinal, and bladder problems. The dried leaves are helpful for cleansing the kidneys and urinary tract. It is a tonic, astringent, and disinfectant.

Red Clover: For centuries, European gypsy cultures have used Red Clover for medicinal purposes. It was also part of Native American remedies. Red Clover promotes cleansing of the blood through antiseptic and antibiotic actions. It supports the elimination of toxins in the urine. As a tonic, Red Clover rejuvenates the nervous system. This herb contains the anti-cancer compound *genistein*.

Juniper: This plant has a long history as a folk remedy. It is used to treat kidney and bladder conditions. Juniper can also ease indigestion and flatulence. This herb is a diuretic, and it has anti-inflammatory and antiviral effects.[31]

The herbs listed above often come in various encapsulated formulas designed to cleanse specific organs or systems. They may also be purchased individually in bulk or tea bags to be prepared as a hot beverage.

You may want to use these various herbs singly or in combination. They can be consumed as an adjunct to the liver cleanse or at a separate time.

Reminder: When taking any kind of cleansing herbs, it is very important to drink a lot of water and to take enough of the Bowel Stimulating Formula to ensure that your bowels keep moving. One of the main reasons for discomfort during a cleanse is dehydration and/or incomplete elimination (which doesn't allow the toxins being released into the system to exit the body efficiently).

HOW OFTEN TO CLEANSE

The first time you cleanse, your schedule might look like this:

> **Week 1-2: Colon Cleanse**
> **Week 3-4: Colon/Liver Cleanse**
> **Week 4-6: Complete System Cleanse**

Once you achieve the level of health you desire, it is wise to do a "maintenance" cleanse twice a year. It is like doing a thorough cleaning of your house, and then occasional light dusting.

It is usually recommended to cleanse during the change of seasons, during the spring and fall. You can choose full cleanse or a modified cleanse.

A modified cleanse for maintenance might look like this:

> **Week 1: Colon Cleanse**
> **Week 2: Colon/Liver Cleanse**
> **Week 3: Complete System Cleanse**

HOW TO ADJUST DIET WHEN CLEANSING

During this time, it is advised to eat a little lighter, but it is not necessary to be extreme.

When you are taking herbs for cleansing, you do not have be perfect in your eating and lifestyle habits. You can still maintain your normal work and social life. Just try to be a little more conscious.

Follow nutritional basics detailed in Chapter 9: *emphasize*—vegetables, fruits, whole grains (brown rice), light protein (fish, tofu); *limit/eliminate*—sugar, dairy, red meat, alcohol, fried foods, and processed, refined foods.

An important point: Please do not think of this as all or nothing. Most "diet" plans support that concept. You might eat pretty healthy for a few days while starting the herbs, and then go to a party and eat and drink a little heavier. That's okay. Keep taking the herbs and just do the best you can.

The program that I have emphasized to patients over the years has been one of consistency and moderation. The last thing you need is to get "gung ho" and try to be "perfect" only to disappoint yourself (and possibly sabotage the whole opportunity for a great cleanse).

Most people who have cleansed following the guidelines detailed above continued to work, maintain family lives, social schedules, business, etc. It is the rare individual who is able to get away for a few months and "cleanse" on a pristine island. If you have that opportunity, then there are more extreme supervised cleanses available at such centers. See "Resources for More Intensive Detoxification" in Chapter 15 for more information.

OTHER SUPPORTIVE HABITS

During a cleanse, it is common to get a bit introspective as you are getting "back in touch" with your balanced self. Activities that complement and assist in cleansing include light exercise such as yoga, spending time in nature, and journaling. Make sure you get enough rest. Some people find that they need more sleep during a cleanse.

Make sure you are enhancing your circulation as you cleanse deeper with herbs. As the toxins are being broken down, we want them to make a quick exit, and optimal circulation greatly assists this process. Massage, hydrotherapy, skin brushing, and light exercise are valuable tools. The next chapter will guide you through choices for improved circulation.

ADDITIONAL HERBAL FORMULAS

■ Candida/Parasite Formula

In Chapter 6, the epidemic of yeast and parasite health-related issues was explored. Since this imbalance is more common than not, it is advisable to use herbs with antifungal and anti-parasitic properties as a preventative approach. Since so many people have health challenges that are yeast and/or parasite related and are not aware of this contributing factor, the use of antifungal and anti-parasitic herbs can bring pleasant surprises—people often notice increased energy and decreased chronic symptoms.

Some natural substances with antifungal and anti-parasitic properties include:

Wormwood: Ancient Greek texts mention the worm-expelling abilities of Wormwood. Today it is used to rid the body of intestinal worms and parasites. Wormwood also stimulates enzymes that promote bile flow. Recent research displays its powerful anti-malarial properties.[32] Wormwood eases liver congestion and promotes more frequent bowel movements.

Black Walnut: Native Americans used tea made with Black Walnut to cure ringworm. The hulls of Black Walnut have antifungal and anti-parasitic effects. Research has proven its effectiveness in destroying candida albicans and other fungi; as well as salmonella, staphylococcus aureus, and other pathogenic bacteria. The bark helps clear liver congestion. This herb assists detoxification by oxygenating the blood. Anti-cancer effects have also been found.

Quassia: This herb is a larvicide that is known to possess anti-amoebic, anti-tumor, and antiviral properties. Quassia has been used to treat indigestion, amoebic dysentery, giardiasis, malaria, and pinworms.

Clove: Derived from a tender evergreen tree from the tropics, clove is effective against several parasites, including intestinal worms.[33] Clove can also help relieve nausea. This herb has pain-relieving and antiseptic abilities.

Grapefruit Seed Extract: This substance has been extensively researched for its extremely potent broad-spectrum antibacterial, antifungal, anti-parasitic, and antiviral compounds.

Caprylic Acid: A long-chain fatty acid derived from coconut, Caprylic

Acid has been proven effective as a strong antifungal agent.

Undecylenic Acid: Similar to caprylic acid in function and potency, Undecylenic Acid is a long-chain fatty acid derived from the castor bean. It has very powerful antifungal properties.

Pau D'arco: This herb contains lapachol and beta lapachone, two components that have been researched to be more potent than ketaconazole, a common antifungal drug with strong side effects.[34]

If you suspect a yeast and/parasite involvement, using a formula with herbs similar to those above might help you feel better. Follow the directions on the package. If you suspect a significant problem, please do not try to treat yourself. See a qualified health professional who is familiar with the yeast and parasite testing and treatment protocol.

▪ Energy Enhancement

After the cleanse, you may want to explore herbs traditionally used to enhance your newfound abundant energy. It is best to consult with a practitioner of Traditional Chinese Medicine, a naturopath, or professional herbalist to see which herbs and dosages are best for you. See Chapter 15.

Unlike the cleansing formulas detailed above which are to be taken for short periods of time during a cleanse, most energy-enhancing herbs are tonics, and are traditionally taken on a more regular basis. It is suggested to take energy-enhancing herbs in formulas rather than as single herbs. You will find the herbs listed below in many of the energy tonics on the market:

Ginseng: This is an herb with a long history of use. It is an adaptogen, assisting the body in handling stress by supporting the adrenals. There has been substantial research on its ability to enhance athletic performance and boost energy. Ginseng stimulates the immune system[35] and has anti-cancer effects.[36]

Astragalus: This herb from China is known for its powerful immune-supportive properties.[37] Astragalus has antiviral properties,[38] protects the liver,[39] and aids in wound healing. It has been used extensively for its ability to combat fatigue.

Fo-ti (Polygonum Multiflorum): This root's anti-aging properties are recognized in Traditional Chinese Medicine.[40] It has been shown to aid in slowing hair loss. Research shows its ability to lower cholesterol, decrease hardening of the arteries, and enhance immune function. Fo-ti has displayed antibacterial action.

Codonopsis: This herb increases stamina and vitality, clears the lungs, and helps build the blood due to its concentrated nutrients. Codonopsis also strengthens weak digestion.

Rehmannia: A Chinese root herb, Rehmannia is used to treat anemia and fatigue.[41] Known for its powerful immune supporting properties, it also helps promote healthy blood-sugar regulation.[42]

Ashwaganda: This herb comes from India and is traditionally used as a rejuvenating tonic. Research shows that Ashwaganda supports immunity by increasing the red blood cell count.[43] It may help counteract the immune suppression associated with chemotherapy.[44] Ashwaganda is powerful antioxidant and is also known for reducing stress and improving learning and memory.

Note/caution: Many herbs marketed for "energy" are simply stimulants. These products will give you an initial boost, but in the long run will drain your energy reserves. Herbs to avoid that are often included in energy-enhancing formulas include Ma Huang, Guarana, and Kola Nut.

A FEW FINAL THOUGHTS ON HERBAL CLEANSING

Herbs provide a wonderful opportunity to experience increased health. This chapter was presented to give you some basic guidelines for herbs traditionally used for cleansing. Using some basic detoxification formulas on the market (that include the herbs detailed in this chapter) will give most people a feeling of increased energy and may improve various health challenges.

It is important to note that many of the herbs should not be taken on a regular basis. Just like with food, we need a variety. If you take the same herbs for a long time, you run the risk of developing an allergy and/or the herb will not have the same beneficial effect as when you first started using it.

If you have a significant health condition, the herbs outlined in this chapter may not be appropriate for you. There are many wonderful practitioners who can assist you in the proper use of herbs to improve your health. See Chapter 15 for references.

WHAT'S AHEAD

The information in *The Detox Solution* so far has explored ways to remove toxins from our environment and our bodies. The principles learned so far will only display the health benefits if the circulation in the body is optimal. The next chapter will offer various techniques to ensure your circulation is the best it can be.

TWELVE

Boosting Detox Through Enhanced Circulation:
Exercise, Hydrotherapy, Skin Brushing, Spa Treatments, Massage, Breath Work & Acupuncture

> When those who enjoy a hot bath inhale the air of the bath, so that the heat of the bath enters their spirits and makes them hot, they are known to experience joy. It often happens that they start singing, as singing has its origin in gladness.
>
> — Ibn Khaldun, 14th Century Arab historian, politician, philosopher

In this chapter, you'll discover additional steps you can take to enhance the benefits you're receiving from the detoxification program. Having optimal circulation is crucial to efficient detoxification. The two circulatory systems—*cardiovascular* and *lymphatic*—carry nutrients to cells and transport toxins away from cells for elimination.

To begin using the ideas covered in this chapter, make sure you incorporate some regular exercise into your life. This is an essential practice and the most important one suggested here. If you do nothing else, do get your body in motion. Some of the initial sections below offer basic background on exercise to help you get started. Then, as you review the rest of the chapter, you'll learn about other practices that you may wish to add to your routine—either on a regular basis or occasionally. However it's not necessary to do every practice that is described in this chapter. How much you do is up to you.

YOUR BODY'S CIRCULATION SYSTEMS

Before describing the practices, let's review what's involved in the circulation that takes place in your body. Basically the two systems—cardiovascular and lymphatic—are different, but interrelated. The cardiovascular system includes the heart, lungs, arteries, capillaries, veins, and blood. The lymphatic system is made of vessels, nodes (such as in the armpits, neck, chest, and groin), ducts, and lymphatic fluid. These two systems run parallel to each other, and share some duties in taking care of the body.

Two functions performed by the cardiovascular and lymphatic systems are to deliver important nutrients to and remove harmful toxins from cells throughout the body. These vital responsibilities are accomplished via the movement of blood and lymphatic fluid. Toxins that are carried away include metabolic wastes, inflammatory by-products, carbon dioxide, and foreign substances.

Though the cardiovascular system has the heart to propel the blood through the vessels continuously, the lymphatic system has no such pump. Instead it relies on skeletal muscles to squeeze lymph vessels during body movement and breathing to promote movement of the lymphatic fluid. When stimulation of the lymphatic system is insufficient, its nourishing, protective, and cleansing functions are impaired. Fatigue and toxicity can result. Also, when blood flow is at a less-than-optimal level (such as in someone who rarely exercises), the natural detoxification process is compromised. The practices in this chapter were selected because they strengthen the circulation of both blood and lymphatic fluid.

Many body processes, not just those directly related to detoxification, are supported by strong circulation of these two important body fluids—blood and lymph. Other processes include those that control inflammation, ward off infections, respond to trauma, and repel disease. Among the life-supporting elements delivered in blood and lymph are oxygen, infection-fighting agents, proteins, enzymes, vitamins, minerals, hormones, sugars, and fats.

EXERCISE

As mentioned earlier, the most important practice in this chapter for supporting detox is to exercise regularly. Exercise promotes both strong blood circulation and increased flow of lymphatic fluid. It also aids detoxification in other ways. Physical activity stimulates the release of toxins through your skin as you sweat. It promotes greater detoxification through the lungs and better oxygenation of the cells. Research has shown that exercise can improve the activity of liver detoxification enzymes.[1] Regular workouts can also reduce fat reserves—principal locations where toxins are stored. Exercise boosts your metabolism too, which helps with overall detox.

Just in case you need more reasons to feel motivated to exercise, recognize that, in addition to detox, working out is one of the best actions you can take to promote your overall health and longevity. Here's a list of just some of the benefits that regular exercise can provide:

- Increases lung capacity
- Boosts your energy level
- Elevates mood and reduces the stress that you're holding in your body
- Improves patterns of sleep and reduces insomnia
- Provides a break from a busy life and allows you to gain perspective
- Boosts immunity to colds, flu, and disease
- Promotes healthy digestion and elimination
- Can support your body's ability to heal
- Assists in maintaining a healthy weight
- Tones your body and improves your appearance
- Reduces your risk of heart disease, high blood pressure, arthritis, cancer, diabetes, and other debilitating chronic illnesses
- Lowers elevated blood cholesterol levels
- Maintains and enhances the functioning of muscle tissue
- Improves flexibility, agility, and range of motion
- Helps build and keep healthy bones and joints
- Slows down the aging process, promoting a youthful glow.

Due to the sedentary nature of many of our lives and jobs today, it's necessary for most of us to make a conscious effort to build regular exercise into our routine. To help yourself stick with it, choose an activity that you'll enjoy. If you already have this area covered, keep moving! Just realize that you don't need to knock yourself out to stay fit. Some people go overboard in the beginning with exercise, become discouraged, and then give up. Don't let this happen to you!

One facet of becoming fit is to ultimately commit to doing some *aerobic* activity each day. This includes any exercise that will raise your heart rate—such as biking, swimming, or brisk walking. The aerobic exercise that I usually recommend to start with is walking. This form of exercise furnishes a great total body workout. You'll find more information on walking on the following page.

TARGET HEART RATES: HOW TO GET YOUR NUMBERS

To check if the intensity of your exercise is producing an aerobic effect, you'll want to determine an appropriate range for your target heart rate. A common approach is to first figure out an approximate maximum heart rate for your age group. This can be accomplished by taking the number 220 and subtracting your age (Example: 220 − 35 years of age = 185). Next, multiply the result by 0.65 to get the low end of your training heart rates (Example: 185 X 0.65 = 120). Then take the original figure and multiply it by 0.85 to obtain the top of the training range (185 X 0.85 = 157). A heart rate anywhere between these two numbers (Example: 120 to 157) is the desired result you'll want to achieve through exercise.

To see if your heart rate falls within this range, take your pulse immediately upon ceasing exercise. Use your index or middle finger to feel your pulse either on your neck or wrist. Count the beat for 15 seconds, and then multiply the result by four. If your pulse is below the range, work out a little harder the next time. If it's above, ease up a bit on the intensity of your workout.

Note that the standard recommendation for the minimum time span and frequency of your aerobic workouts is 20 minutes per session performed three times a week. If you're in great shape and have the time, you might want to expand this to up to an hour each day. And here's some good news for those of you who have been couch potatoes.

Researchers have found that you can also benefit if you split your session up into, say, two or three 10-minute workouts sprinkled throughout your day. So if you're really out of shape, you can start with these shorter sessions and add time gradually toward longer durations. Or, if you're nursing an injury, consult with your doctor and see if you're ready for a low-impact activity such as swimming.

In addition to walking, two other exercise activities that enhance the detoxification process are yoga and rebounding. These are also described in sections below.

▪ Walking

More and more people are discovering the joys of walking. One reason that this exercise works for so many people is its ease of use. You can merely step out the door of your home or office and begin. Still I advise that, as often as possible, you seek out locations that include an experience of communing with Nature—such as a tree-lined street, the beach, woods, or a city park. For other days, a treadmill at home or the gym can help keep you on track. If you can, avoid the treadmill at the gym as your regular walking location because loud music, fluorescent lighting, poor indoor air quality, and obsessive exercisers can make the surrounding environment toxic. And avoid taking in heavy toxins while walking by staying away from busy traffic.

Though walking for exercise is for the most part a straightforward practice, there are some things to consider. First, you'll want purchase a pair of *good walking shoes* that provide adequate support and cushioning. Shoes are available today that are specifically designed for walking—even running shoes have different features that make them less desirable for walkers.

Stretching is an important element of a walking practice. A short and simple stretching routine at the beginning and end of your walk will help you avoid injury. It will also support detoxification by stimulating the lymphatic system and increasing oxygenation. Areas of the body that are particularly important for walkers to stretch include the calves, quadriceps (located at the front of the thigh), hamstrings (at the rear part of the thigh), and back.

Remember to stretch slowly and don't overdo it. You don't want to stretch to the point of pain. Go into the position as far as feels right to you. Avoid bouncing and instead hold the position steadily for 10 to 20 seconds. Release your body gently and slowly. Over time, your body will become increasingly flexible. There are many good books on stretching that you can consult for specific positions. Yoga, which is discussed below, can also be used to help you stay limber.

Once again, to gain the aerobic benefits, you'll want to sustain your movement for at least 20 minutes three times a week. Also, walk at a

---

NEW STUDY SHOWS EXERCISE HELPS LIFT DEPRESSION IN DIAGNOSED PATIENTS

Exercise works just as well in relieving depression as a popular prescription drug, Zoloft. That's according to a new study at Duke University Medical Center. Researchers found that a "modest exercise program" effectively reduced or eliminated symptoms in patients with major depression. And it even seemed to do a better job than Zoloft in preventing symptoms from coming back once the depression had ceased.

This latest study was a follow-up to earlier research in which 156 volunteers participated in a four-month study of exercise, Zoloft, and depression. The new investigation focused on whether the benefits from exercise would continue. Results indicate that participants who stuck with exercise for four months were far less likely to have the depression return than those who just took the drug or utilized a combination of the drug and exercise.[2]

Various forms of exercise could be performed by the participants who went the physical activity route. These included brisk walking, stationary bike riding, or jogging. They exercised for 30 minutes three times a week. This was in combination with 10-minute warm-up and 5-minute cool-down sessions.

It's not known exactly why the exercise was effective. Proving that mood-elevating body chemicals called endorphins were responsible is difficult. Zoloft works by regulating another body chemical, serotonin.

While the reasons were unclear, the results are encouraging. Exercise is a resource most people can take advantage of and its side effects are quite positive!

brisk pace. If you've been inactive, stroll along at your own rate for shorter amounts of time, and increase the speed and duration as you become more fit. Set your goal to eventually be 30 to 60 minutes of brisk walking most days.

Some items helpful to take along on your walk are a sun visor or hat, sunglasses, fanny pack (why carry more than you need?), and a small amount of emergency cash/fun money. Also make sure you bring an adequate but not excessive supply of water. As you amble onward, you'll lose body moisture through sweat. Replenishing your supply by drinking water will prevent dehydration and aid the detoxification process.

For a natural sunscreen, try jojoba oil. Though sunlight is important for health, we must now be extra careful because the erosion of the ozone layer has dramatically increased the rates of skin cancer. Pure jojoba oil is an inexpensive, natural sunscreen, and it's also good for your skin.

Remember to dress comfortably in loose-fitting clothes made of fibers that will allow your skin to breathe. Bring a long-sleeved shirt that you can put on if overexposure to the sun becomes a concern. Layered cold-weather clothing or rain gear can keep you walking in winter and on rainy days.

As you walk, let go of your cares and truly enjoy the experience of movement. Allow your senses to come alive and take in the wonder of our world. Think of your walks as a self-nurturing practice rather than a chore. You can use the time to clear your mind from the thoughts of life's challenges and to allow creative inspiration to flow. Vary your routines and walking times to keep this activity interesting for you.

■ Yoga

In addition to walking, yoga is a wonderful practice that can be done regularly to support your body's natural detoxification processes. It can also improve one's physical fitness, emotional balance, and spiritual outlook. This ancient system of physical postures, breathing exercises, and meditation techniques has been evolving for over 4,000 years. One reason it supports detox is that as you twist, bend, and stretch, your internal organs and spine are gently massaged. Thus cleansing and repair processes are stimulated. Also, integrated deep and conscious breathing brings invigorating and healing oxygen to every cell of the body. In addition, yoga provides an opportunity to cleanse the mind and spirit through meditation and mindfulness.

YOGA'S MANY FORMS

One of the first things you discover when exploring yoga is that there are many different varieties available. Below is a sampling of what you're likely to find here in the States. Note that those just beginning a yoga practice are wise to train with a teacher at first, rather than learning from a book or video. An instructor can catch any mistakes in form before they become an ingrained pattern.

Hatha: This form of yoga is the most familiar type in the West. It focuses on stretching and strengthening the body, and balancing the left and right brain hemispheres. In the United States, hatha yoga classes are widely available.

Sivananda: A gentle form of yoga, Sivananda is deeply spiritual. Basic elements of the system are correct postures, breathing skills, relaxation, positive thinking, and meditation. Positions emphasize strength and flexibility of the spine.

Kundalini: Once available only to a select group, Kundalini was brought to the States in 1969. It too features an integration of spirituality and exercise. In addition to postures, the system includes dynamic breathing, chanting, and meditation. One goal is to awaken spiritual energy.

Bikram: Studios teaching Bikram yoga are especially conducive for detox since room temperatures are kept high (nearly 100°). This is done to mimic the conditions in which the positions were originally performed. Sweating is seen as a way to move toxins out of the body. Twenty-six postures address the proper functioning of body systems.

Iyengar: This form of yoga was designed by prominent yogi, B.K.S. Iyengar, who resides in India and still teaches even in his 80s. The emphasis here is on deeply experiencing the richness of each pose. Positions are held for longer periods than in other types of yoga. Attention is paid to achieving correct muscular and skeletal alignment.

Ashtanga: Growing in popularity, this practice uses postures done in a quick sequence. The core of this system is six series of postures of varying levels of difficulty. Breathing helps you keep up with the rapid pace of this intense form of yoga.

Restorative: This type of yoga focuses on stress reduction, relaxation, and rejuvenation. Restorative yoga is great when you don't want a strong workout, but still want the benefits of yoga, especially increased circulation. This form is also suggested for those who cannot engage in intense physical activity due to limiting health challenges.

Power Yoga: Originating from a book of the same title, rigorous Power Yoga was developed by author Bender Birch who gave a Western spin to Ashtanga yoga. The emphasis here is on strength, flexibility, and continued movement.

Confused about which branch of yoga is right for you? Try a type of yoga that seems to match your fitness level and personal goals. Check out different classes until you find one you enjoy. Be careful not to push too hard too soon.

The focus of this Eastern practice was originally spiritual enlightenment. Today there is a growing recognition that yoga also has much to offer in maintaining health and in healing the body. Among the conditions being studied in relationship to yoga are high blood pressure, asthma, pain and inflammation, symptoms of menopause, arthritis, heart disease, and carpal tunnel. One benefit often mentioned by those practicing yoga is its effectiveness in reducing stress. Many people find that a regular practice of yoga is simply a great way to develop a stronger and more flexible body.

A yoga practice consists of a series of exercises called the *asanas* (postures). Each posture focuses on the integration of the body, mind, and breath. Proper alignment of the spine is essential for the practice. There are literally thousands of asanas to learn, so the development of boredom is unlikely. Results of holding these positions include enhanced blood flow, total body conditioning, mental and physical relaxation, and an energizing of the body. Some of the well-known postures are the cobra, spinal twist, and shoulder stand.

Breath control or *pranayama* is used in yoga to help foster energy flow throughout the body. It also helps to quiet the mind. The form of breath used is often smooth and flowing thus encouraging calmness.

A heightened body awareness is among the many benefits of

performing yoga. Some long-time, serious devotees of yoga are even said to be able to control bodily functions (such as heart rate) that are normally thought of as involuntary.

▪ Rebounding

This form of exercise is particularly good for supporting detoxification. Rebound exercise is basically bouncing movements that are performed on a mini-trampoline. These relatively low-impact movements range from gentle bouncing, to walking in place, to exercising with moves that resemble those of an aerobics class, to stationery jogging. Rebounding's rhythmic bouncing action is great for stimulating the distribution of lymphatic fluid. Performed at an aerobic level, rebounding can also strengthen your heart muscle; over time, it may even improve blood flow when you're at rest! Because rebound exercise effectively promotes circulation and thus aids cleansing of the body at a deep level, it is sometimes referred to as "cellular exercise."

Jumping on a rebounder can be invigorating and fun! It's a convenient form of exercise because you work out in the privacy of your own home. Even a short session can improve your mental outlook and feelings of well-being. Because it boosts circulation, bouncing on a rebounder can be helpful in relieving pain and in healing the body. Rebound exercise is an efficient oxygenator of body tissues. Regular use improves agility and your sense of balance. Some turn to rebounding because it's easier on the joints than many other forms of exercise.

Surprisingly, the biomechanical stimulation that comes from rebounding can be greater than from jogging! For instance, the magazine *Alternative Medicine Digest* reports that a 150-pound person can burn 410 calories an hour when rebounding as compared to 355 while running.[3] This effect comes partly from the way the force of gravity acts upon the body during rebound exercise. At the uppermost part of each jump, you achieve weightlessness, but then you land with two to four times the force of gravity. This increases the weight resistance that is used during the exercise.

There are various types of rebounders available. An excellent quality rebounder is appropriately called the Lympholine. This product appears to be the sturdiest rebounder on the market, offering full-suspension and excellent support. See the Resource section for more information.

As someone committed to daily exercise, I've found that my

rebounder is the only piece of exercise equipment I own that does not collect dust! Various forms of exercise are enjoyable to me; I usually spend my exercise time outdoors either walking, running, cycling, hiking, or practicing yoga. For the times when I'm not able to do my exercise outdoors due to the weather or time constraints, I love exercising on the Lympholine. I play a few of my favorite CDs and enjoy varying my movements to the music. With other pieces of equipment, such as a stairclimber or treadmill, I've found the restriction of movement too limiting. As a result, it seemed I was more focused on the time *(How much longer do I have to do this?)* than on enjoying the routine.

At those times when you can't get outside for a walk, try a 20-minute session on the rebounder. As an adjunct to a walking program, just three to five minutes of rebounding a day will help improve the flow of lymphatic fluid. If you're not going to have a whole 20 minutes or so for a workout, you can still feel a difference with just a few minutes a day. In fact, people who are at desks all day can simply get up periodically and jump for a few minutes to feel refreshed and increase their blood and lymphatic circulation.

■ Movement Unlimited

Movement is essential to optimal health. It is important for your exercise routine not to feel like a chore. You want to enjoy moving your body—not feel like you are doing something you "have to do." In addition to the exercise forms most often considered, there are various forms of **dance** that give you a great workout and can be a lot of fun. Instruction in *salsa, hip-hop, jitterbug, jazz, tap, swing, and belly dancing* is widely available. Also, taking a long **bike ride** or **hike** in a scenic area is often so enjoyable you forget you are exercising. (Quite a contrast from the stationary bike at the gym.)

Internal martial arts are increasing in popularity. **Qi Gong** and **tai chi** are ancient Chinese exercises that combine movement, meditation, and breath. Studies consistently show these Eastern practices to be very effective in decreasing stress, enhancing the immune response, and increasing detoxification. Classes in Qi Gong and tai chi are offered at martial arts studios, community fitness centers, and even some hospitals.

Note to Readers: Be careful not to fall into the trap of thinking "more is better" when it comes to exercise. Be aware of your current fitness level before you engage in any physical activity. Select an exertion amount that is appropriate for you at this point. Jumping into too rigorous an activity can result in injury, and then you may end up sitting on the sidelines for a while. Increase your time and the intensity of your workouts gradually as you become more fit. If you are dealing with a current health concern, check in with your doctor before you start an exercise program.

HYDROTHERAPY

A variety of water therapies *(hydrotherapies)* are available to assist you in your detoxification. These range from saunas, to steam baths, to epsom salt soaks, to aromatherapy baths, to warm body packs. Most of these approaches dramatically increase circulation, and they all encourage cleansing through skin pores as you sweat. Sweating helps bring toxins to the surface of your skin so they can be eliminated. Many of the practices also clear pores of clogged debris—including "dead" cells, amassed oils, and tiny dirt particles—so more toxins can exit through this route. Since our bodies normally eliminate about 25% of all toxins through the skin, you can greatly benefit from further stimulating this type of detoxification.

An important aspect of hydrotherapy is the use of hot and cold temperatures. Heat encourages the deeper flow of blood and lymph throughout the body as vessels dilate. Thus toxins can be removed in areas where the circulation of these fluids had been sluggish. Higher temperatures also boost body functions—including heart rate and metabolism. As temperatures rise, these body processes become more efficient, and thus detoxification is enhanced. If cold is used as a follow-up to heat, circulation is further improved as tissues constrict and move fluids and toxins along.

The hydrotherapies are among the most pleasant practices related to detoxification. In addition to improvements in health related to detox, another benefit many of the therapies bring is deep relaxation. Saunas, steam baths, and aromatherapy baths are wonderful ways of taking time to be gentle and nurturing to yourself. There is nothing you need to do but let go and allow your body, mind, and spirit to relax, cleanse, and heal.

■ Saunas & Steam Baths

The enjoyment of saunas and steam baths is nothing new. Among the most famous and long-time indulgers are the people of Finland; virtually every home in Finland has a sauna. Their traditional saunas have aspects of both the dry saunas and steam baths seen in American health clubs and spas today.

Another famous tradition is that of the Turkish bath, which is more like our steam rooms. The Turkish bath has roots in the Muslim culture where its rituals incorporate religious beliefs. In Muslim countries, visits to a Hamman or bathhouse equipped with a central steam facility were a popular activity for centuries. It is still done there today, though not as widely. Turkish baths, a derivative of the Hamman, have been in use throughout Europe since the mid-1800s and can also be found in the U.S.

Both dry saunas and steam baths are among the most efficient ways of driving toxins out of the body. These approaches can be especially helpful for those individuals who have had extreme over-exposures to toxins, such as on the job or through illicit drug use. In fact, some people who have used these forms of hydrotherapy report that they could actually smell the chemicals that were leaving their bodies. Dry saunas, in particular, have become an essential part of specialized programs dealing with recovery from drug abuse or environmental illness. Research has shown sauna therapy to be effective in the removal of pesticides and heavy metals.[4]

Dry saunas and steam baths are usually kept at temperatures ranging from 140° to 170° Fahrenheit.

SPAS: "The Detox Solution" in Action

A great place to experience the benefits of hydrotherapy, massage, exercise, etc., is a spa. Today, many spas offer detoxification programs and classes to deepen your awareness of the points covered in *The Detox Solution*. Being away from your daily routine, usually in a beautiful location, is a great opportunity to encourage, learn, and incorporate new beneficial lifestyle habits. Spas offer healthy and delicious cuisine, body treatments, aromatherapy, exercise classes, yoga instruction, and more. For more information on spas throughout the world, check out *www.spa.com*, *www.spaindex.com*, *www.spas.about.com*, *www.spamagazine.com*, and *www.healingretreats.com*.

Since you'll be losing fluid as you sit in this high heat, be sure to drink a glass or two of pure water beforehand, and take bottled water in with you to sip. Your body will lose about a pint of water in a quarter hour. Just 10 to 15 minutes is all you should do for starters. Follow this with a cold shower. Use shower water that is as cold as you can tolerate.

Though many people love unwinding in a dry sauna, some favor steam baths. Try both and see which you prefer. You may like both. Indulge in a sauna or steam bath once or twice a week to support your detoxification and general health.

Note that pregnant women should not use saunas or steam baths. These types of hydrotherapy are also not recommended for children. Anyone with a history of abnormal blood pressure or heart disease should consult their doctor first, and proceed slowly. Professional supervision can be necessary for using saunas or steam baths for more intense detox purposes, such as after long-term chemical exposures at work or in drug/alcohol rehab.

■ Aromatherapy Baths

Essential oils derived from plants can also assist the detoxification process. One way to enjoy them is to add the oils to your bath for a pleasurable and detoxifying soak. Doesn't it sound appealing? The Egyptians were among the first to distill plant essences—some 6,000 years ago! Traditionally, natural oils have been used to foster health and well-being. Today sources of essential oils include flower petals, fruit, seeds, nuts, bark, leaves, and roots.

Each essential oil is different in its aroma and effects. For this reason, you'll want to give some thought to which ones you'll choose for your bath. The oils can be used one at a time or in combination, depending upon the results you desire. The sidebar on the next page, "Properties of the Essential Oils," will introduce you to the qualities of some of the most popular essential oils.

When you're ready for your aromatherapy bath, run a tub full of hot water, and then add a six to eight drops of the essential oil (or oils) of your choice. Stir the water with your hand to spread the oil throughout. Relax in the bath for about 10 to 20 minutes. Run more hot water as needed.

Note that essential oils can be stored and used over a period of about one year. They should be kept in a cool, dark place. Make sure the lid is tightly closed when you put the flask away.

PROPERTIES OF THE ESSENTIAL OILS

Each essential oil has its own personality. The list below provides the dominant qualities of some of the essential oils that seem most favored. Note that some essential oils should never be applied directly to the skin. Because these oils are highly concentrated, burning and irritation can result if they are used full strength. Be sure to read the label carefully to see if this is the case with the oil you are using.

Balancing: Angelica, geranium, peppermint, sandalwood, ylang ylang.

Detoxifying: Basil, birch, cypress, eucalyptus, fennel, garlic, geranium, ginger, grapefruit, juniper, lavender, marjoram, olibaum, peppermint, rosemary, rose.

Emotionally Uplifting/Anti-Depressant: Bergamot, chamomile, clary sage, geranium, grapefruit, jasmine, lavender, orange, rose, sandalwood, ylang ylang.

Energizing/Circulation Enhancing: Basil, bay, bergamot, cinnamon leaf, citronella, lemon, lemongrass, patchouli, rosemary, spearmint, thyme.

Pain Relieving: Bergamot, chamomile, lavender, marjoram, rosemary, cypress, wintergreen.

Sedating/Relaxing/Anti-Anxiety: Bergamot, cedarwood, clary sage, frankincense, juniper, lavender, marjoram, rose, sandalwood.

Some companies provide blends of oil that are pre-mixed for specific purposes. As mentioned in Chapter 3, it is important to use high-quality oils derived from organically-grown plants. Companies that offer these products include Jurlique (*www.jurlique.com*) and Simplers (*www.simplers.com*).

▪ Epsom Salt Soaks

A naturally occurring substance, epsom salt consists of magnesium, sulfur, hydrogen, and oxygen. It's sometimes referred to as "magnesium sulfate." The name epsom salt comes from the village of Epsom in England where this mineral was found in spring water in the early

DAILY DETOX IN THE SHOWER

Here's an easy-to-use hydrotherapy technique that you can apply in the shower each day to stimulate circulation of lymph and blood. Simply end your shower by luxuriating a few moments under a downpour of comfortably hot water. Once you're quite warm, follow this up with a rinse of icy water for several minutes. In addition to boosting circulation, you will also feel rejuvenated by this practice!

1600s. By the late 17th Century, word had spread, and the town had become a popular destination for those seeking rejuvenation. Epsom salt is mined in many locations today. You'll find it for sale at most drug stores, health food stores, and supermarkets.

To prepare this type of bath, you'll want to add about 2 cups of epsom salts to comfortably hot water as your tub fills. Agitating the water with your hand will help the salts to dissolve. When the bath is full, step in and make sure you immerse as much of your body as possible. Your bath should last for about 10 to 20 minutes. Add more hot water when necessary.

You'll find that the epsom salt soak will bring about profuse perspiration. To boost this effect, prepare a hot herbal tea (such as peppermint or yarrow) ahead of time that you can sip as you bathe. Drinking the tea will also help you rehydrate.

When you're done with your soak, exit the tub carefully as you might feel slightly light-headed. As the water drains, visualize toxins, worries, and stress floating away. Rinse off your body lightly with lukewarm water, and pat your skin dry.

Because this soak is likely to make you feel drowsy, it's best to take it just before bedtime. The magnesium in epsom salts soothes sore muscles and will profoundly relax you. You're likely to find that you have a very restful sleep, though you will probably continue to sweat. In the morning, rinse off your body again and apply a natural body oil.

An epsom salt soak can be enjoyed once a week.

Note that epsom salt soaks are not recommended if you have abnormal blood pressure or eczema.

▪ ## Warm Body Pack

This last hydrotherapy technique utilizes the simple props of a filled hot water bottle, a bottle of castor oil, a small piece of flannel, a few towels, and a warm blanket. The purpose of the practice is to stimulate blood and lymph flow in the abdomen, enhance liver detoxification, encourage muscle relaxation, and support bowel elimination. It is particularly helpful for those suffering from irritable bowel syndrome, irregularity, or menstrual discomfort.

First, place a towel on the bed where your lower back will fall (to prevent oil from dripping on the sheet). Next, take about a capful of castor oil and apply it to your stomach between your pubic bone and rib cage. Then lie down in bed, and lay the flannel sheet over the oiled area. Put the water bottle on top of the flannel, and cover everything with towels to keep the heat in. Have a blanket handy to throw over you so you won't get chilled. Lie in this position and relax for about 20 minutes. This is a good time to meditate or to practice positive visualization techniques.

When you're through, drink a glass or two of water flavored with a few drops of juice from a fresh lemon. Rest for five or ten minutes before you clean up.

SKIN BRUSHING

A traditional healing practice that is helpful for boosting both blood and lymph circulation is dry skin brushing. As the name implies, this practice simply consists of applying a brush to dry skin with quick, short strokes.

Along with promoting circulation, dry brushing also exfoliates the skin, clearing the pores of dead tissue. With regular application of this technique, your skin will feel softer and smoother over time. It will also take on a healthier appearance—almost a "glow." Your immune system will be stimulated as well. Skin brushing also assists in breaking down cellulite.

To use this technique, you'll need a long-handled, natural-bristle skin brush; these are sold at most health food stores. Don't opt for nylon or synthetic bristles, as they can be too rough on the skin. You'll usually want to time your brushing for just before your daily shower or bath. If you use the dry sauna or steam bath, you could dry brush afterwards before you wash up.

When skin brushing, begin with the sole of one foot. Move up the front and back of one leg, and then end on that side with your buttock. Repeat with the other leg, starting again with the foot.

Next, brush your hands and arms, moving up each side separately as you did with your legs. Begin with the fingers of one hand. Then brush both the palm and the back of the hand. Progress up your arm toward your armpit. Repeat on the other side.

Brush your shoulders, neck, and back, and then move to the chest. As you do your front, move the brush toward your heart. Brush more softly over the breasts and avoid the nipples.

As you finish with your stomach, brush it in a clockwise direction. This will stimulate the digestive tract.

In all, this whole process should take no more than five minutes! It may take some practice to perform it that quickly in a relaxed manner. Shower or bath after the skin brushing is complete.

When your dry skin brushing becomes an established routine, you'll be able to increase the pressure a little bit incrementally. However you shouldn't rub so hard that your skin becomes red. Even at the right pressure, dry skin brushing may seem slightly painful at times. When this occurs, use a lighter stroke but continue onward.

Never share a skin brush, and be sure to rinse it with warm water after each use. Hang the brush in a open area where it can dry out.

MASSAGE

Massage has long been a part of the healing arts. Records show that the Chinese used therapeutic massage as long ago as 3,000 B.C. In fact, many modern systems of massage have evolved from these ancient techniques. Today massage is viewed as an effective way of reducing stress and relieving pain. Alternative practitioners also recognize massage as a practice that supports detoxification in various ways.

For instance, during massage, lymphatic fluid is moved along as fingers do their work. Blood vessels dilate so cardiovascular circulation is also improved. And when body tissue and fat stores are massaged, toxins are released for faster elimination. For these reasons and others, it's a good idea to drink pure water after a massage to minimize the symptoms of increased detoxification; the added fluid allows the body to remove toxins more rapidly.

There are various types of massage to choose from:

Swedish massage is a popular form of soft-tissue bodywork involving vigorous movements. Developed by massage pioneer Peter Ling of Sweden during the early 19th Century, it combines ancient techniques from China with more modern concepts. Swedish massage works well with a detoxification program because facilitating improved circulation of blood and lymph fluid is a major focus. Other goals are to calm the nervous system and generate profound relaxation. To prepare for a Swedish massage, the client usually undresses and is draped with a sheet. Subsequent massage motions—including gliding, kneading, tapping, and friction techniques—work the major muscle groups.

Shiatsu massage comes from Japan and is centered on an Oriental system of channels (meridians) of life energy. It also incorporates acupressure or pressure points. This is a deeper tissue technique than the Swedish system as practitioners utilize their own weight (rather than just muscle strength) to stimulate the meridians. So you'll find that elbows and knees may be used along with fingers and hands to deeply manipulate body tissue. Higher feelings of energy rather than deep relaxation are the main goal here. It's not customary for patients to undress for a shiatsu massage, so wear nonrestrictive, comfortable clothing.

Today there are also professionals who are trained specifically in moving lymphatic fluid through vessels and nodes during a gentle massage. This technique was developed by Emil Vodder in Denmark during the 1930s and is referred to as *Manual Lymphatic Drainage* (MLD). In MLD, touch is centered on circular kneading movements that vary in intensity. Areas closer to the center of the body are worked on first. Motions are repeated in a rhythmic fashion in one location before moving on.

When choosing a professional for any type of bodywork, a primary consideration should be the comfort level you sense with that individual. You should be able to relax and express your needs. If you are already working with an alternative practitioner in another field, he or she may be able to refer you to a bodyworker with solid training and experience.

BREATH WORK

Many people think of breathing as involuntary; they don't realize that our breathing technique can be refined. Yet detoxification and your general health can be greatly improved by a heightened awareness of and greater skill with this function. Once you are trained in better techniques, the healthier patterns can become the automatic way you breathe.

Michiko Rolek, author of *Mental Fitness* and *Black Belt for the Soul*, has spent many years teaching the importance of breathing. She comments, "Breathing keeps us alive. Yet unless we lose our breath running up a flight of stairs, we scarcely notice or appreciate its power. The Eastern arts and sciences, on the other hand, approach the breath with deep respect. It is seen as pure energy, or Chi, a healing force harmonizing mind and body." In Rolek's book, *Mental Fitness,* you'll find various breathing exercises that you can try.

One common problem is shallow breathing; this approach cheats the body of the optimal intake of oxygen that might otherwise be achieved. Shallow breathers take air only into their chest instead of breathing fully into the abdomen. They exhale from the chest as well. Not only does this type of respiration limit detoxification, it can also contribute to anxiety and stress. In contrast, proper breathing (deep respiration) enhances detoxification and promotes relaxation.

Another complication regarding our breath is that recent findings indicate the air itself may have as little as 50% of the oxygen it once contained![5] This was revealed after air bubbles were discovered that had been trapped for years in fossilized amber. Sadly, the oxygen content of our air appears to still be declining. As you see, we really can't afford to compromise the depth of our breathing!

One way proper breathing directly assists detoxification is that the motions involved stimulate the flow of lymph. Stronger, deeper breaths simply result in stronger stimulation of lymph nodes and vessels in the region of the lungs. In this way, a buildup of stagnant lymphatic fluid can be prevented in the area. Also, when you take in more oxygen with fuller breaths, higher amounts of this life-enhancing element are available for distribution to cells throughout the body. This added oxygen in turn can help the body break down and eliminate toxins at the cellular level. Lastly, you'll be expelling more of the toxin carbon dioxide and ridding the lower lungs of other waste gases when you exhale more fully.

Take a moment now to notice the way you normally breathe. Would you describe it as shallow or deep? If you're not sure, lie down on your back in your bed for a quick test. Place one hand on your stomach and one on your chest. Which one moves first? If it is your chest, you're probably not breathing deeply enough.

TRAINING YOURSELF TO BREATHE MORE DEEPLY

Breath work is one way to make sure that you're using more than just the top portion of your lungs. The following simple exercise can help train your body to breathe deeply on a regular basis.

1. Lie on your bed with pillows under your head and knees. Your hands should be resting on your stomach just above the navel.
2. Breathe fully into your abdomen. Notice how your hands rise.
3. Breathe out and assist your body by pushing gently downward with your hands.
4. Repeat the exercise ten times.
5. Lie still for a moment before rising.

Practice this exercise once or twice a day until you feel deeper breathing has become routine for you. In addition to practicing breathing exercises, the practices of yoga and meditation also train the breath to be more efficient.

Proper breathing is important to support the body in many ways besides enhancing detoxification. It can help elevate moods, strengthen the immune system, promote healing, improve the quality of your sleep, and even decrease your risk of cardiovascular complications. Every cell in the body requires a continuous, rich supply of oxygen in order to survive. Yes, oxygen is an essential nutrient. We can only live for a few moments without it!

▪ Acupuncture

Acupuncture has been used for thousands of years to enhance energy flow throughout the body. Research has shown that when needles are inserted into the skin at specific locations, the electrical signals in the body are boosted, enhancing circulation and reducing stress. In addition to encouraging healthy blood and lymph circulation, acupuncture has a unique ability to encourage the flow of *qi*, or life force. Also, studies have consistently demonstrated the effectiveness of acupuncture for detoxification.

▪ Strong Circulation – Part of Basic Maintenance

As you now know, there are many ways that you can assure that your circulation is strong. You can think of these techniques as part of your regular health maintenance "bag of tricks." Just as you wouldn't neglect oil changes and tune-ups for your car, it's wise to make sure that the cells of your body are properly maintained through strong circulation. One of the major duties of circulation is to remove toxins at a cellular level.

WHAT'S AHEAD

Now that many of the areas of physical detox have been presented, we'll move on to the emotional and spiritual aspects of detoxification. While the ways we work with our emotions and Spirit definitely affect the body, they are also important, separate dimensions of detox that deserve special attention. Each one has an entire chapter devoted to it.

In the next chapter, you'll have an opportunity to examine whether you are handling your emotions in constructive or harmful ways. You will discover tried-and-true suggestions for gaining greater emotional wisdom that have worked time and time again for many. Our emotions have such a great influence on whether we experience daily life with joy or apprehension. Using the tools in the next chapter will allow you to experience a greater sense of inner peace and well-being.

THIRTEEN

Emotional Wisdom:
Transforming the Stress Response

When you repress your emotions, you are
working against them. When you express them
harmfully, you are working for them. To experience
them honorably means working with them, so they
can heal and protect you as they were meant to.

— Karla McLaren, author, *Emotional Genius*

In the mid-90s, psychologist Daniel P. Goleman gained attention by
challenging the notion that IQ was the single most important factor
for succeeding in life. In his book, *Emotional Intelligence,* he asserted
that the ability to manage our emotions is actually a much more significant element than mere brain power. Since then, other works—such as
Karla McLaren's recent audio book *Emotional Genius*—have furthered
this line of thought and introduced methods for developing emotional
competency. In this chapter, we will explore how emotional patterns can
either enhance our well-being or contribute to our toxic load. This chapter also supplies helpful background on related subjects, such as the
effects of emotional stress on our bodies. For the purposes of this book,
you can think of using Chapter 13 for an "emotional detox."

Over the years, I have observed that detoxification and emotional well-being are intimately linked. When physical detoxification is

accomplished, it's much easier to explore where you need to grow in dealing with your emotions. This is because your emotional life can often be influenced by such factors as a high sugar intake or symptoms of a toxic overload. Consequently, you will find yourself more in touch with your true feelings after detoxing. You'll also be less reactive to external events. On the other hand, if you habitually experience a lot of negative emotions, the body's natural detoxification pathways (as well as your overall health) will consequently be compromised.

Today many people feel challenged by their emotional responses, and prescriptions for antidepressants and tranquilizers are at an all-time high. In our "faster-than-ever, never-slow-down" society, this should come as no surprise. Over 17 million Americans have taken Prozac (about 35 million people worldwide), and sales for Prozac, Paxil, and Zoloft combined are estimated at $4 billion a year.[1] Do all of these people really need to be on mood-enhancing drugs? Many people have found such medications to be helpful, but this treatment is often not correcting or identifying the person's underlying problems. Often the medications also have uncomfortable and potentially dangerous side effects. We have yet to observe the long-term consequences of these medications. However, when we supply the body, mind, and spirit with the essentials for optimal living, we have a good chance of experiencing healthier moods.

Many people on antidepressants or tranquilizers are concerned about their reliance on such prescription drugs to manage their emotional state. My own patients have asked about alternatives. They express a desire to be the master of their emotions without having to take such strong "happy pills" every day. For others, emotional challenges are dealt with through overeating, substance abuse, or just plain repression and denial. This chapter is included in *The Detox Solution* to offer effective ways to create a healthier emotional life.

Let's start by exploring some basic background about an important aspect of our emotional health—that is, our relationship to and awareness of stress. Stress is a common reason that many people give for turning to medications or negative coping patterns. Since stress is a part of all our lives to some degree, it's important to understand it thoroughly.

EMOTIONAL STRESS & DISEASE

In the book so far, we've explored the effects of stress in terms of physical toxins. You learned that the amount of toxins in our environment and food can far exceed our body's ability to deal with them. Thus these toxins are *stressors* to our system. In everyday life, most people think of an *emotional overload* when they hear the word *stress*. It's this emotional type of stress that we will focus on now.

When do we become *emotionally stressed?* This occurs when *the demands on our resources **appear** to exceed our capacity for achieving balance and well-being*. At these times, our sense of security seems threatened. Emotional stress can then take on physical manifestations that add to the complications of one's life.

In recent years, a rapidly growing field of research called *psychoneuroimmunology (PNI)* has verified the strong effects that thoughts and feelings have on one's physical health. This interrelationship is often referred to as the *mind-body connection.* Thousands of studies have noted the influence of thoughts and emotions on our physical well-being. We've learned that positive emotional influences can help someone heal. Conversely, a pattern of negative or toxic emotions—such as fear, resentment, and anger—can contribute to ill health and disease.

Again, like physical stressors (such as toxic chemicals), emotional stressors can be handled by our bodies when they stay below a certain level. That's because our body is designed to bring us back to a state of equilibrium after an occasional experience of strong negative emotions. However, when the emotional stress is extreme and continues for prolonged periods, we begin to get into trouble.

Hans Selye, an endocrinologist, created a classic three-phase model for what occurs in the body during periods of prolonged emotional stress. First, our system goes into a state of mobilization that Selye termed the *alarm phase.* Also known as the *fight or flight response*, this initial phase readies the body for immediate action. We notice that our heart begins to beat rapidly, our body starts to sweat, and that we feel a surge of adrenaline. Scientists believe this is a built-in response designed to protect us from danger.

If the stress continues, we then enter a second phase called *resistance.* Here the body gets additional assistance to continue to respond to the stress temporarily. This aid comes in the form of cortisol and other stress hormones secreted by the adrenal glands. An individual entering this phase continues to respond to the stressor as a threat, and has not yet utilized techniques to perceive it differently. When the stress

MEASURING THE EFFECTS OF STRESS: The Adrenocortex Stress Profile

When your body has a stress response, levels of the hormone cortisol become elevated in your system. Cortisol is an important chemical that is involved in the body's energy level, immune response, detoxification efficiency, thyroid function, anti-inflammatory response, and cardiovascular performance. Repeated stress reactions—and resulting continued oversecretion of cortisol—can affect health in many ways. Research has shown that unhealthy cortisol patterns are linked to depression, schizophrenia, poor memory, chronic fatigue syndrome, immune suppression, accelerated aging, obesity, hypertension, heart disease, osteoporosis, menstrual problems, thyroid disorders, anorexia nervosa, Cushing's Syndrome, Addison's Syndrome, HIV, and AIDS.[2]

Specialty labs have a test that measures cortisol patterns. It may be referred to as an "Adrenocortex Stress Profile." This test also looks at DHEA levels, another hormone that is intimately involved in the stress response. I have used the test with many patients. It helps me determine how stress responses might be affecting the person's physical health. Having these lab results is useful in tailoring a protocol that is specific for the patient. I highly recommend anyone with a high-stress lifestyle to have this test done and to seek professional guidance for "getting off the fast track" of life. See Chapter 15, "Maximize Your Plan: Working with a Health Professional," for more information on tests that can be performed to evaluate the stress response and its effect on your health.

hormones of the resistance phase are released over too long a period of time, negative physical effects result. Immune response is lowered, changes in the digestive tract set the stage for irritable bowel syndrome and ulcers, blood pressure rises, insulin levels are adversely affected which can contribute to diabetes. With proper stress management, however, the body can instead return to its pre-stressed state.

If we stay in this second phase for an extended period, the stress can lead us to the third and final phase determined by Selye—*exhaustion.* Here the body's resources are depleted. A weakened immune system increases vulnerability to disease. Body functions can fail and specific organs may collapse.

As you can see, living in constant stress can lead to a health disaster. Numerous studies have shown that stress is a major contributor to many diseases. One project, at the University of California at Riverside, analyzed a hundred different studies on the relationship between people's emotional stress and their physical health. It found that being chronically anxious, pessimistic, depressed, or irritated actually doubles one's chances of developing a major disease!

This doesn't have to be your story. Stress can be dealt with in a healthier way. You'll learn how in this chapter. In a moment, we'll identify the specific stressors in your life and then review some emotional management techniques that can be helpful.

EVALUATING THE STRESS IN YOUR LIFE

It's important to be aware of the amount of emotional stress that you're attempting to cope with in your life. Remember how we assessed the physical stressors that were part of your environment and diet? In a similar way, we're now going to identify the specific *emotional stressors* that you're dealing with.

Take the time you need to think about your life and how you respond to external influences. Your responses will go a long way in helping you reduce your stress load.

Emotional Lifestyle Assessment

- Do you enjoy your work/co-workers?
- Do you feel reasonable job security?
- Are you in a supportive family/home environment?
- Do you have opportunities to express and receive love?
- Do you trust that you will always have enough of what you need?
- Do you have sufficient creative expression?
- Does your environment feel like a sanctuary, free of clutter?
- Do you make time for relaxation during the course of your day?
- Do you enjoy deep restful sleep?
- Do you take days off?

- Do you go on vacations?

- Are your relationships harmonious?

- Do you have a circle of friends who you can depend on?

- Are you involved in community activities, such as church, social, or professional organizations, support groups, or volunteerism?

- Are you virtually free of any significant health challenges?

- Have you accomplished a notable personal achievement in the past six months?

If you noticed that many of your answers are an enthusiastic "yes," congratulations! You have created a life that supports you emotionally. On the other hand, if you notice that you have more "no" answers than you would like, this is a good time to evaluate how you can improve the quality of your experience. Awareness of areas that need healing is the first step.

EMOTIONAL EMPOWERMENT

It is truly empowering to eliminate any emotional stressors that you realize need not be a part of your life. At the same time, realize that our *perception* of a circumstance is a major factor in whether or not we experience it negatively. In his famous play *Hamlet,* Shakespeare wrote, "There is nothing bad or good, but thinking makes it so." Our perceptions are so powerful that changing our thinking about something can even turn a negative stressor into a positive one.

Yes, there can be positive stress! Perhaps your frustration about an unfulfilling job or relationship will give you the extra push you need to move on. Instead of allowing your unhappiness to create obsessive thoughts about how bad things are, try using that energy to think of how to make a change. See your emotional messages as clues to what you need to do. Don't permit your feelings to drag you down. Acknowledge them, let them go, and then take action. Remember, responding in this way is not only a step toward creating a happier life. You will also be moving toward living in an emotional state that supports good health. Every thought we have has a powerful effect on the body.

In her booklet, "How to Heal Yourself from Toxic Emotions,"

medical authority Christiane Northrup, M.D., agrees that shifting your response to a stressor is key. She also suggests reducing the *frequency* of your exposure to those stressors that seem unavoidable. The example she gives is visiting in-laws. If a woman is experiencing stomachaches, panic attacks, or headaches when she spends time with her spouse's family, one thing she can consider is simply seeing them less often. Perhaps fewer exposures will give the woman the time she needs to change the way she views these individuals. She could also work on improving her responses to emotional situations and developing coping skills.

LOOKING AT YOUR EMOTIONAL HABITS

In this chapter so far, ideas about the importance of enhancing emotional health have been presented. You now understand the powerful link between your emotions and your physical health. You've identified your own particular stressors, and have some strategies to use to reduce their impact. Now let's dig a little deeper. It's time to assess the quality of your particular set of emotional habits.

Awareness is crucial to emotional management. How long does it take for you to realize that you've had an emotional reaction? Do you know at the time, or only realize it later? Each reader of this book will be at a different level of self-awareness.

Don't rush through the following assessment. It may take you a while to come up with an honest evaluation of your emotional response habits. If so, pay attention to your emotional patterns over the next week, or two, or three. Jot down any insights that arise along the way.

As you observe your responses, note whether your behavior most often fits what is described under Column A or Column B. If you feel it's about even, jot down A/B as your response.

Your Emotional Responses

Column A	Column B
▪ It's hard for me to relax.	▪ I can let go and relax easily.
▪ I often have a short fuse.	▪ I consider myself to be very patient.
▪ I'm easily irritated.	▪ It takes a lot to upset me.

- I don't tend to share my emotions.
- People often leave me feeling let down.
- I make assumptions and get disappointed.
- I'm reluctant to express my needs.
- It's hard for me to say no.
- Addictive behavior patterns —such as overeating, smoking, substance abuse, or overspending—are a part of my life.
- I "like" to stay busy all the time.
- I'm not very organized.
- I blame others.
- I let unaddressed issues linger.

- My thoughts are often negative.
- I don't feel very good about myself.
- It's hard for me to prioritize.

- My mind is too busy.
- I shut people out.
- My feelings overwhelm me.
- I feel compromised in many situations.
- I don't feel safe.

- I express my emotions productively.
- I'm aware of what I can expect from others.
- I make clear arrangements with others.
- I tell people what I need from them.
- I set limits regularly.
- I deal with my emotions directly.

- I balance my life—working, resting, playing.
- I plan and organize regularly.
- I take personal responsibility.
- I handle conflict as it comes up.

- I think in a very positive way.
- I think I'm terrific!

- I easily set priorities each day.

- My mind is often calm.
- I'm very open.
- I can handle what I feel.
- I make sure I take care of myself.
- I feel secure.

- I frequently live in emergency mode.

- I am in control and take proactive steps to manage my life.

If you find that you mostly identified with the statements in Column A, don't be too hard on yourself. You have a lot of room to grow! For those of you with fewer Column A considerations, recognize these as the areas where you need to do the work. In either case, for each A answer, look at the choice given under Column B. Think about how you could be responding differently. Begin to incorporate these new behaviors into your life.

If you had no A responses, think about the ways you can reinforce your positive behavior.

One of the most powerful forces in humankind is that of emotional expression. Emotions have led to destruction, artistic creation, war, peace, killing, healing, fighting, and making love. It's crucial to be aware of our emotional responses in order to live in harmony with others.

INTRODUCING THE "EMOTIONAL RESPONSE SYSTEM"

No matter who we are, there will be situations that challenge our ability to manage our responses. However, learning to manage our emotional reactions is empowering. Here is a seven-step system for keeping an emotional outburst in check. Let's call it our "Emotional Response System." The point is to experience and deal with the emotion without indulging it. Observe how you're feeling (rather than being consumed by it), and take productive action.

▪ During or near the emotional response:

1. **Recognize the shift in your physical state.** Do you feel as if you're about to cry? Are you in a sudden state of alertness? Do you have an aggressive desire to scream at someone or to attack him or her physically? Having this initial awareness will help you to become more of an observer to the situation; you'll eventually feel less consumed or overpowered.

2. **Start to breathe more slowly and deeply.** Gentle abdominal breathing will help you begin to calm down. Most emotional outbursts

are preceded by a period of poor breathing. By spending a few minutes working with your breathing patterns, you will slow down your nervous system. This will give you a chance to reevaluate the situation.

3. **Gain perspective with a *time out*.** Go into another room, step outside, or call a sympathetic friend to vent your feelings. It's virtually impossible to resolve problems when either party is in a charged emotional state. However, time heals and gives us an opportunity to see the truth in any situation. Why not use the blessing of healing time and avoid an emotional outburst?

4. **Spend time in quiet contemplation before confronting anyone.** You could meditate, pray, or spend time in nature. When you quiet your mind, solutions, truth, and clarity naturally unfold.

5. **The power of affirmation can help to change your perception of the situation.** Phrases such as "Things aren't always as they seem," "I am open to seeing this situation differently," or "I choose peace in this situation" allow your awareness to shift. With this new perspective, you create an opportunity for a healthier emotional response. There are always at least two sides to everything.

6. **When you're ready to talk, make sure you listen to the other perspective.** There might be a misunderstanding. Through dialogue, you may be able to develop a plan of action together.

7. **Make every effort to resolve the issue cleanly.** Don't give up until you get a resolution, or feel you've explored all the alternatives.

It feels so much better when we consistently deal with our emotions in a healthy manner. Holding onto our upset without giving it clear thought or taking tempered action is a recipe for continued aggravation. On the other hand, slamming another person with the full force of our emotions can result in a severed relationship. The next time you feel a charged outburst about to pop, try the Emotional Response System. You will notice over time how you will feel empowered with healthy emotional expression, as opposed to powerless over your outbursts.

PREVENTION: IT WORKS WITH EMOTIONAL HEALTH TOO!

There are many tools that you can incorporate into your daily life to help yourself avoid toxic emotional eruptions. Many of the tools listed below will assist you in gaining perspective. Once you start to see potentially upsetting situations as a small piece of your life, it will become easier to respond in a more productive way.

You've probably heard the expression "This too will pass." This is true for most of the situations that challenge us emotionally. Think now of earlier times when you were upset. The chances are great that you have moved on.

Here's a list of twenty-five proactive tools for preventing extreme emotional reactions by creating a balanced relationship with your feelings:

1. **Go within.** It's important to consistently engage in meditation, prayer, or some other form of introspection. These activities will help you tap into your inner resources. You'll find yourself producing creative solutions. You'll also become better acquainted with a Very Important Person (V.I.P.)—you!

2. **Rejuvenate yourself with a nature break.** Many people sit for hours each day in front of a computer, and their energies are slowly drained. Engaging in outdoor activities can replenish you. Don't let yourself become emotionally zapped. Recharge your emotional batteries by strolling through a park, watering your garden, or lying back in the grass and taking in the sky. When you have more time, take a contemplative walk in the woods or by a lake or the ocean.

3. **Watch out for information overload.** According to *The Longevity Strategy*, a book by David Mahoney and Richard Restak, M.D., one issue of the *New York Times* contains more information than the average person in the 17th Century encountered over a lifetime! With the development of the Internet and more electronic media available than ever, it is important to take inventory of just how much information your brain is processing daily. Be selective about how much and what kind of data you allow to permeate your being. In the Judaic tradition, the practice of the Sabbath discourages the use of electronic stimulation. Try a break at least once a week from the newspaper, television, and the Internet.

4. **Let your media influences be uplifting.** It is not just the amount but also the type of information that affects our emotional health. If you find yourself watching the news before you sleep and frequently viewing violent movies, these practices will tend to have a negative

residual effect. On the other hand, if you tend to view programs that are entertaining and uplifting, you will be adding positive influences to your experience.

5. **Make sure you get enough sleep.** It appears that Americans are working more, sleeping less, and feeling more tired than ever. You could be eating healthy and exercising regularly, but if you neglect the basic need of restful sleep, it is virtually impossible to create optimal health. People who skimp on their sleep usually feel emotionally vulnerable. If you have a "to do" list that is too long, cut some items and make getting more sleep a priority.

6. **For an uncluttered mind, create an uncluttered environment.** When our environments are cluttered, we tend to experience more frustration, confusion, or anxiety. Make a point of periodically getting rid of things you don't use. Emphasize beauty in your environment by keeping a vase of fresh flowers where you spend most of your time. If you need help with creating an environment that is conducive to emotional stability, you might consult with a feng shui practitioner. *Feng shui* is an ancient Chinese art of placement for the home or office that emphasizes balance and harmony of surroundings.

7. **Make a commitment to a regular yoga practice.** An underlying purpose of all the branches of yoga is to create a sense of balance and harmony in those who practice it. While your day might have been chaotic and rushed, performing yoga can assist you in finding your peaceful inner Eden. Eventually becoming centered through yoga, you will be able to respond in ways during your day-to-day life that are healthier emotionally. You won't be as easily jostled by challenging situations. In addition, breathing techniques used in yoga can help you release long-held tension. Chapter 12 on circulation includes information on the various yoga disciplines as well as other forms of exercise.

8. **Learn how to set healthy boundaries.** Many people feel "overbooked for life," but forget that they had a choice about making the appointments. When you set boundaries clearly, life doesn't overwhelm you. Perhaps you need to work on your assertiveness skills. Learn to spend more of your life doing what *you* actually want to do, and less of what you *think* others want for you.

9. **Make looking at the positive side a regular habit.** We all know at

least one person who seems to be able to find that silver lining in every storm cloud. We are lifted by their very presence because of this great attitude. This could also be you! To begin to put a more positive spin on life, try to look at the positive aspects of situations at every opportunity. Then when a more challenging circumstance comes up, your brain will be trained to look for the bright side. You'll be less likely to engage in a toxic emotional response.

10. **Just say "no!" to procrastination.** Instead of procrastinating, adopt a "take charge" approach. Procrastination can contribute to low self-esteem and anxiety, as you put off facing something but still worry about it. The pent-up tension can build up so much that it finally bursts! How much easier it is to just deal with it early on! If you find yourself avoiding taking action, explore the real reasons. Then find ways to become motivated about taking responsibility rather than dreading it.

11. **Cultivate a spirit of gratitude.** Being thankful for all that you have is a great habit. Unfortunately, many people focus on what they don't have. It seems that what we concentrate on in life expands, so a negative way of thinking can be a self-fulfilling prophecy. When you start feeling thankful, you'll find you have more and more to be thankful for. This is a very easy, fun, and effective tool for decreasing stressful emotional responses.

12. **Watch the words that you use.** Words that can cultivate toxic emotions include "should," "ought," "stress," "must," "busy," "worry," "he made me feel," "she made me do such and such," etc. Because it is often used to imply victimization, this language can allow us to feel powerless. Open up your options by searching for words of empowerment. These include "can," "will," "want," "choose," "love," and "peace." I often suggest a thirty-day "diet" from the words "worry," "busy," and "stress" for patients having emotional challenges. They learn to find more creative and empowering descriptions of how they are feeling, and their perception of difficulty often transforms. The results have been remarkable, including stress reduction and a greater capacity for joy and inner peace. The biblical phrase, "the Word was made flesh" can be witnessed personally through our choice of language, for we tend to embody what we speak.

13. **Speak well of others.** Avoid gossip. When discussing other people,

think of how you would like to be spoken about. I guarantee that it will feel better to find ways to be happy for others rather than sharing resentments about them. If you find yourself being tempted to say something negative about another person, see if you're bothered by a characteristic you are denying in yourself. When you accept that part of you, your feelings about the other person are likely to change.

14. **Discover mindfulness.** This essentially is the practice of living fully in the moment. One reason that children and animals are so therapeutic and enjoyable to be around is that they focus on the here and now. They're not worried about tomorrow or yesterday. They're just open to the joy of the present.

15. **Create community support for yourself.** Since we *do* live in a very reactive world, you'll benefit from reaching out to others striving to live at a healthier emotional level. You'll find such support at twelve-step programs, churches, meditation groups, etc. You'll also find kindred spirits at self-help workshops and classes.

16. **Foster your emotional growth through books, tapes, websites, and seminars.** There's such a richness of these resources today! For instance, check out O. C. Smith's Mind Power site (*www.ocsmiths mindpower.com*), and the books that are recommended there. After Smith's song "Little Green Apples" became a hit, he began to research positive thinking and the power of the mind. Since then, he has become an internationally-acclaimed motivational speaker, sharing his findings on the amazing potential of the mind. You'll find many useful tips on his site. Smith has also condensed his ideas into an audiotape series called *Mind Power* that is available through his site. Another excellent site loaded with tapes to foster empowerment is Nightingale-Conant (*www.nightingale.com*). An additional way to find ways to increase emotional growth is to browse the psychology and self-help sections of your local bookstores periodically.

17. **Journal your thoughts and feelings.** This practice will serve you in several ways. First, you'll discharge emotional upsets as you write them down on the page. Secondly, you'll have the opportunity to clarify your thoughts and feelings. And last, you'll have a record of your experiences, which will help you decipher your patterns.

18. **Schedule regular exercise on your appointment calendar.** Although

a sure way to lift your spirits is to get your body moving, how often do we abandon exercise for the sake of something that seems more pressing? Writing your exercise appointments on your calendar will help you keep the commitment. Also, choosing a nonstrenuous exercise, such as walking, can help you avoid downtime due to injuries. For more information on exercise, see Chapter 12.

19. **Try kindness.** The Dalai Lama says that kindness is his religion. A kind attitude is so needed in our oftentimes insensitive today. Turn up your compassion meter, and recognize those opportunities where you can make a difference. Stepping into a stranger's or even a loved one's shoes is also one of the best ways of gaining a kinder, gentler perspective.

20. **Develop Gumby's flexibility.** One way we set ourselves up for an emotional upset is by remaining rigid despite changing circumstances. Remember Gumby, the cartoon character? He's the one toy that didn't break because he was willing to bend. Flexibility is an important skill when used wisely.

21. **Be a student of life; look for your lessons.** As you grow stronger emotionally, a helpful approach is to view situations that challenge you emotionally as opportunities to make new choices. Is the salesperson rude? Instead of getting angry, find someone else to help you. Is a loved one inconsiderate? Instead of withdrawing, look for the right time to discuss the behavior. Working through one situation at a time will lead you away from victim behavior and teach you emotional courage.

22. **Practice patience.** One cause of unhappiness is a reluctance to wait for things to develop at their own pace. We can even steal some of our own joy in receiving by acting impatient about outcomes. Doing your best right now will further your best interests more than worrying about when something will happen. Next time you find yourself growing impatient, relax and let the tension go. Trust in the process of life.

23. **Build healing rituals into your life.** What rituals soothe your soul? Is it a weekly bubble bath by candlelight? A break-of-dawn stroll through your neighborhood? A quiet moment over herbal tea at the end of the day? Take the time to nourish yourself emotionally by practicing healing rituals regularly rather than falling into counterproductive, self-destructive activities.

24. **When making decisions, don't forget your heart!** To create a happy life, we must understand what is true for us individually. We have this knowledge when we take the time to listen to our heart. It's important to resist external pressures to make decisions based solely on the values of others. What is it that you *really* want for yourself? What are your values? What are your personal priorities?

25. **Enjoy and note your progress.** As you notice that circumstances you used to feel upset by no longer have a hold on you, you will begin to enjoy emotional empowerment. When you truly realize that your emotions can be great teachers instead of overwhelming enemies, life takes on a whole new meaning.

SOMETIMES PROFESSIONAL HELP IS NECESSARY

Some people find that they need professional help in accessing, sorting through, and working with their feelings. Their emotions may be somewhat blocked or perhaps cause confusion. Others seek assistance in developing behaviors that will better serve them. Professional counseling can also be called for at those times when you are facing a specific emotional crisis such as a death, life-threatening illness, or job loss.

There's great diversity in the therapy field, so you'll find that you have lots of options if you seek professional emotional support. One of the most important elements is going to be the *person* you choose, regardless of the orientation of their training. Whether you select a psychiatrist, psychotherapist, behavioral counselor, spiritual coach, or hypnotherapist, you'll want to pick someone who can get through to you, help you see where you're going

QUALITIES OF SUCCESS from Ralph Waldo Emerson

"To laugh often and much; to win the respect of intelligent people and the affection of children; to earn the appreciation of honest critics and endure the betrayal of false friends; to appreciate beauty; to find the best in others; to leave the world a bit better whether by a healthy child, a garden patch, or a redeemed social condition; to know even one life has breathed easier because you have lived. This is to have succeeded."

off track, and send you off after each session in the direction of growth.

A particular specialty may have more to offer you, depending on your goals. Think through how you want to grow. If you want to identify the underlying reasons for self-defeating patterns, long-term psychotherapy may be best. If you prefer shorter term support to drop a particular emotional crutch—such as smoking or overeating—hypnotherapy can be a good choice. If you need to work on becoming more assertive or in developing communication skills, a counselor with a behavioral approach might fit you well. Or if you hope to develop a deeper spiritual base and to experience more joy, a spiritual counselor may be right for you.

Often used as an adjunct to psychotherapy, *Neuro-Emotional Technique (NET)* is a powerful tool to release subconscious patterns that keep us from experiencing a positive emotional outlook. NET is used by psychotherapists and other health practitioners, and is effective in clearing negative response tendencies, including phobia and fear patterns. See Chapter 15 for more information.

On a related note, *massage* is another way to work through and release unresolved emotional tension. If you investigate massage as an option, you'll find that some types have more of an emphasis on incorporating emotional growth with bodywork. One such branch of massage, known as the Rosen Method, blends gentle touch with verbal communication to release suppressed emotions. For more information on the Rosen Method, go to *www.rosenmethod.org* on the web. For background on body-centered massage, see Chapter 12.

TRADITIONAL CHINESE MEDICINE & THE EMOTIONS

For over 5,000 years, the Chinese have known that emotions affect our health.

In Traditional Chinese Medicine (TCM), there is a sophisticated system of evaluating whether holding onto emotions such as anger, sadness, fear, and worry may be contributing to ill health. TCM offers very effective treatments for emotional balancing through the use of herbal formulas, acupuncture, meditation and internal martial arts techniques such as Qi Gong and Tai Chi. As a Chinese medicine practitioner, I have witnessed the improvement of the emotional health of many, mostly without the need for prescription medication. For more information on TCM, see Chapter 15.

WEEKEND GROWTH SPURTS

Weekend retreats or full-day seminars can be a fun way to learn emotional management techniques. One sponsor of such programs is the Heartmath Solution of Boulder Creek, California (*www.heart math.com*). During the weekend program, Heartmath teaches a scientifically-proven technique of reducing the stress response. Participants learn how to continue to monitor their improvements when they return home. This group offers innovative programs in eighteen cities; they address stress management, emotional intelligence, and relationship transformation.

FLOWER ESSENCES

A therapy that makes a remarkable contribution to emotional healing is the use of flower essences. These essences provide tremendous assistance on the journey to emotional well-being. Although flower essences have been used for thousands of years, their official development as a therapy is attributed to Dr. Edward Bach, an English physician who observed the emotional and spiritual dimensions of healing.

"True healing involves treating the very base of the cause of the suffering," Bach said. "Therefore no effort directed to the body alone can do more than superficially repair damage. Treat people for their emotional unhappiness, allow them to be happy, and they will become well."

Flower essence practitioners have reported profound shifts in the emotional well-being of their clients who have used this therapy. The essences are safe for most children, adults, and even animals. They are so helpful in transforming toxic emotions. The essences seem to increase our awareness of the true nature of the emotional stress response. They can assist your efforts to work through life's challenges in order to arrive at a place where you can regularly experience love, joy, peace, and harmony.

The following list is just some of the many flower essences that are available. Notice how they influence us in different ways.

▪ The Major Flower Essences & Their Qualities

Aspen: Replacing fear of the unknown with trust and confidence.

Cerato: Trusting intuition; transforming doubt and uncertainty.

Chicory: Experiencing unconditional love instead of codependency.

Holly: Opening the heart to love; releasing jealously, anger, and suspicion.

Honeysuckle: Being fully in the present; letting go of the past.

Impatiens: Increasing patience; letting go of irritation.

Mimulus: Transforming everyday fears and worries into confidence.

Mustard: Aiding in the reduction of depression.

Pine: Helping to heal guilt, self-blame, unacceptance of oneself; provides self-acceptance and self-forgiveness.

Rock Water: Increasing flexibility and the willingness to live in the flow; decreasing rigidity.

Scleranthus: Improving one's decision-making ability; decreasing confusion and hesitation.

Walnut: Letting go of influences from others; having the courage to follow one's destiny.

Water Violet: Helping to release an unnecessarily independent "I don't need anyone" attitude; encourages community.

White Chestnut: Promoting a calm, clear mind; reduces chattering, busy mind.

Wild Oat: Helping to clarify one's life purpose and direction.

Wild Rose: Supporting the will to live; experiencing joy in life.

Willow: Letting go of old resentments and anger; allowing acceptance and forgiveness to dominate emotions.

Just as there are thousands of flowers, there are thousands of flower essences. There are some great websites to help you further familiarize yourself with these empowering healers. These include: *www.flower essence.com*, *www.pacificessences.com*, and *www.starfloweressences .com*. It is best to work with a flower essence practitioner.

NUTRITION & OUR EMOTIONS

We have all experienced the effects of food and mood. Whether it comes from an overdose of sugar or caffeine, or going too long without eating, the powerful influence of food on our body chemistry is unquestionable. Following the dietary tips in Chapter 9 will support emotional health, but sometimes special assistance is necessary. Food allergies and nutritional deficiencies can lead to depression, anxiety, and emotional instability. See Chapter 15 if you feel input from a health professional on nutrition would help you achieve emotional balance.

People who are feeling overwhelmed emotionally often crave foods that give them a temporarily calming feeling. This might include sweets, carbohydrates, and/or fats, and usually it comes in the form of junk food. While these foods have a chemical effect that raises serotonin levels (producing a temporary antidepressant effect), this type of eating can further complicate the problem, for it ultimately results in mood swings.

Basic nutritional tips for supporting emotional health includes the information presented in Chapter 9, with special emphasis on the following: (1) reduce or eliminate your intake of caffeine, sugar, and alcohol; (2) eat a balance of protein and carbohydrates so your blood sugar remains stable; (3) avoid processed foods as much as possible; (4) drink at least nine 8-ounce glasses of water daily.

HERBS CAN HELP

There are many herbs available that can assist in reducing emotional stress. It is wise to seek the advice of a health practitioner who has a thorough understanding of herbal medicine and emotional health. If you are on prescription medication, do not add herbs to the mix without consulting a professional. The interactions could be dangerous.

An herb that has been receiving a lot of attention for its calming properties is called *kava*. A number of clinical studies have found that this South Pacific botanical is an effective alternative to conventional anti-anxiety medication—without the dangerous side effects. Other herbs commonly used to reduce tension include *chamomile, valerian, and passionflower.*

LIVING WITH EMOTIONAL WISDOM

Now that you have a basic understanding of how to reduce emotional stress in your life, there are just a few more thoughts to leave you with.

Try viewing your emotions as investments. Having consistent emotional patterns of anxiety, impatience, and irritability can be viewed as poor investments. Expressing joy, love, and peacefulness are wise investments. Unlike the New York Stock Exchange, you can virtually guarantee a return when you cultivate healthy emotional patterns.

As you've learned, being aware of our perceptions is an important aspect of emotional management. Scientists have found that we evaluate situations as we perceive them emotionally first, not how we think about them. Emotions travel faster than the speed of our thoughts! When we are managing our emotions in a healthy way, we know that our feelings about a situation are based on our perceptions. This enables us to get some emotional distance before jumping to conclusions.

It is always important to acknowledge your true feelings. Stay in touch with how you feel about various aspects of your life. Sometimes it is appropriate to share these feelings with others, sometimes we just keep them to ourselves. Keeping a feeling to ourselves is different than repressing them in a denial pattern. Feelings that are held in and not acknowledged often come out later in life; they can build up over time and can create tendencies to repeatedly express rage, fear, and worry.

Emotions are wonderful teachers when we are in touch with them. The point of this chapter is not solely to remove the toxic effects of emotions (unbalanced emotional reactions). The intention is to emphasize that healthy emotional expression is one of life's greatest gifts. Healthy emotional expression ignites the fire of your soul. It is so empowering to experience the inspiration that results from positive emotional expression.

Have fun noticing your progress as you move ahead on your emotional journey. Notice how you are replacing negative emotional patterns with positive ones. It's quite rewarding when you recognize that situations or people that used to "push your buttons" don't seem to have much of an effect anymore. Is the situation or the person different? Not necessarily. If you have been applying the concepts presented in this chapter, it will be because you have replaced those "buttons" with an increased awareness of truth. Since the buttons no longer exist, they can't be pressed.

The time spent in the indulgence of anger, fear, worry, greediness, self-pity, and victimization is time that could be spent experiencing love, joy, peace, compassion, forgiveness, and creative expression. Aren't these positive experiences what we were created for? *Any moment not spent in love is a wasted moment.* Enjoy this precious time in your life. You won't get a second chance to experience *today.*

With time, you will grow to higher levels of emotional competency. You'll move from just coping to stretching to new capacities and heights of experience. Your focus will change from stress management to living life to the fullest. A calm center will empower you with the knowledge that your peace of mind can never be stolen. Though you may get upset from time to time, you will quickly return to being centered. You'll know that you're the one who is in charge of you. All you really need is the intention to create healthy emotional expression and the willingness to see the truth in every situation.

You may not always feel that you can control specific circumstances in your life, but remember that the way in which you respond is *your choice.*

WHAT'S AHEAD

Next we'll explore the spiritual dimension of our lives. It's interesting to note that many basic spiritual principles that we hear about today have been part of the major religions for centuries! In Chapter 14, we'll review some of the most powerful spiritual ideas and the ways spirituality can enrich your experience on a daily basis.

F O U R T E E N

Reclaim Your Spirit:
Illuminating Beliefs, Thoughts, Words & Actions

> Don't be anxious about your life . . .
> Look at the birds in the air.
> They don't sow or reap or harvest,
> and yet your Heavenly Father feeds them.
> Who can add anything to his
> lifespan through being anxious? . . .
> First seek his kingdom and his goodness,
> and all these things shall be yours as well.
>
> Matthew 6

A book that examines all of the toxic influences that come into our lives would be incomplete without including the factors that block the growth of our spiritual awareness. In the last chapter on emotional wisdom, you learned how to train yourself to respond consciously to situations rather than in an emotionally reactive way. As you develop a healthier relationship with your emotions, it will be easier to transform spiritually.

Just as we looked at emotional patterns in Chapter 13, we will now consider how you are living spiritually. Spirituality has many dimensions. This chapter covers such topics as connecting internally with your Spirit, the impact of your belief systems, and the importance of thoughts, words, and actions in directing your spiritual path. It will also present powerful spiritual principles. The goal of the chapter is to help you to identify non-supportive practices and beliefs and to learn how to choose those that enrich your Spirit. Just like the rest of the book, this chapter is not just about eliminating what is toxic; it is also about discovering what is beneficial. Life is a precious gift to be celebrated. When you move into the flow of Spirit and live with purpose, you can discover more joy and fulfillment.

Certainly there are many different spiritual paths and belief systems. This chapter will include the basic spiritual principles that are most common and the most dynamic. Many come directly from religious traditions, while others are more visible in the works of non-traditional sources. Those readers who are already affiliated with a religion may be pleasantly surprised to discover that they can go deeper into spirituality within their own community. Most religions have rich spiritual traditions that go beyond the weekly services and congregational activities. If you do not identify yourself with a specific religion or spiritual tradition but also want to deepen your spiritual life, you may find several ideas in Chapter 14 that are worth contemplating.

Today there is a resurgence of interest in spirituality. More opportunities for spiritual renewal are available today than ever before. Let's begin now to look at some of the possibilities. At the end of the chapter, you will find a reading list for further exploration. It is my hope that this chapter will serve as a springboard for spiritual transformation.

AWAKENING THE SPIRIT WITHIN

"Only in quiet water do things mirror themselves undistorted.
Only in a quiet mind is there an adequate perception of the world."
— Hans Margoius

In modern life, it is easy to feel that you have become a "human doing" rather than a "human being." Because the world often encourages us to lead overly busy lives, it's important to consciously remind ourselves to *slow down*. Practices such as meditation and prayer help us discover our inner stillness and the vibrant Spirit that lies within us.

Spirituality is not something that is stagnant; it is a process that is ever-evolving and must be cultivated. Through increasing our awareness, we can learn to connect to our "soul" whenever we choose. What is the "soul"? As Webster defines it, the soul is *"the immaterial essence... an active or essential part... a moving spirit."* It is the part inside of you that knows that all is well. The part that feels connected to your purpose and very existence. Do you have soul expression regularly or rarely?

The benefits of connecting with the soul include tapping into one's true nature. Living in alignment with truth results in increased happiness, contentment, fulfillment, and inner peace. Most spiritual traditions teach that cultivating a link to your inner awareness is the secret to living a joy-filled life. A developed inner guidance lets you know whether you should continue down the same path or if it's time to move in a new direction.

You can lose a job, possessions, etc., but your Spirit can never be taken away from you. However, it is common to ignore our spiritual needs or lose touch with our deepest reality. By awakening the Spirit within, you can gain control of your life rather than allowing external factors to determine your direction. You develop a sense of knowingness that will help you make the right decisions.

The emphasis on the external world—jobs, money, and status—has caused confusion as it presents the illusion that happiness resides outside ourselves. When we live in this illusion, we never have enough. I recently had a conversation with an accountant whose clients consisted of mostly millionaires. In his over forty years of practice, this seasoned professional told me that he *never had a client who **believed** he had enough money*! When we lose contact with the true source of our abundance, we can easily develop fear of limitation.

Connecting to the Spirit within can bring an awareness of empowerment. A healthier perspective is developed, resulting in greater satisfaction in life. Instead of feeling empty from the insatiable pursuit of material things or external recognition, you can have access to information leading you to choices that are best for you and those around you. You can draw from the unlimited bank account of the kingdom of heaven within you.

MEDITATION: THE MIRACLE OF SILENCE & STILLNESS

"All our troubles in life come because we refuse to sit quietly for a while each day in our rooms." — Blaise Pascal

"Silence is the root of our union with God and with one another. In the silence, we are filled with the energy of God Himself that makes us do all things in joy. We need to find God, and God cannot be found in noise and restlessness. God is the friend of silence. See how nature— trees and flowers and grass—grow in silence. See how the stars, the moon, the sun, how they move in silence. The more we receive in silence, the more we can give in our active life."

— Mother Teresa

A wonderful way to connect with your soul and to reclaim your Spirit is by learning to listen to the inner silence and by developing an awareness of deep stillness through the practice of *meditation*.

Meditation is a practice that calms the mind while increasing awareness. When you begin to practice meditation, one of the first things you notice is its relaxing quality. Meditation helps us de-stress and calm down on a physical level. In fact, psychotherapists sometimes recommend meditation to their patients as an anxiety-reducing tool. The practice of meditation is also a way to clear our minds of the constant chatter that blocks our perception of the more essential messages. It forces us to pay attention to our individual truth. Regular meditation is good for our health too. Compared to the national average, meditators have been found to need 56% fewer hospitalizations than non-meditators.

Choose a time for meditation when you will not be interrupted. Take the phone off the hook, and turn off the radio or TV. Alert those who share your living space that they should not interact with you for a specified period of time. You may want to set a timer to alert you when your chosen meditation time has elapsed. Select 20 minutes for your initial sessions, lengthening the time as desired.

Whenever possible, you'll want to be in a peaceful environment when you meditate. You may decide to sit in an uncluttered pleasant room by a window or in a garden in the backyard. If you'd like, you could create a specific space in your living environment for your meditation practice, decorating it with items that delight your soul. (See section titled "Actions: Creating Sacred Space" which comes later in this chapter.)

The position for practice that beginning meditators often start with is to simply sit along the front of a chair with your back straight and your head centered above the spine. Your feet should be planted flatly on the floor or ground. Or you could sit forward on a cushion on the floor or ground, crossing your legs once you are comfortable.

The following is a simple meditation that could be used by beginners as well experienced meditators:

1. Assume your chosen sitting position (see above). Close your eyes.
2. In your mind, silently repeat a word or phrase (often referred to as a "mantra," which means sacred word) that helps you identify with your soul. You may choose the name of a deity or a word that represents an aspect of Spirit. Repeat "Let go. Let God," "Peace," "Jesus," "Yahweh," "Shalom," or the sound "Om" each time you exhale. The use of a mantra is to help clear your mind of busy thoughts. If your mind wanders from the phrase, word, or sound, gently bring your focus back to it.
3. You will probably notice as you begin your meditation practice that your mind might not be calm. It takes time and practice for the mind to slow down, and meditation is one of the best ways to cultivate a peaceful mind. When you have thoughts during your meditation, think of them as clouds passing by. Don't judge them, hold on to them, or "try" to get rid of them. Just observe them and let them flow. Return to your attention to your mantra.
4. Relax and become comfortable just sitting as you are. Your breathing should be full, with the air going down deep into your abdomen. Exhale slowly.
5. Continue the practice for 20 minutes. You may want to start with 5 or 10 minutes as you develop your practice, with a goal building up to 20 minutes once or twice a day.
6. Open your eyes and sit quietly for a moment or two before you move onto your day. Some people like to end with a prayer, blessing, or moment of gratitude.

This is just one example of a basic meditation. There are so many different types that you could practice—Zen, Christian Contemplative, Kabbalah, Transcendental, Qi Gong, etc. Whichever you choose, it can be a path to inner peace.

When you're trying a new technique, it's helpful to use audiotapes to guide you along. A good source is *The Meditation & Prayer Catalog* from Sounds True of Boulder, Colorado (*www.soundstrue.com*). In the catalog, you'll find tapes such as "Meditation for Beginners" by Jack

HAPPINESS AS AN ART

Many people see happiness as elusive. But in his book, *The Art of Happiness,* the Dalai Lama (the spiritual leader of Tibet) tells us that happiness is a reasonable goal—one that can be achieved through the retraining of our minds. What is necessary, he points out, is a "transformation of our attitude," of "our entire outlook and approach to living."

To demonstrate the importance of our attitude, the book includes two stories. The first is about a man who contracted HIV, but after an initial adjustment, began to appreciate and enjoy life at a higher level than ever before. The second story tells of a woman who gained an unexpected windfall, but after a short time, found herself no happier than she was before the money came in. The Dalai Lama concludes: "the essential point is that happiness is determined more by one's state of mind than by external events."

In addition to taking on the right attitude, the Dalai Lama teaches that we must also identify the factors that truly lead to happiness and increase them, as well as becoming aware of negative factors and phasing them out of our lives. Here are some happiness-contributing factors that the Dalai Lama highlights:

The ability to want and appreciate what we now have
A receptiveness to the joy of life
An awareness of avoiding that which would bring
    momentary pleasure but longer-term pain
Being compassionate, warm-hearted, and kind
The tendency to look for the good in others
Conducting our lives so that we have many forms
    of connections with others
Facing our problems head-on so that we learn
    what we must do
Developing a relationship with our emotions in which
    we do not prolong our suffering
Skill in shifting perspective and seeing a situation or
    an "enemy" in new ways

> *A willingness to learn from suffering and garner the gifts*
>
> In this book, the good news that the Dalai Lama delivers is that *happiness is an art*, rather than a random event happening only in the lives of the chosen few. The choice is ours.

Kornfield, "Kabbalah Meditation" by Rabbi David Cooper, "The Contemplative Journey" by Father Thomas Keating, "Loving-Kindness Meditation" by Sharon Salzberg, and "The Present Moment" by Thich Nhat Hanh.

One of the fastest growing categories of books today is that of spirituality and religion. The desire for ways to achieve deeper meaning in life has resulted in the creation of resources. Take some time to browse these sections at your local bookstore.

Of course, the web has a wealth of information to help you to explore various spiritual practices. The site *www.beliefnet.com* covers virtually every religion and spiritual tradition and practices associated with each. The World Community for Christian Meditation is represented at *www.wccm.org*, the Kabbalah is extensively explored at *www.kabbalah-web.org*, and *www.buddhism.org* can link you to the diversity of various Eastern traditions. Using the search engines with a word such as "meditation," "prayer," or the tradition of your choice will lead you to a virtual world of support for your spiritual practice.

RAISING OUR CONSCIOUSNESS: TOXIC VERSUS SUPPORTIVE BELIEFS

"We become what we believe."
— Oprah Winfrey

In order to grow spiritually, we need to examine our belief systems and how they are reflected in our lives. Belief systems are the underlying principles that we refer to in order to make day-to-day choices and assessments. Certain belief systems are toxic to us because they are not based in truth. These toxic beliefs are stressful to the soul—our internal truth monitor.

Some people rely on belief systems that cause them to feel badly about themselves because of past actions and behaviors. Many erroneously think that guilt is a way to promote positive change. However this attitude only creates a downward spiral. When people use belief systems that are self-punishing and do not serve the highest good for all, at some level they are not aware of the Ever Present Loving Spirit Within Them. A way to bring more light into the darkness is to raise your consciousness by examining the beliefs that rule your days.

Let's look at some common *life-draining beliefs* that influence people's lives and repress them spiritually:

> *I will be happier when I have a better job, a different*
> *   relationship, a bigger house, etc.*
> *Life is hard.*
> *It is normal to feel stressed most of the time.*
> *Others are to blame for my unhappiness.*
> *I can control the changes in my life and resist those*
> *   that don't seem comfortable.*
> *Self-deprivation is good.*
> *I can force things to happen.*
> *Just getting by is the best I can hope to accomplish.*
> *Holding onto anger and resentment is natural.*
> *You have to struggle to survive.*
> *Everyone judges me; why shouldn't I judge others?*
> *I will have inner peace if I just get a few more dollars*
> *   in the bank.*
> *Happiness, peace, and joy come from others.*
> *The only time to connect to God is when you are in*
> *   trouble and need help.*
> *Each one of us is alone and unsupported in this world.*
> *I have to work hard for everything I want.*
> *My actions are a series of mostly unrelated activity.*
> *It is helpful to worry about what you want and*
> *   need in life.*
> *Vulnerability is our natural state.*
> *I can't expect my needs to be met.*

In contrast, consider these *life-affirming beliefs*:

I trust that all that I need will be supplied.
A moment where love is not expressed is a
wasted moment.
I attract exactly what I need.
Happiness is a choice that I can make right now.
I know that life presents challenges so I will have
opportunities to grow.
I take responsibility for my actions.
Change is part of the magic of life.
I can live happily in the flow of life.
I express unconditional love daily.
Living life to the fullest requires being willing to
learn and change.
In order to be free, I must forgive.
Inner peace is mine for the asking.
My happiness, peace, joy, and love are generated
from within.
I am blessed to be part of the Divine plan of creation.
I feel the presence of God expanding within me daily in
the form of love.
There is a sacred purpose to my actions.
I am so grateful for everything. I count my blessings daily.
I feel protected.

As the Dalai Lama reminds us, it is not our circumstances but our responses to them that determine the quality of our lives. Belief systems can influence us deeply because they affect how we perceive or interpret a situation. For instance, if we see challenges in life as opportunities to grow, life will naturally move us along to a higher level of awareness as we open up to new possibilities. But if we resist change, we can feel that we are merely victims of circumstance, accepting all the negativity of the situation.

Of course, some experiences in life will be more challenging than others. In certain situations, it will take more work in order to see the gifts. But if our belief system is based on our existence in a world that meets our needs through the grace of God, we are more likely to come through the challenge with blessings rather than scars.

In order to get in touch with your personal belief systems, it helps to begin to pay attention to your thoughts as you walk through your day. Are they more reflective of the first list, the life-draining beliefs, or the second list, the life-affirming ones? If you find that your beliefs tend to be self-defeating, try incorporating some of the beliefs from the second list into your life. This shift can be an important step toward a richer experience of life and a deeper spiritual awareness.

GOD WITHIN: THE RICHNESS OF TRADITION

"Late have I loved you, O Beauty ever ancient, ever new, late have I loved you! **You were within me,** *but I was outside, and it was there that I searched for you. In my unloveliness I plunged into the lovely things that you created.* **You were with me, but I was not with you."**
— St. Augustine

With the kingdom of heaven residing within us twenty-four hours a day, seven days a week, going to religious services once a week is usually not enough to truly satisfy the Spirit. In order to more regularly experience the fruits of the Spirit in your life, increasing your awareness on a daily basis is encouraged. This does not mean that your days must be stripped of all pleasure or that you have to choose a monastic lifestyle of material deprivation. What is helpful is to start and end the day with a prayer or meditation that affirms the Spirit within you, and to allow that awareness to be cultivated throughout the day. We can find reminders of this Divine Presence within in various Scriptures from world religions.

▪ From Christianity
"You won't see signs of the coming of the kingdom of God. It won't be a matter of saying 'here it is!' or 'There!' Look, the kingdom of God is within you."
"Do you not know that you are God's temple and that God's Spirit dwells in you? For God's temple is holy, and you are that temple."

▪ From Judaism
"Just as God fills the whole world, so the soul fills the body. Just as God sees, but is not seen, so the soul sees, but is not itself seen. Just as God feeds the whole world, so the soul feeds the whole body. Just as

God is pure, so the soul is pure. Just as God dwells in the innermost precincts of the Temple, so also the soul dwells in the innermost part of the body."

■ From Buddhism
"If you think the Law is outside yourself, you are embracing not the absolute Law but some inferior teaching."

■ From Hinduism
"God bides hidden in the hearts of all."

■ From Confucianism
"What the undeveloped man seeks is outside; what the advanced man seeks is within himself."

■ From Islam
"When I love him, I am his hearing by which he hears; his sight by which he sees; and his foot by which he walks."

■ From Sikhism
"Ever is He present with you—think not He is far: By the Master's teaching recognize Him within Yourself."
"Why wilt thou go into the jungles? What do you hope to find there? Even as the scent dwells within the flower, so God within thine own heart ever abides. Seek Him with earnestness and find Him there."

Cultivation of the awareness of this Divine Presence within us has not been emphasized in the past century. Yet that awareness is what has been at the heart of the spiritual life of saints and sages throughout the ages. Most people claim to believe in God, yet many are not aware of the wonderful tools available to enrich their faith and to enhance every aspect of their lives. More and more people all over the world are expressing a hunger for something more than uninspiring services and dogma. The great religions all have very strong mystical traditions, and we are witnessing a renaissance of these practices, influenced by the increased interest in meditation and contemplative spiritual practices.

There are also ways to develop your spiritual life with ideas from the non-traditional spiritual arena. The intent of this chapter is not to promote any particular religious or spiritual practice, but to encourage you to see the beauty and spirituality that is common in all traditions and to find a practice that brings you peace.

Note: Some readers may not be comfortable with the words "God" or "religion." Your experience of religion may have been associated with lots of guilt, shame, and rules. Although these qualities are not at the roots of the great religious traditions, in some cases the messages that have been relayed did not hold the emphasis of a Loving Presence. It is often helpful for those who have experienced "religious abuse" to revisit their roots and see if their pain has sprung from a misrepresented teaching. There is quite a movement in most traditions to bring back the mystical elements, where the emphasis is on love, not judgment.

There are many paths to Spirit—both traditional and nontraditional. The important thing is to choose what works in your own life, to find a practice that allows you to experience the fruits of the Spirit such as joy, peace, patience, and faith. There is always room in God's heart for everyone whose path is based on love.

BASIC SPIRITUAL PRINCIPLES FOR THE ILLUMINATED LIFE

In the clinic, patients are assisted in their spiritual development through the offering of workshops that explore meditation, prayer, and other important tools for the journey. Many have shared that they observe their health concerns are related to a lack of purpose, direction, balance, and inner peace in their lives, and they notice improvements as they incorporate a regular spiritual practice. A recent report from the National Institute of Healthcare Research supports this observation. Combining the results of twenty-nine studies, researchers found that people who attended religious services or used spiritual principles as coping mechanisms had longer lives than those who didn't include this activity in their lives.[1] An earlier report from the Mayo Clinic found that optimists, on average, live longer than pessimists.[2]

There is so much to say on the subject of spirituality, as there are so many spiritual principles that we might explore. Below you will find a list of basic principles that are common to most spiritual traditions:

Grace: Grace simply refers to the purity of the blessings of life. When you connect with the spirit of Grace, you are living in the flow of life and in the presence of God and are willing to receive blessings. Grace is living in the present moment. By allowing blessings in your life, you can live in a state of grace.

Surrender/God's Will: This concept has to do with the understanding that we are all part of the whole. It explores our interconnectedness. Surrendering to God's Will is not about surrendering to a gray-bearded man up in the sky who wants you to do something that is not good for you. It is about getting out of the ego, the part of you that feels separated, and to start living with purpose. It is actually about surrendering *to* what is best for you, to what will bring you true peace and happiness. It is astounding how many people hold onto ideas, beliefs, and behaviors that bring them misery. Without surrender to Spirit, your life will be all about the ego, and you will not be happy. But if you are willing to become a living instrument of God's ideals of love, honesty, fairness, humility, and peace, more joy will flow into your life. You will begin to see your part of the whole, and your purpose on the planet will make more sense. Surrender is one of the essential gifts of spiritual transformation.

Balance: People are realizing that they need all types of experiences and that they must make room for them. It's so easy to be consumed by the work ethic. Yet we need to make time for intimacy, contact, and connection. And we must also attend to our Spirit. Keep in mind that it's possible to go out of balance in any area. You could even pray too much, neglecting the attention that a loved one requires. Balance is crucial to joyful living.

Connection: Many people feel isolated and separate. Our society actually promotes this feeling by encouraging us to focus on our individual goals for more money, more things, etc. However, when you grow in Spirit, you come to see that we are all connected. Our actions affect one another. We are all in this world together.

Gratitude: Assuming an attitude of gratitude allows us to become aware of the richness of our world. We get in touch with the wonder of life and the magic of our existence. The habit of counting our blessings allows us to experience the little miracles that happen each day. Gratitude might be for a sunny day, a delightful meal, a good friend, a successful job assignment, or even a comfortable pair of shoes. We are truly blessed!

Forgiveness: When you forgive, you are willing to see the good in other people and do not judge them based on one lone act. While you do not condone what they did, you send them love and wish them the best. You then let go of the issue. Forgiveness is good for the soul. In contrast, hanging onto resentment and anger is destructive to your physical and spiritual health. Talking things through can help you understand each other.

Simplicity: Simplifying our lives brings greater spiritual freedom. If we hold onto things we no longer need, they become a burden. We begin to serve the things rather than having the things serve us. Also, so often, we feel pushed to buy more and more, yet do not appreciate what we already have. Simplicity gets us in touch with how much we really need. This knowledge comes from our inner guidance.

Beauty: We are surrounded by beauty, yet it is often overlooked. But when you make a point to see the beauty in this world, you are enriched. You see the rose, the elegant architecture of a museum, the clouds, and a friend's sparkling eyes. Why would we care to live if we did not enjoy the earth's beauty? By allowing beauty to come into our consciousness, we feed our soul.

Choosing Love: According to the Bible, *God is Love*. The world can always use a little more love, a little more kindness. Next time you encounter a challenging situation, ask yourself, "What would be the most loving way that I could respond to this situation?" The way we relate to others is a strong reflection of the richness of our Spirit. However, it is important to love yourself first. It is impossible to truly love others if you don't love yourself first, for you can't give what you don't have.

Purpose: We all have a purpose to fulfill in our lives. If we use our inner guidance to make career choices, we will find life to be a lot more satisfying. To be living in a spiritually purposeful way doesn't mean that you have to be a monk or a priest or a nun. You could be a fireman or a mom. Whatever choice you make, use your gifts. You want to be doing something that connects to who you are and allows you to be of service to others.

These spiritual principles are timeless and have lasting value. It enriches our Spirit to tune into them. We can compare our mind, our consciousness, to a radio. If we tune into the radio station of Truth, our life will be a reflection of this. Without a clear signal of aware-ness, we may only reflect the static we are attracting. Once again, the choice is ours.

BEYOND BELIEFS:
OUR THOUGHTS, WORDS & ACTIONS

Your being reflects the sum total of your thoughts, words, and actions. For your thoughts become your words which become your actions. If your thoughts, words, or actions are not generated from a loving place or do not affirm your abundance, then you are limiting your life force. This will affect your physical, emotional, and spiritual health. In the next sections, we will explore how we can use our thoughts, words, and actions to lift ourselves up spiritually.

■ Thoughts: Our Intention

Developing an awareness of your intentions is a crucial step. Because once you have chosen a certain intention, you will attract the circumstances that will help it unfold. Actually, we tend to have a num-ber of major encompassing intentions for our lives as well as numerous ones that relate to our moment-by-moment experiences. A basic over-all intention might be "to survive;" a momentary intention, "to get home before the movie starts on Channel 11."

When you choose intentions that have a spiritual basis, they enrich your experience. Try consciously choosing one major spiritually based intention. You might consider it to be similar to choosing the title for your life's story. For instance, one of your major intentions some time back might have been "to make a lot of money." Yet, in the process, you may have discovered that the job you have to do to bring in all that cash is coming at too high a price to other areas of your life. You could change your major intention now to something like "to know God" or "to celebrate life." Celebrating life could translate into changing to a slightly lower paying job that preserves your peace of mind and pro-vides a sense of purpose.

Having a strong intention is like having a road map. You've chosen your course in life. In contrast, if you don't consciously make a choice, you can end up somewhere that you don't want to be.

The concept of "priorities" goes along well with intentions. You may encounter a situation where you will have to determine which of your intentions is the most important. Say you are asked to do something unethical on the job. What would your priority be? To keep the job or honor your integrity? Honoring yourself could mean making a hard decision; yet in the long run, you would be a lot better off spiritually. Honoring your integrity is always a healthy priority.

■ Thoughts: Mindfulness

"Beginning the day, I see that life is a miracle. Attentive to each moment, I keep my mind clear like a calm river."
— Thich Nhat Hanh, *a Zen master who was nominated for the Nobel Peace Prize by Martin Luther King, Jr.*

Mindfulness is simply a practice of "living in the moment." You conduct your daily activities with love and a total sense of awareness. You know that each activity is the most important thing to be doing in that moment. With mindfulness, you live with love, purpose, and joy. This creates hours, days, weeks, and, eventually, a lifetime of joy—a stream of consciousness of peace.

In contrast, many of us place our thoughts on the argument we had the night before or the impression we'll make at a gathering the next day. Our thoughts can be anywhere but in the present moment. How often have you driven your car during a hectic time of your life and arrived home without any memory of the trip? Your mind was not present but instead it was focused on the other situations you are dealing with. This is the opposite of mindfulness. At these times of distraction, you miss out on your entire present experience as you play out worrisome scenarios in your mind.

In the spiritual classic, *The Practice of the Presence of God*, the 17th Century Christian mystic known as Brother Lawrence details his mindful cultivation of the awareness of God in every moment, whether it was a moment of meditation, eating, walking, or even dishwashing. He lived each moment as a moment of prayer, of sacred awareness of the preciousness of life.

Take a few moments now to practice being in the moment. You may find counting your exhalations silently or out loud to be a good way to quiet your mind. Begin to pay attention to all the details of your environment. Notice the sounds, colors, and smells. Feel the breeze blowing in through the open window. Note where the light from the lamp falls and where there is shadow. As you observe, know that you can choose to be mindful in any moment or any situation. Isn't it great to feel so fully alive?

For further information on the practice of mindfulness, you can also explore the writings of Zen monk Thich Nhat Hanh. His works include *Peace in Every Step: The Path of Mindfulness in Everyday Life; The Art of Mindful Living: How to Bring Love, Compassion and Inner Peace into Your Daily Life* (audio); and *Teachings on Love: How Mindfulness Can Enhance Your Intimate Relationships* (audio).

■ Words: Increasing Awareness of Our Language

Examining the words we use in our everyday lives is a way to enliven the Spirit. For you may be surprised to discover that many of your words are toxic. Our language becomes toxic when it is based on judgment, resentment, cynicism, and anger. Alternately, words that nurture the Spirit are compassionate, loving, forgiving, hopeful, and joyful.

One of my patients mentioned to me that it seems as if people constantly brag about how tired and stressed out they are. I also regularly hear people say how stressful their work or life is. We need to find creative words that take us away from feeling victimized. Choosing new language can help us move in a new direction toward a more peace-filled existence. While this takes discipline, it will be well worth the effort.

If you find yourself talking about how stressed or tired you are, think about making changes so you can begin to describe your life in a new way. If you say, "Things are going great," or respond with "Wonderful!" when someone asks you how you are, you will gradually find yourself moving in that direction and feeling better.

On a related note, language is often used in a judgmental way toward others. Many psychologists believe that when individuals use words to blame other people, it is usually a reflection of some way that they are blaming themselves. The truth is that the more we use words to love and forgive others, the more we can love and forgive *ourselves*.

Every word that we choose is either a blessing (expressing Spirit) or a denunciation (expressing negativity). As Helen Keller once said,

"Keep your vision to the sunshine, and you will not see your shadow." If you continue to affirm the good, this is what will you will tend to encounter. When you choose to say, "What a beautiful day!" that is what you will see. Give thanks through your words for everything— even things that may not seem so great—and see what you learn.

■ Words: Affirmations & Affirmative Prayer

*"Whatever you are thinking about is what you are affirming as the reality in your life. When you start to affirm positive words and thoughts you begin the process of self-empowerment and your life automatically becomes better. It is not important what happens to you in life, but rather **what happens in you**. You determine the truth of your being. Affirm your wonder, your magnificence, your perfection and your wholeness at all times. Set your sights high and affirm your good."*

— O.C. Smith, in *Mind Power*

Many messages that we receive from society express fear and lack, or promote the idea that we need people or things outside ourselves to be happy. Therefore, it is important to surround ourselves with more positive input. Two proactive ways to do this are through the use of *affirmations* and *affirmative prayer.*

First, let's look at affirmations. As you become more acquainted with the words you share with others as well as your own thoughts, you are likely to notice negative statements you are saying to and about yourself. You may note thoughts such as "I can't do this," "This is too hard," "I am stupid," etc. You may hear yourself saying, "Finding the right relationships is impossible," "I never hear about jobs that I want," or "I'm not going to be able to lose this weight," etc. Replacing these self-defeating thoughts and speaking with language that is more supportive will be good for your soul. The thoughts and words you choose will be the seeds of your life's harvest.

Since we just explored the idea of being careful about our expressed words, let's focus now on affirmations specifically. These strong, positive statements will assist you in realizing your potential. They are powerful tools to help train yourself to experience a more joyful life. Take a moment now to think of various areas of your life where you could use some support. This might be regarding your work, friendships, hobbies, love relationships, family, etc. Now create some short concise statements that will support you in moving toward your goals. Some examples would be: "I relate well to men (or women)," "I know how to accomplish my goal," "My mother and I work easily through our conflicts," etc. Write the affirmations down and choose one to state outloud when you first awake and before going to sleep. Repeat it to yourself throughout your day. Change the affirmation once a week.

The following life-encompassing affirmations from the Old and New Testament can be soul-healing and peace-generating. They can assist you in coming into alignment with your Spirit. Consider using one of them as an ongoing affirmation:

I am far from oppression and fear does not come near me. (Isa. 54:14)

I have the peace of God that passes understanding. (Phil. 4:7)

I have no lack for my God supplies all of my needs according to his riches. (Phil. 4:19)

I am greatly loved by God. (Col. 3:12; Rom. 1:7; Eph. 2:4)

Affirmations are uplifting and easy to incorporate into your life. For more information on working with affirmations for spiritual and physical healing, refer to *You Can Heal Your Life* by Louise Hay.

Prayers that affirm The Divine Presence will also help you to strengthen your Spirit. These affirmative prayers may be ones that were created by others or you may want to produce your own either spontaneously or with forethought. While you're making your choice, keep in mind that there is a marked difference between an affirmative prayer and a begging prayer. When someone begs for something in their prayer, there is often an underlying fear that they may not deserve it. It's important to recognize life's true abundance. There is no need to beg for what you already have. Just ask that you can see the Truth more clearly. Prayer is the desire to unite our will with God's, to see the truth, and to let go of illusion.

The following affirmative prayer is one of my favorites because it is so complete. It comes from the Unity tradition, a nonsectarian educational organization with roots in Christianity, Quakerism, Theosophy, and Hinduism. If you are uncomfortable with the word

God, you may insert Loving Source, Spirit, etc., whenever you wish to express your connection with the Creative Loving Intelligence that Governs the Universe.

Prayer for Protection

The Light of God surrounds me.
The Love of God enfolds me.
The Power of God protects me.
The Presence of God watches over me.
The Mind of God guides me.
The Life of God flows through me.
The Laws of God direct me.
The Power of God abides within me.
The Joy of God uplifts me.
The Strength of God renews me.
The Beauty of God inspires me.
Wherever I am, God is!
And all is well.

I love this prayer because it does not imply any separation between God and us. It affirms the Divine Presence Within. It is a wonderful way to start and end the day. What a powerful practice to set the tone for the day in the morning and encourage peaceful sleep in the evening. Sure beats the accident/traffic reports in the morning and the death and destruction reports on the nightly news!

■ Actions: Random Acts of Kindness

If you are having difficulty creating a connection to the Spirit, there are also actions you can take that will help you feel the Divine Love of God flowing through you. One type of action is to begin practicing random acts of kindness. Here are some ideas:

Allow another driver to pull into your lane, and then wave with a smile.

When a clerk at a cash register appears glum, find a way to cheer him or her up.

Help someone who is struggling with his or her grocery bags or luggage.

Give an extra large tip to a waiter or other helper.
Call or visit someone you know who might be down or lonely.
Be patient with someone who responds slowly.
Smile, smile, smile, smile!!

Practicing random acts of kindness is fun—it helps break down barriers. These actions are part of the solution to ending feelings of isolation and separation among people. Note that there are certainly larger actions you could take as well. Mentor a challenged student. Clean up trash on the beach. Sing in a group that performs in nursing homes. What you want to do is find something that you can contribute that fits your skills and passions.

When you put the Spirit within you into action, you will more fully feel Its presence. Remember, it needs to be nurtured. You might compare the Spirit or soul to a small flame that needs more wood. Soon it can turn into a large brilliant blaze. By practicing acts of kindness—both large and small—you train yourself to respond with kindness. In more challenging situations, you'll find yourself looking for the kinder, more peaceful response.

Here is a tip for handling larger challenges in your interactions with others. Take a few deep breaths and try repeating the affirmation, *"I choose peace in this situation."* This phrase will help you feel centered, and your inner guidance will enable you to select a peaceful, creative response as opposed to a volatile, destructive one.

Once again, we are the culmination of our choices.

■ Actions: Creating Sacred Space

Since so much of our time is spent in chaotic environments that are clogged with people, traffic, or streaming media, it is important to create a space in your home that is uncluttered and peaceful. This is the place where you'll want to do your meditation or to have your quiet time alone. When you don't have such sacred space, it can be difficult to cultivate an inner stillness and peacefulness.

In choosing the location for your sacred indoor space, listen to your intuition. Which space is conducive to comfort and relaxation? Do you have pleasant associations with it? Once you've made your selection, clear the location of unnecessary items until it no longer feels "busy." You may also want to add things that offer a feeling of peace and harmony. They might be items from the outdoors such as colorful stones or minerals, shells or other items gathered from the beach, etc. Attractive banners or wall-hangings can add to the ambiance too. Consider the correct lighting as well, making sure it isn't overly harsh or too soft. Burning some pleasant essential oils in the area may help you relax and enhance your mood.

Humankind has long sought sacred space, a physical place where the Divine can be experienced. In addition to indoor spaces, there have also been sacred outdoor sites throughout history. So you might want to also find a serene location outside where you can do some of your centering work. This could be a grassy area near a lake or a spot on the beach by the ocean. Scout for a location where you are least likely to be disturbed by other people.

By selecting your sacred space, you make room for your Spirit to come alive. You create an alternative to the daily chaos so you can get in touch with who you are and who you can become.

■ Actions: Experiencing Spirit through our Senses

Some people separate the spiritual from everyday life, believing that spiritual experiences must appear in a magical, mystical, super-natural format. We often think of the so-called "sixth sense," of ESP (extra-sensory perception), as the way the Divine speaks. Some experts do not validate the existence of a separate "sixth sense." Rather they view so-called ESP as a heightened awareness incorporating the basic five senses.

When the five basic senses of sight, smell, taste, hearing, and touch are not frequently experiencing joy and other fruits of the Spirit, it is natural for us to feel separate. When we make choices that allow us to experience beauty on a regular basis with our senses, it is easier to be aware of the Divine Presence within us.

Many people seem to feel closer to God in Nature. One reason is because the senses are taking in the pure beauty of creation.

In contrast, it's difficult to feel connected to Spirit when:

■ You spend the whole day indoors with no fresh air or sunshine.

■ The only touch you have experienced is your own fingers on a computer keyboard.

■ You have spent a day at the office listening to office gossip instead of beautiful music.

- The only smells of the day you can recall include photocopy machine vapors and exhaust fumes, with no hint of fresh flowers or homemade cookies.

- You come home to a sterile lifeless environment.

- You just popped a mediocre dinner into the microwave for your evening meal.

- You plan to settle in for the evening to watch a movie or TV show that glorifies violence, infidelity, abuse, or some of the other lowest common denominators.

What we take in each day makes up who we become. You can read all the self-help books you want, but if you don't spent time taking in the vast beauty of this world, it will be hard to believe in the true abundance of life. Take time every day to nourish your Spirit through all of your senses: taste, sight, smell, touch, and sound. This way you are choosing experiences that truly support your Spirit.

I am blessed to live a mile from the beach in Santa Monica, California, which is adjacent to Los Angeles. After a long day of writing, researching, or seeing patients in the clinic, I often walk along the beach at sunset. No matter how I am feeling, which is usually pretty good, I become absolutely elated as I am walking and witnessing some of the most beautiful sunsets in the world. I see the magnificence of the horizon with my eyes, hear the waves crashing with my ears, smell the refreshing salt air, touch the grains of sand with my bare feet, and taste a refreshing beverage that I usually carry on my walk. What never ceases to amaze me is that as I take my two-mile walk along the beach, I will only pass by ten or twenty people enjoying this profound splendor. Where are the millions of people that live nearby?

Some ideas to experience beauty through the senses include:

- Plant some flowers in the ground or in pots near your front door.

- Enjoy some tasty, nutritious food.

- Relax in bath water scented with essential oils.

- Listen to beautiful, soul-soothing music (not jarring noise).

- Read poetry outloud.

- Run your fingers through the hair of a lover.

- Pet your cat or dog, enjoying the softness of the fur.
- Take a walk through the woods or by the ocean.
- Read a soul-expanding book or watch an inspiring movie or TV program.

Our spirits become starved when they are constantly bombarded with mediocrity. Seek out quality and pleasure in life. You deserve the best!

CELEBRATION WITH SACRED SOUND

Be not lax in celebrating
Be not lazy in the festive service of God
Be ablaze with enthusiasm!
— Hildegard von Bingen, *14th Century*
mystic, healer, musician

One of the most powerful ways to shift our state is through musical expression. If we hear a song about a jilted lover, we may identify with the grief. If we constantly listen to music that implies that happiness can only come from outside ourselves in the form of a romantic relationship, we risk deepening that illusion. On the other hand, if we hear musical expression that represents truth, it can shift awareness to one of faith, hope, and enthusiasm in a matter of seconds. As has been presented throughout the book, we are the result of many choices and experiences. As music has such a deep imprint on our belief system, let us choose carefully music to uplift our soul.

Music that is uplifting to the spirit takes many forms—from Sanskrit and Gregorian Chants, Gospel and Soul, to Classical, Motown, and even Rock and Roll. When Neil Diamond sings "Turn on your heartlight, let it shine wherever you go," I think of the Spirit Within. The Beatles' "All You Need is Love" says it all.

An excellent way to transform Spirit-limiting beliefs into messages of peace, abundance, and trust is to listen to the extraordinarily talented singer and songwriter, Rickie Byars (*www.rickiebyars.com*). Her CDs "In the Land of I AM" and "I Found a Deeper Love" are extremely transformational and beautiful musical masterpieces. See the Resource section for more empowering music recommendations.

THE WAYS OF PEACE

"Overcome evil with good, Falsehood with truth, And hatred with love." — Mildred Norman, *The Peace Pilgrim*

From 1953 to 1981, a woman known as "the Peace Pilgrim" walked over 25,000 miles for peace. Her goal was to teach humankind the ways of peace—goodness, truth, and love. Today Mildred Norman's teachings live on through a remarkable book *The Peace Pilgrim: Her Life and Work in Her Own Words.* The title is available at bookstores and also at the website *www.peace pilgrim.com* (where the entire book is available free of charge).

Many say that the Peace Pilgrim was a living model of her principles. She left this world in 1981. The following list is what Norman called "Symptoms of Inner Peace":

*A tendency to think and act spontaneously rather than
   on fears based on past experiences
An unmistakable ability to enjoy each moment
A loss of interest in judging other people
A loss of interest in interpreting the actions of others
A loss of interest in conflict
A loss of the ability to worry
Frequent overwhelming episodes of appreciation
Contented feelings of connectedness with others and nature
Frequent attacks of smiling
An increased susceptibility to the love extended by others
   as well as the uncontrollable urge to extend it.*

The Peace Pilgrim felt that inner peace was a do-it-yourself project, but she wanted to point the way. Her energy is said to have been boundless. Her example gave hope to many who wanted to also find the universal energy Norman believed to be available to all.

DON'T NEGLECT THE SPIRIT!

"We are spiritual beings having a human experience."
— Deepak Chopra, M.D.

No one is too busy to "fit" spirituality into their lives. Although many pack their days with activities that are often not soul-fulfilling, we are never actually separate from Spirit. When we choose activities that are not life-enriching, it is like putting the wrong kind of gas into our cars. If we create this imbalance, we often end up quieting spiritual unrest in unhealthy ways—with substance abuse, workaholism, etc. Just as good health is something to be cultivated, a life worth living includes attention to developing a peaceful inner Spirit. This is a good beginning for creating a healthy spiritual life.

In our consumer-driven society, it seems almost impossible to experience true happiness and peace without some type of spiritual practice. Father Thomas Keating, in *The Heart of The World*, sums up this concept eloquently:

"You can survive, of course, without moments of interior silence, while you cannot survive without eating or sleeping; but a question could be raised about the **quality of your survival.** *If this spiritual need is not appeased, it will take revenge in strange ways, such as an uncomfortable hunger. We may find ourselves trying to cover up the remembrance of this hunger in order not to feel its pangs. A lot of compulsive behavior—drugs, sexual (abuse), hyperactivity, work for work's sake— can be means of escaping from the awareness of this hunger. Nature seems to have provided us with the need of interior silence. We seek it as we seek returning to a place of security, warmth, and love."*

Remember the days when exercise was thought of as something obese people should do for weight loss? I remember. As an athlete in my youth, the neighbors would often question me about my running, wondering why I was exercising since I wasn't fat! Hard to believe that not very long ago the awareness that exercise is necessary for the health of every individual was not common as it is today. Over the years, volumes of research have reached the masses convincing them of this seemingly obvious fact. Similarly, it won't be too long before we look at the recent times where people thought prayer and meditation were only for nuns, priests, and religious people. As research is consistently showing that a spiritual practice is beneficial to everyone, people are witnessing their own need for a more authentic spiritual expression.

Cultivating awareness allows you to live life to its fullest, most joyful expression. Spirituality is not just about avoiding being bad by following "the rules" and/or feeling guilty or unworthy because you broke them. Instead a healthy Spirit is one that is joyfully celebrating existence. As we have just explored, the Spirit becomes joyful when it is supported by truth and joyful beliefs, thoughts, words, and actions.

As we live in a land of instant coffee, up-to-the-minute stock quotes, and an Internet that allows us to access information and to purchase almost anything within seconds, it is important to remember that a spiritual life cannot be bought and is not instant. It is like a garden that needs to be cultivated. It needs regular watering, feeding, and weeding. It cannot be rushed; in fact, patience is one of its gifts.

As you cultivate a rich spiritual life, you will notice more serendipity, grace, interconnectedness, and meaning. Life will seem to flow more easily. Instead of swimming against the tide, you'll be moving in a loving, supportive current. Instead of blocking the flow of Spirit with limited thinking and behavior, *"Seek ye first the kingdom of heaven, and all things will be added onto you."*

WHAT'S AHEAD

So far, you have been presented with tools to evaluate what you may be encountering physically, emotionally, and spiritually. Choices to better support your experience of life and health have been offered. Following the advice in the book alone may be enough to transform whatever challenges you are experiencing; however, professional help might also be necessary. Chapter 15 provides the details about the wide range of health practitioners available to assist you on your journey.

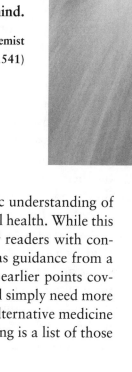

FIFTEEN

Maximize Your Plan:
Working with a Health Professional

The art of healing comes from nature
and not from the physician.

Therefore the physician must start from
nature with an open mind.

— Paracelsus, Swiss-born alchemist
and physician (1493-1541)

The Detox Solution can provide you with a basic understanding of what the body, mind, and spirit need for optimal health. While this will be enough for many people, there will be other readers with conditions that require more focused attention as well as guidance from a health professional. The detox program and all the earlier points covered in the book will still apply, but these readers will simply need more care. Many of their conditions will respond well to alternative medicine and supervised detoxification programs. The following is a list of those ailments that can benefit from such approaches.

- Addictions: drugs (recreational and prescription), alcohol, tobacco
- ADD/ADHD

- AIDS
- Allergies
- Alzheimer's disease
- Arthritis

- ■ Asthma
- ■ Autism
- ■ Autoimmune conditions
- ■ Back pain
- ■ Cancer
- ■ Candidiasis
- ■ Chronic fatigue
- ■ Digestive disorders
- ■ Gynecological concerns
- ■ Headaches
- ■ Heart disease
- ■ High blood pressure

- ■ Infections
- ■ Infertility
- ■ Insomnia
- ■ Kidney problems
- ■ Liver conditions
- ■ Osteoporosis
- ■ Parasitic infections
- ■ Prostate problems
- ■ Reproductive difficulties
- ■ Respiratory ailments
- ■ Viral conditions
- ■ Weight problems

Following the basic advice in *The Detox Solution* is likely to result in improvement of many of the conditions listed above. However, there are wonderful resources today for obtaining professional assistance and a program of care that is tailored just for you. You'll find many excellent resources in this chapter.

It's wonderful that individuals are taking more responsibility for their health these days, but it's also important to recognize when professional assistance can help you reach your goals more efficiently. Too frequently I see patients who come to me after exerting a lot of effort on their own or following the advice of unqualified people. Even if they've made many wise decisions, it's often been in a fragmented way. They have their bags of ginkgo, vitamins, powders, and potions. Many of their decisions to buy these items were from various articles they'd read over time. More often than not, patients bring their supplements to me and ask me what to do with them because "they forgot what they were taking them for." Many times they have made good decisions, but their understanding of how all the products fit in their total plan for healing was missing. They didn't have a road map marked with the most direct route to healing. They needed qualified professional advice.

This is an exciting time to be living. There's more health information and resources available now then ever before. However nothing can replace the human element when it comes to the healing process. The experience of the health professional you choose is key. An effective practitioner with good references and experience with your particular problem can really make a difference. Credentials, a fancy office, and pictures of celebrities on the wall are nice, but *a track record of success with your health concern is the most important factor.*

You may find that an alternative health professional can help you without input from a practitioner from Western medicine. Or you may want care from both the complementary and traditional fields. The resources in this chapter are oriented toward practitioners who are knowledgeable in alternative medicine, and it includes physicians also trained in Western medicine. Note: Even if you choose to stay with an exclusive Western medicine practitioner, the suggestions in *The Detox Solution* can enhance your health and possibly reduce your need for medication and surgery.

CHOOSING A HEALTH PRACTITIONER

Selecting the right practitioner is essential to the quality of your healing experience. The time you set aside for choosing a health professional is a great investment. One of the best ways to find someone is by asking people you know—friends, relatives, or co-workers—who they go to for care. Excellent resources for alternative practitioners are also provided in this chapter.

Before you decide who you will see, it's a good idea to call the offices of a few professionals and talk to their office manager. You can find out if the basic approach of the practitioner seems like a match to your needs. Also ask about the amount of time that's usually spent with a patient. In general, holistic practitioners tend to spend more time with patients and to place more emphasis on health education. If you've only been to Western health care professionals in the past, you may be surprised by the amount of attention you receive during your visits to alternative practitioners.

Often an initial visit is the time when you determine whether or not the professional is the right person to treat you. Here are some questions to keep in mind during the appointment:

What is their belief system about healing? Do they seem to encourage their patients to become a co-creator of health? Does the practitioner come across as a health coach and educator? Or do they act condescending or superior and discourage questions?

Do they look for the root cause of your problem? Or do they simply attempt to eliminate the symptoms without investigating the condition further?

Are you encouraged to develop daily habits that will support your health? Or is the discussion limited to a specific treatment protocol?

Do you feel that you can build a good rapport with this professional? Are your styles compatible?

Does the practitioner listen and really hear what your concerns are? Or does the professional seem to be following their own agenda without really dealing with your original complaint?

Do you feel the uniqueness of who you are is considered in assessing your health challenge? Or is the approach more generic and superficial?

Is the practitioner a model for good health? Does he or she seem to "walk the talk"? Or can you tell that this person neglects self-care?

What is your experience in spending time at this office? Is it a healing environment? Do you feel cared for? Or are you just another patient marching down a busy assembly line?

Building a good relationship with the health professional is a two-way process. The patient carries responsibility for what takes place as well as the practitioner. To address your health concern, write down questions ahead of time and prioritize your concerns. During your initial visit, you can begin to get to know the practitioner by asking why he or she decided to work in the health field.

Working with a holistic practitioner demands more cooperation on the part of the patient. It will require that you become educated about your condition and also participate in making decisions about your care. Remember, these practitioners are operating from the premise that your body heals itself and they are assisting by providing life-supportive therapies. This differs drastically from the Western paradigm that primarily seeks to alleviate symptoms with the use of synthetic substances.

In regard to "symptom management," it is important to note that repressing symptoms is quite different from actual healing of the body. For instance, clearing a breakout of the skin by applying a prescribed medicated ointment might help a patient feel better about his or her state of health. However, if that skin eruption is caused by food allergies, the underlying problem is not being addressed. The deeper problem can possibly degenerate into a more serious condition if left to fester.

Am I suggesting that we should abandon all prescription medication in favor of natural approaches? No! There are times when the health professional will want to manage symptoms as they work on the underlying cause. However, when you start *healing the body* rather than merely managing symptoms, the need for many medications decreases. Then you and your doctor can adjust the dose accordingly or eliminate the medication when appropriate.

Finally, remember that not every holistic health professional will have detoxification experience. The categories listed below are those that usually include detoxification in their scope of practice. If you have one of the conditions mentioned at the beginning of this chapter, you may find that a supervised detoxification program is an important part of your healing journey.

DIRECTORY OF HEALTH PROFESSIONALS

■ Multidisciplinary Resources

Several organizations can provide the names of health professionals in various disciplines. These practitioners will include alternative health professionals as well as M.D.s who have been trained in using detoxification as a healing tool. The references below can direct you to practitioners in your area who are more likely skilled in detoxification. (Note: The other sections below explore each discipline separately.)

Energetix, 92 Waycaster Circle, Dahlonega, GA 30533
(888) 464-7630 • *energetix@mindspring.com*
www.energetixdirect.com
This organization provides referrals to the public to physicians of various disciplines who are extensively trained in detoxification protocols. Energetix also provides information to health professionals as to where specialized training in clinical detoxification is available.

Healthcomm/Metagenics Inc., P.O. Box 1729, Gig Harbor,
WA 98335 • (800) 692-9400 • *www.healthcomm.com*

Price-Pottenger Nutrition Foundation, P.O. Box 2614, La Mesa,
CA 91943-2614 • (800) 366-3748 • *www.price-pottenger.org*

■ Traditional Oriental Medicine/Acupuncture

The practice of Oriental medicine originated in China over five thousand years ago. Its modalities include the use of herbal medicine, nutrition, massage and acupuncture. Practitioners of Oriental medicine are called Licensed Acupuncturists. If the idea of facing needles is disconcerting (although they are virtually painless), it's important to realize that seeing an acupuncturist does not mean that such a treatment is a must. A licensed acupuncturist is often a doctor of Oriental medicine and has approximately 4,000 hours (four years) of training in medicine; some of these practitioners use herbs and nutrition exclusively rather than needles.

The World Health Organization has cited 104 conditions that acupuncture can treat including addictions, pain, arthritis, migraines, depression, insomnia, and immune challenges. With regards to detox, acupuncture has been valuable in the treatment of illnesses due to exposure to radiation, pesticides, toxic chemicals, and air pollution, as well as for smoking withdrawal and drug and alcohol detox.

National Acupuncture and Oriental Medicine Alliance
14637 Starr Road Southeast, Ollala, WA 98359
(253) 851-6896, fax (253) 851-6883 • *www.acuall.org*

American Association of Oriental Medicine,
433 Front St., Catasauqua, PA 18032,
(888) 500-7999, fax (610) 264-2768 • *www.aaom.org*

National Certification Commission for Certification of Acupuncture and Oriental Medicine, 11 Canal Center Plaza, Suite 300, Alexandria, VA 22314, (703) 548-9004, fax (703) 548-9079 • *www.nccaom.org*

www.acupuncture.com
Comprehensive website of resources and information.

■ Physicians with Acupuncture Training

There is also an association of medical doctors who have received training in acupuncture. These physicians have at least 200 hours of acupuncture education. This curriculum usually does not include background in herbs or Oriental medicine, although some medical doctors have delved into these areas on their own.

American Academy of Medical Acupuncture,
5820 Wilshire Boulevard, Suite 500, Los Angeles, CA 90036
(323) 937-5514 • *www.medicalacupuncture.org*

■ Homeopathy

"Homeopathy cures a larger percentage of cases than any other method of treatment." — Mahatma Gandhi

Homeopathic medicine uses minute amounts of natural substances to stimulate the body's defenses in a very specific way. The basic principle is "like heals like," as the substances stimulate similar reactions in the body as the illness and therefore promote healing. This approach to medical treatment was quite popular from the mid-19th Century to the early 20th. Homeopathy advocates included Thomas Edison, Mark Twain, and John D. Rockefeller. Now the homeopathic pharmaceutical system has made a comeback, with millions of people currently using these natural treatments worldwide.

At many U.S. pharmacies, homeopathic medicines can be purchased over-the-counter. It is generally safe to try homeopathic products sold in this manner for minor ailments, i.e. for colds, flus, sleeplessness, etc. For more chronic conditions, consult a homeopathic practitioner. More than 3,000 health professionals currently practice homeopathy in America.

Some of the conditions well suited for treatment with homeopathy include allergies, fatigue, headaches, digestive disorders, arthritis, autoimmune diseases, premenstrual tension, and back pain.

National Center for Homeopathy, 801 North Fairfax Street, Suite 306, Alexandria, VA 22314, (877) 624-0613, fax (703) 548-7792 • *www.homeopathic.org*

Homeopathic Educational Services, 2124 Kittredge St., Berkeley, CA 94704, (510) 649-0294, fax (510) 649-1955
www.homeopathic.com

Santa Monica Homeopathic Pharmacy, 629 Broadway
Santa Monica, CA 90401, (310) 395-1131, fax (310) 395-7851
www.smhomeopathic.com

▪ Chiropractic

Chiropractic is another medical system that emphasizes the importance of removing obstacles in order to promote healing. To this end,
chiropractic seeks to remove nerve interference by adjusting the spine.
When the body gets proper nerve supply, organs and systems can function better. Joints in other areas are adjusted also to promote proper
positioning and to prevent pain, weakness, and malfunction. Many chiropractors do more than body adjustments and additional musculoskeletal treatments. They are often board-certified in nutrition and
can offer a wide range of holistic services. You'll need to inquire.

Over 15 million people go to chiropractors each year. Common
conditions treated by these professionals include backache, joint pain,
sports injuries, and trauma. Other ailments that respond well to chiropractic care are arthritis, gastrointestinal disorders, respiratory problems, high blood pressure, menstrual difficulties, heart symptoms,
chemical addictions, and depression.

American Chiropractic Association, 1701 Clarendon Blvd.
Arlington, VA 22209, (703) 276-8800, fax (703) 243-2593
www.amerchiro.org

International Chiropractors Association, 1110 N. Glebe Road,
Suite 1000, Arlington, VA 22201, (703) 528-5000,
fax (703) 528-5023 • *www.chiropractic.org*

▪ Naturopathic Medicine

Naturopathy utilizes a wide variety of healing practices to support the body's own healing processes: nutrition, homeopathy, herbal
medicine, therapeutic exercise, physical therapy, lifestyle counseling,
and pharmacology. It draws on time-proven principles from long-
standing health traditions, such as Ayurveda and Traditional Chinese
Medicine. These principles include the power of nature and the
importance of finding the underlying cause for ill health.
Naturopathic physicians (N.D.s) are considered to be primary care

providers. Many naturopaths are well trained in the principles of detoxification.

Naturopaths are licensed currently in 11 states including Hawaii, Alaska, Washington, Oregon, Utah, Montana, Arizona, Connecticut, New Hampshire, Vermont, and Maine. Naturopathic medical schools offer four-year programs that follow three years of standard pre-medical education. The four-year curriculum includes approximately 4,500 hours of academic and clinical training.

Naturopathic treatment is particularly suited for chronic health problems.

American Association of Naturopathic Physicians
8201 Greensboro Drive, Suite 300, McLean, VA 22102
(703) 610-9037, fax (703) 610-9005 • *www.naturopathic.org*

Naturopathic Medical Network • *www.pandamedicine.com*

■ Medical Doctors

Some Western-trained physicians take more of an active interest in alternative medicine. They make an effort to learn about nutrition, the prevention of disease, and other developments in the field. While it can still be challenging for a patient to integrate both alternative and Western resources into a healing program, it is becoming more common to do so. The doctors belonging to the organizations below are open to both approaches. It seems likely that more doctors will join their ranks in the years ahead.

American College for the Advancement of Medicine
23121 Verdugo Drive, Suite 204, Laguna Hills, CA 92653
(714) 583-7666 • *www.acam.org*

American Holistic Medical Association, 6728 Old McLean
Village Dr., McLean, Virginia 22101, (703) 556-9728
www.holisticmedicine.org

American Preventive Medical Association, 9912 Georgetown Pike,
Suite D-2, Great Falls, VA 22066, (703) 759-0662
Fax (703) 759-6711 • *www.apma.net*

■ Environmental Medicine

The Detox Solution has presented toxic factors that can be eliminat-ed from your diet, environment, etc. In a similar way, physicians in the field of environmental medicine look at how dietary and environmental elements could be contributing to a patient's ill health. Chemicals, dust, molds, pollen, and foods are examples of what the physician might con-sider. Sometimes it's determined that an ailment is specifically triggered by such a factor or a condition may have been further aggravated by it. If you need additional support to deal with environmental factors impacting your health, consult a physician specializing in this area.

Environmental medicine is a growing field. It is helpful for allergies, chemical sensitivities, arthritis, heart problems, gastrointestinal disor-ders, headaches, insomnia, psychiatric problems, respiratory condi-tions, and skin eruptions.

American Academy of Environmental Medicine
7701 East Kellogg, Suite 625, Wichita, KS 67207
(316) 684-5500, Fax (316) 684-5709 • *www.aaem.com*

■ Orthomolecular Medicine

In orthomolecular medicine, disease is prevented or treated through the administration of optimal amounts of substances naturally present in the body. Biochemical abnormalities are corrected with vitamins, amino acids, minerals, electrolytes, fatty acids, etc. Components of this branch of medicine include dietary recommendations, supplementation, medici-nal herbs, homeopathy, detoxification, chelation, and ozone therapy.

There's a lot of potential in this exciting field. Among the ailments currently treated are depression, schizophrenia, panic attacks, mood swings, cancer, hypertension, heart disease, low blood sugar, menstrual problems, and seizures.

International Society for Orthomolecular Medicine
16 Florence Avenue, Toronto, Ontario, Canada M2N 1E9
(416) 733-2117, Fax (416) 733-2352 • *www.orthomed.org*

■ Chelation Therapy

In this form of therapy, chelating agents are administered intra-venously or orally to remove toxins from the tissues. Chelation therapy has been used for removal of heavy metals from the body (such as mercury, lead, or aluminum) and as an effective means of combating hardening of the arteries. In cases of atherosclerosis, it can serve as an alternative to heart bypass surgery and/or angioplasty. Approximately 1,500 physicians currently practice chelation therapy in the United States.

American Board of Chelation Therapy, 1407 1/2 N. Wells Street, Ground Floor, Chicago, Illinois 60610, (800) 356-2228, Fax (312) 266-3685

American College of Advancement in Medicine
23121 Verdugo Drive, Suite 204, Laguna Hills, CA 92653
(949) 583-7666 • *www.acam.org*

■ Biological Dentists

Dental problems—such as cavities, infections, and root canals—can have a great impact on our health. I have seen many patients who have "tried everything" in both alternative and Western medicine finally resolve their health issue when they dealt with their dental concerns. Often they were coping with a seemingly unrelated condition such as fibromyalgia, chronic fatigue, a skin disorder, or an immune condition. In many cases, there was mercury in their system, low-grade infections in the mouth (sometimes from old root canals), and/or a deterioration of the jaw. These conditions are not typically detected with the testing methods used by non-biological dentists.

Harold Ravins, D.D.S., is a biological dentist and dental acupuncturist with over forty years' experience. He is the Director of the Center for Holistic Dentistry in Los Angeles. Dr. Ravins has consistently observed that a major and frequently overlooked factor in chronic illness is the health of the teeth and gums. He comments, "The mouth is our direct link with the outside world, and often low-grade infections as well as allergies and sensitivities to dental materials go undetected. This results in a constant drain on the immune system."

Biological dentists treat the whole person, and understand how the health of the teeth relates to the health of the body. You can see these professionals for the replacement of mercury fillings with nontoxic materials. (See mercury toxicity information in Chapter 3.) Often these dentists have excellent referrals to other alternative health practitioners in their area.

Environmental Dental Association, 9974 Scripps Ranch Blvd., Suite 36, San Diego, CA 92131, (800) 388-8124

International Academy of Oral Medicine and Toxicology
P.O. Box 608531, Orlando, FL 32860-8531
(407) 298-2450, Fax (407) 298-3075 • *www.iaomt.org*
This academy certifies dentists in safe amalgam
(mercury fillings) removal.

▪ Nutritionists

Sometimes it is helpful to seek the guidance of a qualified nutritionist to determine the food and supplement program that is best for you. Since what we eat plays such a major role in our state of health, dietary adjustments often support efforts to heal various ailments. A professional nutritionist will discuss your health history and probably ask that you keep a food diary to track your habits. Laboratory tests are also utilized.

The IAACN is one of the best sources to find qualified professionals in the nutrition field. This organization offers ongoing training to keep practitioners up-to-date on the latest research findings.

International and American Association of Certified Nutritionists
16775 Addison Road, Suite 102, Addison, TX 75001
(972) 407-9089, Fax (972) 250-0233 • *www.iaacn.org*

▪ Osteopaths

An osteopathic medical doctor (D.O.) receives virtually the same training as a medical doctor (M.D.). However, in addition to traditional Western medicine training, osteopathic medicine recognizes the importance of structural balance of the musculoskeletal system. Osteopaths are specially trained to assess how musculoskeletal imbalances might be contributing to a health challenge. They utilize various forms of physical manipulation to correct these conditions.

D.O.s are licensed as physicians in all 50 states. Among the conditions effectively treated by osteopaths are joint and spine problems, arthritis, chronic pain, chronic fatigue, digestive disorders, psychological dysfunctions, headaches, respiratory challenges, and menstrual difficulties.

American Osteopathic Association, 142 East Ontario Street Chicago, Illinois 60611, (312) 202-8284, Fax (312) 202-8200 *www.aoa-net.org*

American Academy of Osteopathy, 3500 DePauw Boulevard, Suite 1080, Indianapolis, Indiana 46268-1136, (317) 879-1881, Fax (317) 879-0563 • *www.academyofosteopathy.org*

■ Special Detox Plans

When you visit the health professionals listed above, you may be offered a detoxification program that uses specialty products. One product many practitioners use is called *Ultra Clear.* This is a food-based powder created from hypoallergenic (and tasty) ingredients; it is made into a nutritionally supportive and detoxifying beverage by mixing the powder with water or juice. While I have not advocated the use of fasting for detoxification, Ultra Clear is part of a medical program that has been tested and used successfully for over a decade by thousands of practitioners. You can obtain more information on Ultra Clear and related products at *www.ultrabalance.com.*

The toxic concerns addressed throughout this book are very real. Many of you will feel better just by eliminating toxins on your own and following advice given in *The Detox Solution.* However, for others, it can be helpful to know that additional support like Ultra Clear is available. While you may find good quality products to enhance your cleansing in most health food stores, Ultra Clear is an example of a product used in clinical detoxification programs and available only through practitioners.

■ Resources for More Intensive Detoxification

The Environmental Health Center is an excellent resource for someone who has had a more serious exposure to toxins, such as long-term work alongside a synthetic chemical on the job. While just about anyone interested in detox would probably benefit from the services provided by William Rea, M.D., and his associates, this center has expertise in handling extremely ill patients.

Environmental Health Center, William Rea, M.D.
8345 Walnut Hill Lane, Suite 220, Dallas, TX 75231-4262
(214) 368-4132, Fax (214) 691-8432 • *www.ehcd.com*

The Tree of Life Rejuvenation Center is a retreat center under the guidance of Gabriel Cousens, M.D., a leading expert in the field of detoxification. At the Tree of Life, participants in the program receive a thorough evaluation and personalized recommendations to heal various health challenges. The Center provides organic cuisine and offers yoga, meditation, and instruction on how to access natural healing forces for complete body, mind, and spiritual renewal.

Tree of Life Rejuvenation Center, P.O. Box 1080
Patagonia, AZ 85624, (520) 394-2520, fax (520) 394-2099
www.treeoflife.nu

■ Testing

If you have a chronic condition, you may have had many tests run. Hopefully they have been conclusive and your treatment is working. However, in many cases, people who are ill are told they are "normal" and it's all in their head. That is partly because the tests that are offered aren't always comprehensive or on target. Sometimes false negatives and positives occur. Other times the results do not give the practitioner any indication of a successful, safe treatment to employ. The following is a description of some of the tests that have been the most helpful to patients.

Parasite Profile: Many cases of conditions caused (or at least aggravated) by parasitic infestations go undetected by traditional parasite testing. Why? Well, there are so many more parasites that might be present than traditional testing looks for. For accurate results, it is helpful to use labs that specialize in parasite testing. See *www.para sitetesting.com*. A parasite infestation may have serious ill health effects. The presence of parasites can create autoimmune reactions and erode the state of the digestive tract. The obvious symptoms of a parasitic infection include diarrhea, abdominal pain, fever, rashes, and blood in the stools. Not so obvious symptoms include indigestion, hormonal imbalances, immune deficiency, asthma, allergies, joint/muscle pain, and chronic fatigue. Remember, most medical doctors are not parasite experts, and many conditions caused by parasites can easily be misdiagnosed.

Candida (Yeast) Overgrowth Detection: This is another common occurrence that contributes to so much chronic illness. Most labs aren't looking for candida. If they don't test for it, they won't find it. Specialty labs can detect the presence of this health-zapping fungus so it can be treated efficiently. The use of antibiotics, contraceptive pills, and refined sugar has caused the amount of yeast in many people to get out of control. Symptoms of a yeast overgrowth include depression of the immune response, gastrointestinal disorders, brain fog, emotional instability, hormonal imbalances, skin disorders, and repeated infections.

Comprehensive Digestive Stool Analysis: This test evaluates the effectiveness of your digestive processing and absorption, and assists in diagnosing particular problems. You can find out about enzymes, parasites, yeast, and the population of beneficial and harmful bacteria from this type of analysis. Poor digestive functioning has wide-ranging negative impacts on our well-being from our emotional outlook, energy level, day-to-day feelings of comfort, and the presence or lack of disease. There is much to be learned from this type of analysis.

Intestinal Permeability Testing: Along with digestion of food and absorption of nutrients, the intestines also guard us from ill effects from toxins and microbes. However, a number of factors can reduce the effectiveness of the intestinal barrier in blocking the entry of potential injurious elements into our system. These factors include excessive alcohol consumption, stress, toxic exposures, deficient diet, and ill health. An increase in the permeability of the intestinal wall, known as "leaky gut syndrome," can contribute to food allergies, inflammatory bowel disease, autoimmune disease, malabsorption of food, and accelerated aging.

Allergy Testing: This type of testing can determine if you have allergies to foods and inhalants. Allergies to elements in food and the environment are linked to various conditions including asthma, arthritis, depression, anxiety, chronic fatigue syndrome, eczema, migraines, indigestion, muscle/joint soreness, skin disorders, irritable bowel, colitis, water retention, difficulty losing or gaining weight,

and decreased immune response. NAET (*www.naet.com*) is an innovative non-invasive testing technique that has a high success rate in
diagnosing and treating allergies.

Heavy Metal Screening: Although skeptics think the whole heavy metal
issue is hogwash, this type of lab testing has been a saving grace for
many patients. There are labs that test for heavy metals (mercury,
lead, nickel, cadmium, etc.) using hair and/or blood samples. Hair
sample testing is used extensively for suspected mercury toxicity.
Heavy metal screening is also used to monitor detoxification treatment. Note: Heavy metals can accumulate in the body over time.
Symptoms differ per the heavy metal involved, but in general
include fatigue, depression of the immune response, headaches,
liver disorders, emotional/psychological reactions, cardiovascular
concerns, neurological disorders, learning problems, gastrointestinal distress, and increased cancer risk.

Adrenocortex Stress Profile: Many conditions originate or are made worse
by our emotional response to stress. Chapter 13 presented techniques
to transform stress and tension into peace and a relaxed disposition.
There are actually lab tests that can monitor your progress. When you
have lived a life of constant stress, the effects will show up as an
imbalanced level of cortisol and other adrenal hormones. An adrenocortex stress profile can detect the imbalances that may be present.
Symptoms of a stress overload include fatigue, weight loss, blood
sugar imbalances, general weakness, muscle and/or joint pain, gastrointestinal disorders, frequent colds or flu, high blood pressure,
menstrual problems, depression, insomnia, and accelerated aging.

Heart Rate Variability (HRV): This is another test to measure how well
your body can handle stress. HRV is a measurement of your sympathetic (the "fight or flight" response) and parasympathetic (the "relaxation" response) nervous systems. HRV is valuable to determine the
influence of emotional stress on illness, and can also be used to measure improvements when stress reduction techniques are employed.

Natural Killer Cell Test (Assessing the Ability to Fight Cancer): It is ironic that when a person receives Western medical treatment for cancer
(surgery, chemotherapy, and/or radiation), the body's immune function is rarely monitored. This is a time when a strong immune system
is needed the most. The natural killer function test offers a way to see
how the immune function is operating with regards to fighting can-

cer. This is a test that can be taken during or after cancer treatments, or as a way to assess your immune system before a diagnosis and possibly take steps to prevent illness. Immune function testing is an area of diagnostics that has grown tremendously over the last several years. Besides the natural killer function test, there are now many other tools available to diagnose and treat diseases and disorders and to monitor the effectiveness of your immune response.

Oxidative Stress Testing: Depending on your current state of health and other factors, you will be more or less able to handle the effects of free radicals. The oxidative stress test can help determine the amount of free radical stress your cells are challenged with, as well as the antioxidant reserves present in your body. These findings are used to assess the impact of free radicals on liver detoxification. Oxidative stress accelerates aging and fosters the development of degenerative diseases.

Organic Acid Analysis: This analysis can help to determine how well the body is clearing toxins. It is often used to see how efficiently prescription medications are being cleared from the system. It can also be used to identify a fungal overgrowth or bowel bacteria imbalance. Abnormal levels of homocysteine, a marker for heart disease, can be detected. The organic acid analysis is a urine-based test.

Amino Acid Analysis: Certain individuals have difficulty processing amino acids from the foods they eat or in manufacturing others made in the body. This can lead to deficiencies in some amino acids and excesses of others. Amino acids are needed for proper cellular detoxification. This test can tell you whether your supplies are at healthy levels. Data also reveals insight into the health of your liver and kidneys. Two of the primary amino acids assessed are cysteine and taurine.

Vitamin and Mineral Assay: One of the best approaches to evaluating the levels of vitamins and minerals in your system is to do assays. In these assessments, levels of white blood cells, red blood cells, and enzymes are checked in blood samples. Since these elements are used to produce various nutrients, the assessments are quite revealing. Other tests measuring vitamin and mineral levels are also available including those that analyze hair and urine samples. Testing one's vitamin and mineral status is important for people with chronic illness. Results can be helpful for designing a supplementation program.

Essential Fatty Acid Analysis: As you learned in the nutrition chapter, many people are deficient in fatty acids. This is often because people do not eat enough of the right kind of fats. Fatty acids are important to our cell membranes, brains, nervous system, heart, and vascular system. A deficiency can lead to chronic toxicity. If you have a toxic overload which is affecting your nervous system, an essential fatty acid analysis may show how efficiently your body is repairing the damage. The test is also requested in cases of chronic illness or ongoing inflammation. Fatty acid deficiencies are present in many disease states. A fasting whole blood sample is used.

Detoxification Profile: So many chronic conditions have liver toxicity as an obstacle to healing. Though this condition may be present, blood tests can claim the liver numbers to be "normal." Routine blood tests look for two liver enzymes (SGPT and SGOT) that indicate liver inflammation, but they do not test the liver's ability to detox. A detoxification profile examines saliva, blood, and urine to determine the ability of the liver to convert and clear toxic substances from the body. The numerous symptoms of a challenged liver include joint pain, fatigue, immune problems, respiratory difficulties, skin eruptions, food allergies, poor memory, mental confusion, sore throat, sinus congestion, weight gain, and frequent infections.

Indican Testing: This urine test screens you for the presence of dysbiosis, an imbalance of bacteria in the bowel. Indican is a toxin that comes from putrefaction in the colon; this substance goes back into the bloodstream and eventually to the kidneys to be excreted in the urine.

Biological Terrain Assessment (BTA): This cutting-edge test evaluates the "terrain" of the body biochemically. It assesses how fertile the terrain of your body is for health or illness. This remarkable system can pinpoint the weak areas of the body with regard to detoxification. It is also helpful in recognizing disease states much earlier than traditional measures. Results reveal information on the current functioning of your liver, kidneys, digestion, and lymphatic system. The BTA test can detect the presence of fungal, viral, or bacterial infections; deficiencies in vitamins, minerals, and antioxidants; and shortages in oxygen at the cellular level. Blood, saliva, and urine are used.

Dark Field Microscopy: In this approach to analyzing the vital fluid of life, blood can remain alive and active; therefore tests provide more extensive information regarding the health of the blood and the body it came from. In contrast, traditional techniques—stains and the electron microscope—use blood that is essentially killed in the process of observation. In dark field microscopy, the blood is stained with light frequencies. At the same time, the background is kept dark so that a contrast is created. Results from a dark field microscopy are often utilized in conjunction with other tests. It is used to both detect imbalances, degenerative conditions, and potential weaknesses. With dark field microscopy, you can see immediately with your own eyes the factors that may be interfering with healing such as fungi, parasites, and poor protein digestion.

EAV Testing: In this method of testing the body's energy system, low voltage electric charges are introduced into the body. Afterwards levels of current are assessed at various acupuncture meridian points on the hands and feet. This assessment is based on readings from a meter that checks the skin's resistance or conductivity to the electric charges. Low readings can show where the body is likely to be having difficulty fighting an imbalance by its own means. This type of testing is also used to evaluate the proper course of treatment. It can help identify areas that may be especially affected by toxins. Results can also indicate sensitivities to certain heavy metals. EAV testing can be used to determine the compatibility of supplements such as vitamins and herbs as well as assessing their effectiveness in the protocol.

Adipose Tissue Testing: Toxins that enter our system can be stored in adipose (fat) tissue. In particular, adipose tissue samples can reveal the amount of pesticides that have been absorbed into our body. A pesticides panel may look for residues of a dozen such chemicals at a time. Fat tissue also stores fat-soluble vitamins and reflects our intake of essential fatty acids.

TEST LABORATORIES

The types of screening technologies that are available become more varied and specific each year. Here's a list of some of the labs with testing related to toxic exposures, immune response, nutrient status, gastrointestinal health, and other relevant areas. If you think a particular test is necessary, most labs can provide referrals to practitioners who can order the test.

Accu-Chem Laboratories, 990 N. Bowser Road, Suite 800
Richardson, TX 75081, (972) 234-5577, Fax (972) 234-5707
www.accuchemlabs.com
This lab tests blood and urine for signs of environmental and occupational chemical exposures. Toxins include pesticides, solvents, and heavy metals.

Antibody Assay Lab, 1715 East Wilshire, Suite 715
Santa Ana, CA 92705, (714) 972-9979 • *www.aalrl.com*
After a toxic exposure, tests for blood antibodies, immune status, and chemical detection can all be done at AAL. They also screen for hormones, allergies, candida, and vitamins.

Doctor's Data, P.O. Box 111, West Chicago, IL 60186
(800) 323-2784, Fax (630) 587-7860 • *www.doctorsdata.com*
Doctor's Data provides hair, blood, and urine analysis to evaluate toxins, specifically heavy metals. They also perform amino acids analyses. Their data is very helpful in monitoring the detox progress.

Great Smokies Diagnostic Laboratory, 63 Zillicoa St.
Asheville, NC 28801-1074, (800) 522-4762 • *www.gsdl.com*
A leader in diagnostic testing, Great Smokies provides assessments for gastrointestinal health, immunology, nutritional status, endocrinology, oxidative stress, detox, etc.

Immunosciences Lab, Inc., 8730 Wilshire Blvd., Suite 305
Beverly Hills, CA 90211, (310) 657-1077, Fax (310) 657-1053
www.immuno-sci-lab.com
Immunosciences focuses on tests where the immune system is a crucial element in ill health. Their emphasis is on complex diseases. This lab covers allergies, autoimmune diseases, cancer, chronic fatigue, immunology, immunotoxicology, and intestinal health.

Meridian Valley Clinical Laboratory, 515 W. Harrison Street, Suite 9, Kent, Washington 98032, (253) 859-8700, Fax (253) 859-1135 • *www.tahomaclinic.com*
Providing state-of-the-art services to the alternative health community, MVCL focuses on steroid hormones, nutritional biochemistry, food/inhalant allergies, and stool analysis.

MetaMetrix Medical Laboratory, 5000 Peachtree Industrial Boulevard, Norcross, Georgia 30071, (800) 221-4640
Fax (770) 441-2237 • *www.metametrix.com*
This full-service lab specializes in toxic element panels, organic acid analyses, allergy/antibody testing, antioxidant assessments, and nutritional status.

National Medical Services, 3701 Welsh Road, Willow Grove, PA 19090, (215) 657-4900, Fax (215) 657-2972
www.nmslab.com
For over 25 years, National Medical Services has provided an extensive line of tests. These include blood and urine screens for pesticides, solvents, and heavy metals.

Pacific Toxicology Laboratory, 6160 Variel Avenue, Woodland Hills, CA 91367, (800) 328-6942, Fax (818) 598-3116 • *www.pactox.com*
This lab monitors blood and urine samples for toxic exposures. Chemicals include solvents, pesticides, heavy metals, styrene (used to produce plastics and drugs), and toluene (used to produce chemicals; found in vehicle fuels and paints).

Parasitology Center, Inc. (PCI), 903 S. Rural Road, #101-318 Tempe, AZ 85281, (480) 767-2522, fax (480) 767-5855
www.parasitetesting.com
A leading parasitology lab, PCI offers diagnostic services that include testing of fecal, blood, tissue, and skin specimens to locate parasitic organisms. The facility looks for parasites of the intestinal tract and organ systems, including the skin. Their expertise includes the identification of parasites that cause infestation after environmental exposures.

Peak Energy Performance, 4680 Edison Avenue, Colorado
Springs, CO 80915, (800) 331-2303, Fax (719) 572-8081
www.peakenergy.com
PEP's primary offering is a blood test to determine the least toxic
replacement dental materials for the individual. PEP also creates supplemental programs for people in detox.

SpectraCell Laboratories, 515 Post Oak Blvd. 830
Houston, Texas 77027, 800/227-5227 • *www.spectracell.com*
This lab specializes in assessing nutrient status by testing levels of
vitamins, minerals, antioxidants, amino acids, fatty acids, etc.

Though a few lab tests are available to individuals, most must be
ordered from a health professional. Working with a health practitioner can give you a better understanding of the results. The professional
will also be aware of the tests that apply most closely to your health
condition.

ADDITIONAL THERAPIES

While you might choose an acupuncturist, medical doctor, chiro-
practor, naturopath, or osteopath to be your primary health care practitioner, there are supplemental therapies that assist the healing process.
Here are some to consider.

▪ Massage Therapy
In massage, your soft tissue is manipulated to help restore balance
to your body and mind. It's a great way to pamper yourself and to let
go of stress and tension. As the practitioner kneads, presses, and
strokes parts of your body, circulation of blood and lymphatic fluid
improve. Many health concerns, including headaches, digestive disorders, arthritis, and minor aches and pains, respond well to massage. To
learn more about the different types of massage that are available, see
the Chapter 12.

American Massage Therapy Association, 820 Davis Street,
Suite 100, Evanston, Illinois 60201-4444, (847) 864-0123
Fax (847) 864-1178 • *www.amtamassage.org*

■ Psychology

There are times when the challenges of life can feel overwhelming. It can help to reach out to a professional to discover possibilities for coping more effectively. Psychologists are experts in human behavior and the workings of the mind. Consulting with such an expert can often lead to insights you may not be able to gain on your own. Look for someone with experience in your type of concern—whether it is a troubled marriage, substance abuse, career confusion, assertiveness, health challenges, or a recent death.

American Psychological Association, 750 First Street NE
Washington, D.C. 20002-4242, (202) 336-5500 • *www.apa.org*

■ Spiritual Healing

Letting go of toxic belief systems is a core component to healing. There are various disciplines whose focus is on clearing such contributing factors to illness as anger, fear, holding onto the past, doubt, etc. They encourage the Spirit to come alive with experiences and expressions of love, forgiveness, trust, and peace. This enhances your ability to transform and heal patterns that do not serve your highest good.

The Institute of Applied Ontology, 1411 Dresden Drive
Atlanta, GA 30319, (404) 231-1470, fax (404) 231-1049
www.applied-ontology.com

Ron Roth's Celebrating Life Institutes for Spiritual Healing
P.O. Box 428, Peru, IL 61354, (815) 224-3377
Fax (815) 224-3395 • *www.ronroth.com*

Unity, 1901 NW Blue Parkway, Unity Village, MO 64065-0001
(816) 524-3550, fax (816) 251-3554 • *www.silentunity.org*

Science of Mind/Religious Science, 3251 West Sixth Street
Los Angeles, CA 90020, (213) 388-2181, Fax (213) 388-1926
www.scienceofmind.com

Caroline Myss/Caroline's Shop, 141 Gooding Street
La Salle, IL 61301, (877) 507-MYSS (6977) • *www.myss.com*

■ Energy Medicine

Interest is growing in using the body's natural energies for maintaining and restoring health. This field of therapy works with both the patient's energy and the flow of energy from the practitioner to the patient. While energy medicine is being explored in a number of medical disciplines, one of the best-known branches is *Reiki*—a hands-on therapy for recharging, realigning, and rebalancing human energy. Reiki has its roots in the Tibetan healing arts. Another powerful hands-on therapy is known as *Healing Touch*.

A third discipline in the field of energy medicine is *Jin Shin Jyutsu*, a therapy that interprets energy imbalances as blockages caused by deeper emotional or spiritual issues. Jin Shin practitioners use the assessment tools of observation, asking questions, touch, and checking the patient's pulse to locate energy blockages. Jin Shin was developed from ancient techniques used in Buddhist and Taoist temples of China.

The International Center for Reiki Training
21421 Hilltop Street, #28, Southfield, MI 48034
(800) 332-8112, Fax (248) 948-9534 • *www.reiki.org*

Healing Touch International, 12477 W. Cedar Drive, Suite 202
Lakewood, CO 80228, (303) 989-7982, fax (303) 980-8683
www.healingtouch.net

Jin Shin Jyutsu, 8719 E. San Alberto, Scottsdale, AZ 85258
(480) 998-9331, fax (480) 998-9335, *www.jinshinjyutsu.com*

■ Yoga

As you learned in the circulation chapter, yoga is a form of exercise that incorporates stretching and physical activity with breathing techniques and mindfulness. Some people have the misconception that yoga is not a serious workout. The truth is that some branches of yoga are quite rigorous. All forms of yoga aid detoxification by stimulating the flow of blood and lymphatic fluid. For explanations of the various branches of yoga, see Chapter 12. Following is an organization of health professionals who use yoga as a therapy for healing.

International Association of Yoga Therapists, P.O. Box 2418
Sebastopol, CA 95473, (707) 928-9898 • *www.yrec.org*

■ Meditation

This is a centering practice that directs your attention inward to an internal quiet realm. You are lead to this place of inner stillness by focusing on the breath or a mantra (a word or short phrase which is repeated silently in your mind). The result is a quieting of the chattering in your head and the development of a relaxed state of being. In this tranquil state, you can discover valuable insights. You also rehearse a feeling of relaxation that can later be accessed at stressful times.

There are many types of meditation. The site below describes a variety of meditations to explore. There are meditation groups in most cities to provide you with practical instruction and group support.

The Meditation Society of America
www.meditationsociety.com

■ Colonics

As you learned earlier, waste can accumulate along the walls of the large intestines. Colonics is a form of therapy that uses the infusion of warm filtered water to unburden the colon of this material. This is a more extensive version of an enema, in that it cleanses the entire colon rather than just the area of the rectum. Colon hydrotherapists are trained to monitor the temperature and pressure of the water during the procedure. Colonics can rid the body of toxins and improve the functioning of the large intestine.

International Association for Colon Therapy, P.O. Box 461285
San Antonio, TX 78246-1285, (210) 366-2888
iact@healthy.net • *healthy.net/pan/pa/iact/index.html*

■ Candida (Yeast) Treatment

So many people with chronic yeast problems have been told that they're fine and that their condition is "all in their head." William Crook, M.D., was one of the health pioneers who confirmed that these patients' concerns are very real. His writings, including the book *The Yeast Connection,* have broken new ground. Crook has an informative website on the candida issue which offers booklets with referrals to physicians with expertise with this condition.

International Health Foundation, P.O. Box 3494
Jackson, TN 38303, 901-660-7090 *www.candida-yeast.com*

■ Biofeedback

In biofeedback, a therapist places sensors on the patient's body that provide readings that are fed to a nearby monitor. Feedback is given on skin temperature, muscle tension, and/or brainwave function. As the patient watches the feedback monitor, he or she learns to make various changes in their body which have a healing effect. People experiencing stress-related disorders (panic attacks, generalized anxiety) can improve their relaxation skills using biofeedback. It also has applications in cases of migraines, stroke, and Attention Deficient Disorder.

Biofeedback Certification Institute of America
10200 W. 44th Avenue, #310, Wheat Ridge, CO 80033
(303) 420-2902, Fax (303) 422-8894 • *www.bcia.org*

Biofeedback Network • *www.biofeedback.net*

Heartmath • *www.heartmath.com*
This organization offers excellent workshops on stress reduction.

■ Neuro-Emotional Technique (NET)

From the NET point-of-view, unhealthy emotional responses can be the result of blockages in our sympathetic nervous system. Due to emotions that have been absorbed into the physiology of the body, these responses may become a "locked-in" pattern. By using muscle testing, body reflex points, and somatic reactions, the NET therapist can help a patient recall a negative emotion, and then make body adjustments to resolve the imbalance. NET is used by psychotherapists and health practitioners to support their patients' healing. The technique is used to clear programmed negative response tendencies, including phobias and fear patterns.

NET Incorporated, 510 Second Street, Encinitas, CA 92024
(800) 888-4638 • *www.netmindbody.com*

■ Allergy Desensitization Technique (NAET)

A remarkable technique to desensitize allergens (without shots) is called NAET (Nambudripad's Allergy Elimination Techniques). It was developed by Dr. Devi S. Nambudripad, author of *Say Goodbye to Illness*. I have used this treatment in my clinic with remarkable success. It is drug-free and non-invasive, and the session itself is rather relaxing. In NAET, allergies are cleared one at a time, using the body's energy and the nervous system. NAET can often be helpful as allergies contribute to a long list of health ailments. These ailments include fatigue, dizziness, eczema, hayfever, itchiness, muscle spasms, respiratory infections, gastric disturbances, etc.

Official NAET Website • *www.naet.com*

■ Flower Essence Practitioners

Emotional and mental dimensions of well-being are dealt with by these practitioners with the help of a line of essences derived from the flowering parts of plants. The original thirty-eight infusions were created by Dr. Edward Bach in the 1930s. Now many other decoctions are available. The quality of each flower essence is used to promote a positive effect. Sometimes combinations of essences are blended together.

Flower Essence Services, P.O. Box 1769, Nevada City, CA 95959 (530) 265-0258, Fax (530) 265-6467 • *www.floweressence.com*

■ Hypnotherapy

In hypnotherapy, both physical and psychological problems are addressed through the power of suggestion. By placing the patient in a hypnotic state, the therapist is able to reach the deepest levels of the mind to tap its healing power. In this relaxed state, the mind is more open to suggestions. Applications for hypnosis include fears and phobias, stress reduction, unwanted habits such as smoking, pain relief, skin conditions, anesthesiology, allergies, insomnia, and improved performance in career or sports.

National Board for Certified Clinical Hypnotherapists
1110 Fidler Lane, Suite L1, Silver Spring, MD 20910
(800) 449-8144, Fax (301) 588-9535 • *www.natboard.com*

American Board of Hypnotherapy, 2002 E. McFadden Ave., Suite 100, Santa Ana, CA 92705, (714) 245-9340 • *www.abh.cc*

DON'T OVERLOOK THE BASICS!

While consulting a professional is sometimes necessary, it's important to remember to cover the basics when dealing with your health concerns. The Surgeon General and other health authorities consistently state that disease is often related to poor nutrition, stress, toxins, etc. Common sense tells us that if we remove such obstacles to healing and incorporate great nutrition, pure water, sunshine, love, a sense of purpose, and a positive attitude into our living that our overall health will improve.

I cannot overemphasize that we need to choose ongoing support for our well-being over symptom-oriented health treatments. Not doing so is like trying to remodel a house built on a shaky foundation. The efforts may result in an initial isolated improvement, however the entire structure will still be weak. But if you strengthen the overall foundation first, the specific areas are likely to need less attention than they would have. This idea has been a principle underlying the steps recommended in *The Detox Solution.*

WHAT'S AHEAD

To assist you with your journey to higher levels of health, the final chapter will recap the major steps suggested in *The Detox Solution.* You'll also find motivation to help you stay on the right path or to get back on track if you've gone astray.

SIXTEEN

Detox for Life:
The Twelve-Step Plan for Optimal Physical, Emotional & Spiritual Well-Being

> Life is a song – sing it.
> Life is a game – play it.
> Life is a challenge – meet it.
> Life is a dream – realize it.
> Life is a sacrifice – offer it.
> Life is love – enjoy it.
>
> — Sai Baba

The *Detox Solution* is intended to be used as a guidebook to design your personalized program for achieving higher states of well-being. One of my main goals in creating the book was to pull fragmented ideas on health from various sources and combine them in a cohesive, informative format. It is my hope that you will turn to *The Detox Solution* often as a resource. The abundance of information found here is meant to enlighten, not to overwhelm.

If you were already on a journey of self-help for wellness before you found this book, then *The Detox Solution* has probably given you some new pieces to add to your repertoire. Or if you hadn't really given much attention to the role that you play in your own health, perhaps this book has served as a wake-up call. Either way, the book is here to support your efforts and to help you achieve success. Remember to always choose the solutions that fit your situation and your individual needs.

To help you work with the program presented in *The Detox Solution,* I've carved out a dozen of the major points included in the book; you can think of the program as a "12-Step Plan." For your easy reference, these 12 steps are summarized in this final chapter, "Detox for Life." For more detailed information, refer to the Index and the appropriate chapters.

THE 12-STEP PLAN

#1. Be committed to the gradual replacement of toxic substances in your world with nontoxic, beneficial ones. By now, you're aware of the unprecedented amount of toxicity that our bodies are attempting to deal with. When you first learn about all the toxic influences, it can feel a bit daunting to think about making changes. The best approach is incremental. By repeatedly switching one toxic element for a healthy new choice, you make step-by-step progress. Along the way, you begin to reap the benefits of your efforts, as you continue to feel and look better and better!

#2. Consume a healthy diet and drink plenty of water each day. Both of these habits will support your body's ongoing detoxification. They will also have a huge impact on your state of health today and in the future. Emphasize *organic* vegetables, fruits, and protein when selecting foods for your meals. In terms of the proper balance of protein, carbohydrates, and fat, find the ratio that is right for *your* body. Remember that food is a common source of toxins, so assess your diet regularly to make sure it stays as toxin-free as possible. To determine your water needs, here's an easy tool—simply use half your body weight as a goal. For example, a woman weighing 140 pounds would require 70 ounces of water daily. A man at 180 pounds would need 90 ounces. Next, divide your result (the total daily ounces) by 8 to determine the number of glasses of water to drink a day.

#3. Use enzyme and probiotic supplements regularly. So much of what we eat today is totally devoid of digestive enzymes. The reasons behind this phenomenon include depleted agricultural soils, genetic engineering, food processing, irradiation, pasteurization, current cooking techniques including microwaving, etc. The situation is compounded when the enzymes we do have are diverted to deal with toxins (such as pesticide residues) or zapped by stressful lifestyles. Enzymes are needed to process the nutrients—vitamins, minerals, etc.—provided in food. You should look for an enzyme supplement that includes the following types: protease, amylase, lipase, lactase, cellulase, invertase, maltase, and alpha-galactosidase. Specific digestive enzyme products are recommended in the Resources section.

Probiotic supplementation can be important because modern eating habits and antibiotic use often throw the body out of balance. It can be helpful to supplement with beneficial bacteria to restore the internal flora. A proper bacteria population in the intestines is necessary for both digestion and your overall health. Important beneficial bacteria to consider include *lactobacillus acidophilus, bifidobacteria bifidum, lactobacillus bulgaricus, lactobacillus salivarius, lactobacillus sporogenes, and lactobacillus plantarum*. Again, see the Resources section for specific product recommendations.

#4. Take a high-quality multiple vitamin and mineral supplement daily. Due to the modern refined diet, poor quality soil, our heavy toxic load, internal toxicity, enzyme deficiencies, etc., we're just not getting all the nutrients we need from our food today. Because both vitamins and minerals are essential, you'll want to take a daily multiple covering both. Since the 1980s, numerous studies have documented the health benefits that come from a daily multiple supplement. These include support for your immune system, fewer colds and flus, more emotional balance, a lower risk of serious diseases such as cancer, greater physical energy, and enhanced mental alertness. In general, a daily multiple helps your body run better. To select the multiple that's right for you, discuss your health goals with the supplement advisor at a health food store or pharmacy. Also, see Chapter 10 for recommended amounts of the various vitamins and minerals.

#5. Also include antioxidant-rich phytonutrients as part of your routine. In recent years, scientists have discovered that plant foods contain chemicals that can improve overall health and prevent disease. These substances have been dubbed "*phytonutrients.*" Many of the phytonutrients act as antioxidants—destroyers of harmful, reactive molecules in our bodies. Phytonutrients also block and cart away carcinogens, detoxify toxins, boost the immune system, and retard aging. Over 12,000 phytonutrients have been discovered so far, and many more are expected to be identified. Phytonutrient supplements are an easy way to make sure you're taking in a selection of the most important types. Specific products are listed in the Resources section.

#6. Maintain healthy bowel movements. While constipation is a common experience, many people are not aware that their bowel movements should be more frequent. You want to have at least one comfortable and full bowel movement a day—this usually occurs first thing in the morning. Optimally, a goal would be two or three a day. There are many simple steps you can take to support the healthy functioning of your intestines. These include drinking an adequate amount of water. Also, be sure that you have enough fiber in your diet—one great source is fresh organic vegetables. Using enzyme and probiotic supplements will help keep things moving too. Regular exercise contributes to regularity as well. So does relaxation; our gut is very sensitive to tension and emotional upset. On the flip side, avoid hard-to-digest protein (such as fatty red meat), refined highly processed foods, overeating, consuming meals when emotionally upset or rushed, and snacking late at night. A well-functioning bowel is an important ingredient that will contribute in many ways to a higher state of physical well-being.

#7. Twice a year, consider an herbal cleanse. The suggested times are in the spring and fall. There are many misconceptions about the best ways to do cleanses. People often think that a periodic juice diet is enough. Again, I want to make the point that herbal cleanses should be done only after you've removed some of the toxic influences from your environment and life and replaced them with positive ones. Only then are you ready to clean out the residues that previous toxic exposures have left in your body. In Chapter 11, there's a checklist for the steps to take before you consider doing herbal cleanses. The chapter also presents *a progressive series of herbal cleanses* which target specific areas of the body. This regimen begins with the colon, and then moves on to a liver cleanse, and then a complete system cleanse (including the kidney, lymph, lungs, and skin). See Chapter 11 for more detailed information and the Resources section for product recommendations.

Note that in general I do not recommend unsupervised fasting as it can release toxins too quickly into your system; there is, however, an excellent product described in Chapter 15 called Ultra Clear, which is used as a part of a professionally-supervised liquid detoxification protocol.

#8. **Choose exercise that is enjoyable to you.** Try to exercise at least 30 minutes every day. Physical activity supports detoxification by promoting strong blood circulation and increasing the flow of lymphatic fluid. It also stimulates the release of toxins in sweat. Regular workouts reduce fat reserves and boost your metabolism. Your mental outlook will improve too and you'll feel less stressed. Healthy digestion and elimination are also supported by exercise. There are so many benefits that you can gain from exercise; see Chapter 12 for further details on what physical activity contributes to a healthy life.

Walking is an easy exercise to incorporate into almost any lifestyle. Try to get outside for your walks on most days, and fill in with treadmill strolls in bad weather or late at night (if safety is a concern). Or you might discover that you enjoy another aerobic activity more—biking, rollerblading, swimming, etc. To stay limber, add in some yoga workouts too. (Be sure to start out at your fitness level; don't overdo it.) Rebounding—jumping on a small trampoline—is another fun way to become fit, and its rhythmic motion stimulates the flow of cleansing lymphatic fluid. Whatever your choice, the goal is to *keep moving!*

#9. **Include lots of joyful activities in your life.** Laugh, play, and have fun. Remember that the activities you choose to engage in are another important influence on your physical, mental, and spiritual well-being. Joyful activities are certain to be a more positive influence than life-draining ones. Also, if you're not having fun in life, aren't you missing the point of it all? *Life is meant to be enjoyed.* Note that having a playful attitude will help your relationships as well. Laughing, acting silly, and being playful add energy to relationships. You'll also be having a better time with yourself. So lighten up! Don't be so serious; allow yourself room to learn. No one is keeping a score card. Begin to take on a more playful attitude and enjoy more of all the wonderful things life has to offer. Louis Armstrong was right; it truly is *a wonderful world!*

#10. Take time to rest. We were not designed to be on a constant tread-mill. Nurture yourself with quiet time and get plenty of sleep each night. Sometimes it's necessary to stop and assess how you are running your life. Do you seem to have every moment scheduled? Or do you allow yourself some breathing space? You do a disservice to yourself when you say yes to most requests. Set priorities and establish some boundaries. Don't let the "time bandits" of work, home, and personal demands steal the private time you need for rejuvenation. It can be helpful to actually schedule some decompression time onto your calendar. At the beginning of the day, you might write in some time for: (1) a morning meditation session; (2) a mid-afternoon nap; (3) an evening bubblebath. You won't be the only one who benefits when you take some time out for you. In the long run, you'll have more to offer others because you'll tend to be refreshed and content.

#11. Share more of your feelings as you learn about expressing emotions in healthy ways. What you feel will be expressed somehow; it's wise to choose to do so consciously and positively. A positive approach to dealing with your feelings will be supported by healthy relationships. Make it a point to seek others who work on dealing with their feelings and conflicts in constructive ways. Also, take time to heal the challenged relationships you have with others. People usually do the best they know how to do. Perhaps you can be a positive influence on a friend who could deal better with their emotions. Even if you eventually recognize that the relationship is destructive and you need to move on, you'll know that you attempted to make a difference. Live positively and joyfully with others, not as a victim of your relationships.

#12. Be committed to continued spiritual growth. Studies have shown that people who turn to spiritual practices as a way to process the challenges they face tend to live longer and be healthier. So here are seven steps you can take to grow spiritually. (1) Each day, learn something new about your true self or the world (universe) at large. Being in a state of wonder and discovery is good for the soul! (2) Periodically, list ten things that you are grateful for. Write down at least ten items, but it's also okay if your list is longer! (3) Practice forgiveness and let go of resentments. It will not only help your relationships; forgiveness also supports good health. Conversely, long-held resentments are rough on the body. (4) Live creatively in the present moment. Don't let the magic of the present slip past you because your mind is caught up in worry or regret. Wake up! Take in the sights, sounds, and aliveness of now! (5) Make some time for meditation; it will help you assess your feelings and also relax your mind and body. (6) Examine the beliefs that rule your life. Often these beliefs have control without our conscious awareness. Be a student of truth so you can replace toxic beliefs with ones that serve your highest potential. (7) Reinforce your spiritual growth with affirmations. A great one is: *Everything in my life is an opportunity to bring me closer to who I am, so I can experience more joy, more love, more prosperity, more wisdom, and more inner peace.*

As you work through the program in *The Detox Solution,* be gentle with yourself.

Just as suboptimal health takes time to develop during the degeneration process, rebuilding health in regeneration will not occur overnight. This type of gradual approach may require an attitude adjustment. We are so used to quick fixes in our society. Western medical care and its drugs and surgery are part of the mass "let's have it now!" mentality. It's time to try a new paradigm; working with ourselves and our natural rhythms rather than trying to impose an accelerated schedule from outside of it. The truth is that healing and rejuvenation are not like instant coffee. Like a great tea, allow your new healthy habits time to steep for a while to get the best results.

The information in *The Detox Solution* has been presented with the intention of providing tools to assist you in achieving a richer, fuller life. Overall what you want is to be on a path to optimal well-being rather than one headed toward slow self-destruction. You are in charge of you; make the best choices for yourself! You are important!

Many of the changes that you'll be making go beyond those that most directly affect your physical well-being. You'll find that your life will start to take on a new feeling as you replace old, toxic activities with new healthier ones. You will begin to gain a deeper appreciation for the good things in life as you engage yourself in pastimes that feed your soul. These may include taking a yoga class, playing a musical instrument, volunteering in a tutoring program, painting a landscape with watercolors, walking by the ocean or a lake at sunset regularly, attending inspiring spiritual or religious services, etc. Whatever you choose, be sure to make the choices that feel right to you.

As you continue to make choices that serve you best, you will notice how the outside world will tend to reflect the peace and harmony that you have created within yourself. As Mahatma Gandhi once said, *"Be the change you wish to see."*

RESOURCES

■ Food Safety Issues

Mothers for Natural Law
www.safe-food.org

Pesticide Action Network
www.pan-international.org

Environmental Working Group
1-202-667-6982
www.ewg.org
www.foodnews.org

■ Supplements for Detoxification Support:
Herbs, Vitamins, Minerals, Amino Acids, Leaky Gut Formulas,
Probiotics, etc.

Dispensed by Health Professionals Only

Apex Energetics
1-800-736-4381
www.apexenergetics.com

Energetix
1-800-990-7085
www.goenergetix.com

Lifestar
1-800-858-7477
www.lifestar.com

Metagenics
1-800-692-9400
www.metagenics.com

Natren
1-800-992-3323
www.natren.com

NF Formulas
1-800-547-4891
www.nfformulas.com

PhytoPharmica
1-800-553-2370
www.phytopharmica.com

Pure Body Institute
1-800-952-7873

Thorne Research
1-800-228-1966
www.thorne.com

Tyler Encapsulations
1-800-869-9705
www.tyler-inc.com

Available Commercially

Arise & Shine
1-800-688-2444
www.ariseandshine.com

Gaia Herbs
1-800-831-7780
www.gaiaherbs.com

Herbal Magic
1-800-684-3772
www.herbalmagic.com

HerbPharm
1-800-348-4372
www.herb-pharm.com

Illumination Naturals
310-451-1143
www.illuminationnaturals.com

Megafood
1-800-848-2542
www.megafood.com

Natren
1-800-992-3323
www.natren.com

Nature's Secret
1-888-297-3273
www.naturessecret.com

Renew Life
1-800-830-4778
www.renewlife.com

Sonnes Organic
1-800-544-8147
www.sonnes.com

Source Naturals
1-800-815-2333
www.sourcenaturals.com

■　Enzymes

Illumination Naturals
1-310-451-1143
www.illuminationnaturals.com

Energetix *(health professionals only)*
1-800-990-7085
www.goenergetix.com

Bio-Energy Systems
1-800-929-8328
www.bioenergysystems.com

Rainbow Light
1-800-635-1233
www.vitamins.quinstreet.com

■ Environmentally Safe Pest Management Products

Beneficial Insectory
1-800-477-3715
www.insectory.com

The Green Spot, Ltd.
1-603-942-8925

■ Nontoxic Building Materials

Eco-Home Network
1-323-662-5207
www.ecohome.org

Environmental Building News
1-802-257-7300
www.ebuild.com

Natural Home Magazine
www.naturalhomemagazine.com

■ Spas/Centers for Detoxification

Chopra Center for Well Being
La Jolla, CA
1-888-424-6772
www.chopra.com

Raj Maharishi Ayurveda
Health Center
Fairfield, IA
1-800-248-9050
www.theraj.com

Environmental Health Center
Dallas, TX
William Rea, M.D.
1-214-368-4132
www.ehcd.com

Tree of Life Rejuvenation Center
Gabriel Cousens, M.D.
Patagonia, AZ
1-520-394-2520
www.treeoflife.nu

Hippocrates Health Institute
West Palm Beach, FL
1-561-471-8876
www.hippocratesinst.com

We Care Holistic Health Center
Desert Hot Springs, CA
1-800-888-2523
www.wecarespa.com

Optimum Health Institute
San Diego, CA
1-800-993-4325
www.optimumhealth.org

▪ Spa Directories

www.healingretreats.com   *www.spamagazine.com*
www.spa.com   *www.spas.about.com*
www.spaindex.com

▪ Artists Who Perform Music for Meditation and/or Inspiration

(available in CD or cassette format at most music stores)

Yolanda Adams
Johann Sebastian Bach
Ludwig van Beethoven
Hildegard von Bingen
Helena Buscema
Rickie Byers
Celtic Requiem
Krishna Das
Enya
Kirk Franklin
Robert Gass
Michael Hoppé
Loreena McKennitt
Wolfgang Mozart
R. Carlos Nakai
Aaron Neville
Chris Rice
Secret Garden
Jana Stanfield
Tim Wheater

▪ Toilet Step

Renew Life
1-800-830-4778
www.renewlife.com

▪ Phytonutrient/Chlorophyll Products

Illumination Naturals
1-310-451-1143
www.illuminationnaturals.com

DeSouzas
1-800-373-5171
www.desouzas.com

Organic by Nature
1-800-362-8482
Green Kamut Corp.

Energetix *(health professionals only)*
1-800-990-7085
www.goenergetix.com

■ Lympholine (Trampoline)

Life Source International
www.home.earthlink.net/~lymphforlife
1-888-391-3719

■ Air/Water Filters &Nontoxic Household Items

Advanced Water Systems
1-800-710-7873

www.allergyresources.com
www.cutcat.com

www.gaiam.com
www.gazoontite.com
www.realgoods.com
www.seventhgen.com

■ Saunas

Health Mate Saunas
1-800-946-6001
www.healthmatesauna.com

■ Juicers/Dehydrators

www.discountjuicers.com

■ Chinese Herbs *(for health professionals only)*

Lotus Herbs
1-800-478-4325
www.lotusherbs.com

Health Concerns
1-800-233-9355
www.healthconcerns.com

Far East Summit
1-888-441-0489
www.fareastsummit.com

■ Informational website

www.alternativemedicine.com

RECOMMENDED READING

■ Toxins, the Environment & Your Health

Baker, Sidney MacDonald, M.D. *Detoxification & Healing*. New Canaan, CT: Keats, 1997.

Bennett, Peter, N.D., and Stephen Barrie, N.D., with Sara Faye. *7-Day Detox Miracle*. Rocklin, CA: Prima Publishing, 1999.

Carson, Rachel. *Silent Spring*. New York: Fawcett World Library, 1962.

Colborn, Theo, Dianne Dumanoski, and John Peterson Myers. *Our Stolen Future*. New York: Dutton, 1996.

Dadd, Debra Lynn. *Nontoxic, Natural & Earthwise: How to Protect Yourself and Your Family from Harmful Products and Live in Harmony with the Earth*. Los Angeles: Jeremy P. Tarcher, 1990.

_____. *The Nontoxic Home & Office: Protecting Yourself & Your Family from Everyday Toxics and Health Hazards*. Los Angeles: Jeremy P. Tarcher, 1992.

Dispenza, Joseph. *Live Better Longer: The Parcells Center 7-Step Plan for Health and Longevity*. New York: HarperCollins, 1997.

Fagin, Dan, and Marianne Lavelle. *Toxic Deception: How the Chemical Industry Manipulates Science, Bends the Law and Endangers Your Health*. Monroe, ME: Common Courage Press, 1999.

Fincher, Cynthia E., Ph.D. *Healthy Living in a Toxic World*, Colorado Springs: Pinon Press, 1996.

Golan, Ralph, M.D. *Optimal Wellness*. New York: Ballantine Books, 1990.

Haas, Elson M., M.D. *The Staying Healthy Shopper's Guide*. Berkeley: Celestial Arts Publishing, 1999.

Jensen, Bernard, D.C., and Mark Anderson. *Empty Harvest: Understanding the Link between Our Food, Our Immunity, and Our Planet*. Garden City Park, NY: Avery Publishing Group, 1990.

Pizzorno, Joseph, N.D. *Total Wellness: Improve Your Health by Understanding the Body's Healing Systems*. Rocklin, CA: Prima Publishing, 1996.

Rogers, Sherry A., M.D. *Tired or Toxic?* Syracuse: Prestige Publishing, 1990.

Steinman, David. *Diet for a Poisoned Planet: How to Choose Safe Foods for You and Your Family*. New York: Ballantine Books, 1990.

Steinman, David, and R. Michael Wisner. *Living Healthy in a Toxic World: Simple Steps to Protect You and Your Family from Everyday Chemicals, Poisons, and Pollution*. New York: Perigee, 1996.

■ Enzymes

Cichoke, Anthony J., D.C. *Enzymes & Enzyme Therapy: How to Jump Start Your Way to Lifelong Good Health.* New Canaan, CT: Keats Publishing, 1994.

_____. *The Complete Book of Enzymes*, Avery Publishing Group, Garden City Park, NY, 1999.

Howell, Edward, M.D. *Enzyme Nutrition: The Food Enzyme Concept.* Wayne, NJ: Avery Publishing Group, 1985.

Lee, Lita, Ph.D., and Lisa Turner, with Burton Goldberg. *The Enzyme Cure: How Plant Enzymes Can Help You Relieve 36 Health Problems.* Tiburon, CA: Future Medicine Publishing, 1998.

Loomis, Howard F., D.C., F.I.A.C.A. *Enzymes: The Key to Health*, Vol. 1, The Fundamentals. Madison, WI: 21st Century Nutrition, 1999.

Lopez, D.A., M.D., R. M. Williams, M.D., Ph.D., and M. Miehlke, M.D. *Enzymes: The Fountain of Life. Charleston*, SC: The Neville Press, 1994.

Santillo, Humbart, B.S., M.H. *Food Enzymes: The Missing Link to Radiant Health.* Prescott, AZ: Hohm Press, 1991.

■ Intestinal Health

Berry, Linda. *Internal Cleansing.* Rocklin, CA: Prima Publishing, 1997.

Jensen, Bernard. *Dr. Jensen's Guide to Better Bowel Care: A Complete Program for Tissue Cleansing through Bowel Management.* Garden City Park, NY: Avery Publishing Group, 1999.

Trenev, Natasha. *Probiotics: Nature's Internal Healers.* Garden City Park, NY: Avery Publishing Group, 1998.

Webster, David. *Achieve Maximum Health: Colon Flora, the Missing Link in Immunity, Health & Longevity.* Cardiff, CA: Hygeia Publishing, 1995.

■ Candida & Parasites

Crook, William, M.D. *The Yeast Connection Handbook.* Jackson, TN: Professional Books, 1999.

Gates, Donna. *The Body Ecology Diet.* Atlanta: B.E.D. Publications, 1993.

Gittleman, Ann Louise. *Guess What Came to Dinner: Parasites and Your Health.* Garden City Park, NY: Avery Publishing Group, 1993.

■ Liver Health

Cabot, Sandra Cabot, M.D. *The Liver Cleansing Diet.* Scottsdale, AZ: S.C.B. International, 1997.

Hobbs, Christopher, L.Ac. *Natural Liver Therapy.* Capitola, CA: Botanica Press, 1986.

■ Nutrition

Atkins, Robert C. *Dr. Atkins' New Diet Revolution*. New York: Avon, 1999.

Batmanghelidj, F., M.D. *Your Body's Many Cries For Water*. Falls Church, VA: Global Health Solutions, Inc., 1997.

Blonz, Edward R. Ph.D. *The Really Simple No Nonsense Nutrition Guide*. Berkeley, CA: Conari Press, 1993.

Cousens, Gabriel, M.D. *Conscious Eating*. Berkeley, CA: North Atlantic Books, 2000.

Erasmus, Udo. *Fats that Heal, Fats that Kill*. Burnaby, Canada: Alive Books, 1993.

Gittleman, Ann Louise, M.S. *Your Body Knows Best: The Revolutionary Eating Plan that Helps You Achieve Your Optimal Weight and Energy Level*. New York: Pocket Books, 1997.

Ross, Julia, M.A. *The Diet Cure*. New York: Penguin Group, 1999.

Sears, Barry, Ph.D. *Enter The Zone*. New York: HarperCollins, 1995.

■ Cookbooks

Brotman, Juliano, *Raw: The Uncook Book*. New York: Regan, 1999.

Calbom, Cherie, and Maureen B. Keane. *Juicing for Life*. Avery Publishing Group, 1992.

Clement, Brian. *Living Foods for Optimal Health*. Rocklin, CA: Prima Publishing, 1998.

Colbin, Annemarie. *The Natural Gourmet: Delicious Recipes for Healthy, Balanced Eating*. Ballantine, 1991.

Fallon, Sally. *Nourishing Traditions*. San Diego: ProMotion Publishing, 1995.

Pitchford, Paul. *Healing With Whole Foods*. Berkeley, CA: North Atlantic Books, 1996.

Sahelian, Ray, and Donna Gates. *The Stevia Cookbook: Cooking with Nature's Calorie-Free Sweetener*. Avery Publishing Group, 1999.

Shannon, Nomi, and Brian Clement. *Raw Gourmet*. Burnaby, Canada: Alive Books, 1998.

Wolfe, David. *The Sunfood Diet Success System*. San Diego, CA: Maul Brothers, 2000.

■ Phytonutrients

Schecter, Steven R., N.D. *Fighting Radiation & Chemical Pollutants with Foods, Herbs & Vitamins*. Encinitas, CA: Vitality Ink, 1990.

Seibold, Ronald L., M.S. *Cereal Grass: What's In It For You!* Lawrence, KS: Wilderness Community Education Foundation, 1990.

■ Herbal Medicine

Buhner, Stephen Harrod. *Herbal Antibiotics: Natural Alternatives for Treating Drug-Resistant Bacteria*. Pownal, VT: Storey Books,1999.

Duke, James A. *The Green Pharmacy*. New York: St. Martin's Press, 1998.

Vukovic, Laurel. *14-Day Herbal Cleansing*. Paramus, NJ: Prentice Hall, 1998.

■ Detoxification Plans

Bland, Jeffrey, Ph.D., with Sara Benum, M.A. *The 20-Day Rejuvenation Diet Program*. New Canaan, CT: Keats Publishing, 1997.

Chaitow, Leon, M.D. *The Body/Mind Purification Program*. London: Gaia Books, 1990.

Haas, Elson M., M.D. *Staying Healthy With The Seasons*. Berkeley, CA: Celestial Arts, 1981.

Haas, *The Detox Diet*. Berkeley, CA: Celestial Arts, 1996.

Silver, Helene. *The Body-Smart System: The Complete Guide to Cleansing and Rejuvenation*. Sonora, CA: Healthy Healing Press, 1994.

■ Detoxification and Children's Health

Crook, William, M.D. *Help for the Hyperactive Child: A Practical Guide Offering Parents of ADHD Children Alternatives to Ritalin*. Jackson, TN: Professional Books, 1991.

Rapp, Doris, M.D. *Is This Your Child's World? How You Can Fix the Schools and Homes That Are Making Your Children Sick*. New York: Bantam, 1996.

■ Emotional/Spiritual Health

Bach, Edward, M.D. and Wheeler, F.J., M.D. *The Bach Flower Remedies*. New Canaan, CT: Keats, 1979.

Benson, Herbert, M.D. *The Relaxation Response*. New York: Avon, 1976.

Breathnach, Sarah Ban. *Simple Abundance: A Daybook of Comfort & Joy*. New York: Warner Books, 1995.

Childre, Doc and Howard Martin. *The Heartmath Solution*. New York: HarperCollins, 1999.

Chopra, Deepak, M.D. *The Seven Spiritual Laws of Success: A Practical Guide to the Fulfillment of Your Dreams*. San Rafael, CA: Amber-Allen Publishing, 1995

Dalai Lama, et al. *The Art of Happiness: A Handbook for Living*. New York: Riverhead Books, 1998.

Davich, Victor N. *The Best Guide to Meditation*. Los Angeles: Renaissance

Books, 1998.

Dyer, Wayne. *You'll See It When You Believe It*. New York: Avon, 1990.

Gass, Robert. *Chanting: Discovering Spirit in Sound*. New York: Broadway Books, 1999.

Gawain, Shakti, *Living in the Light*. Novato, CA: New World Library, 1998.

Goldsmith, Joel. *Practicing the Presence: The Inspirational Guide to Regaining Meaning and Sense of Purpose in Your Life*. San Francisco: Harper, 1991.

Hay, Louise. *Heal Your Body*. Carlsbad, CA: Hay House, 1988.

Holmes Ernest, and Willis Kinnear. *Thoughts Are Things*. Deerfield Beach, FL: Health Communications, 1999.

Goleman, Daniel P. *Emotional Intelligence*. New York: Bantam, 1997.

LeShan, Lawrence. *How to Meditate*. New York: Bantam, 1974.

Millman, Dan. *The Way of the Peaceful Warrior*. Tiburon, CA: H.J. Kramer, 2000.

Morris-Spieker, Michelle. *The Cherished Self: How to Give Back to Yourself When You're Living A Life That Takes All You've Got*. San Juan Capistrano, CA, 2000.

Mother Theresa. *Mother Theresa: In My Own Words*. Liguori, MO: Liguori Publications, 1997.

Murray, Michael T., N.D. *Stress, Anxiety & Insomnia*. Rocklin, CA: Prima Publishing, 1995.

Myss, Caroline, Ph.D. *Anatomy of the Spirit: The Seven Stages of Power and Healing*. New York: Random House, 1997.

Norman, Mildred. *Peace Pilgrim: Her Life and Work in Her Own Words*. Santa Fe, NM: Ocean Tree Books, 1998.

Pearsall, Paul, Ph.D. *The Heart's Code: The Findings About Cellular Memories and Their Role in the Mind/Body/Spirit Connection*. New York: Broadway Books, 1998.

Pert, Candace, Ph.D. *Molecules of Emotion: Why You Feel The Way You Feel*. New York: Scribner, 1997.

Rolek, Michiko J. *Mental Fitness: Complete Workouts for Body, Mind, and Soul*. New York: Weatherhill, 1990.

Roth, Ron, Ph.D. *The Healing Path of Prayer*. New York: Three Rivers Press, 1999.

Ruiz, Don Miguel. *The Four Agreements: A Practical Guide to Personal Freedom*. San Rafael, CA: Amber-Allen Publishing, 1997.

_____. *The Mastery of Love*. San Rafael, CA: Amber-Allen Publishing, 1999.

Shinn, Florence Scovel. *The Writings of Florence Scovel Shinn*. Marina del Rey, CA: Devorss, 1988.

Thich Nhat Hanh. *Peace Is Every Step*. New York: Bantam, 1992.

Williamson, Marianne. *A Return to Love: Reflections on the Principles of a Course in Miracles*. New York: HarperCollins, 1996.

Yogananda, Paramahansa. *Autobiography of a Yogi*. Los Angeles: Self-Realization Fellowship, 1979.

▪ Dental Health

Briener, Mark A., D.D.S. *Whole Body Dentistry*. Fairfield, CT: Quantum Health Press, 1999.

Huggins, Hal, D.D.S. *It's All In Your Head: The Link Between Mercury Amalgams and Illness*. Garden City Park, NY: Avery Publishing Group, 1993.

Walker, Morton, D.P.M. *Elements of Danger: Protect Yourself Against the Hazards of Modern Dentistry*. Charlottesville, VA: Hampton Roads, 1999.

▪ Alternative Medicine

Bienfield, Harriet, L.Ac. *Between Heaven and Earth*. New York: Ballantine, 1992.

Gerber, Richard, M.D. *Vibrational Medicine*. Santa Fe, NM: Bear & Co., 1988.

Goldberg, Burton. *Alternative Medicine: The Definitive Guide*. Puyallup, WA: Future Medicine Publishing, 1994.

▪ Longevity

Chopra, Deepak, M.D. *Ageless Body, Timeless Mind: The Quantum Alternative to Growing Old*. New York: Three Rivers Press, 1998.

Mahoney, David, and Richard Restak. *The Longevity Strategy: How to Live to 100 Using the Brain-Body Connection*. New York: John Wiley & Sons, 1999.

Perls, Thomas T., M.D., M.P.H., Margery Hutter Silver, Ed.D., and John F. Lauerman. *Living to 100: Lessons in Living to Your Maximum Potential at Any Age*. Basic Books, 2000.

Walford, Roy L. M.D., *The 120 Year Diet*. Simon & Schuster, 1986.

REFERENCES

Chapter One

1. Irons, V. Earl. *The Destruction of Your Own Natural Protective Mechanism.* Cottonwood, CA: 1990.
2. Marshall, Robert J., Ph.D. "No Healing Without Quality Food," *Well Being Journal*, May/June 1999.
3. " Study: Fewer Antibiotics Prescribed," *Intelihealth Newsletter*, September 8, 2000.
4. Ibid.

Chapter Two

1. Liska, DeAnn J., Ph.D. "The Detoxification Enzyme Systems," *Alternative Medicine Review.* Vol. 3, no. 3, 1998.
2. Diamond, W. John, M.D., W. Lee Cowden, M.D., and Burton Goldberg. *An Alternative Medicine Definitive Guide to Cancer,* p. 559. Tiburon, CA: Future Medicine Publishing, 1997.

Chapter Three

1. *www.pesticidewatch.org*
2. Dispenza, Joseph. *Live Better Longer: The Parcells Center 7-Step Plan for Health and Longevity,* p. 49. New York: Harper Collins, 1997.
3. Sobel, HL, et al. "Lead Exposure from Candles," *Journal of the American Medical Association.* Vol. 284, no. 2, p. 180, 2000.
4. Anderson, R, et al. "Acute Respiratory Effects of Diaper Emissions," *Archives of Environmental Health.* Vol 54, no. 5, pp. 353-358, 1999.
5. Murray, MT and JE Pizzorno. *Encyclopedia of Natural Medicine.* Rocklin, CA: Prima Publishing, 1991.
6. Gittleman, Ann Louise. *How to Stay Young and Healthy in a Toxic World,* p. 67. Los Angeles: Keats Publishing, 1999.
7. Steinman, David, and R. Michael Wisner. *Living Healthy in a Toxic World: Simple Steps to Protect You and Your Family from Everyday Chemicals, Poisons, and Pollution,* p. 25. New York: Perigee, 1996.
8. Ibid.
9. Lowengart, RA, et al. "Childhood Leukemia and Parent's Occupational and Home Exposures," *Journal of the National Cancer Institute.* Vol. 79, pp. 39-46, 1987.
10. *Biodiversity and Your Food.* Center for Biodiversity and Conservation, American Museum of Natural History, 1998.

11. Colborn, Theo, Dianne Dumanoski, and John Peterson Myers. *Our Stolen Future*. New York: Dutton, 1996.
12. Steinman, David, and Samuel S. Epstein. *Safe Shopper's Bible*, p 376. New York: Hungry Minds, 1995.
13. Walker, Morton. "Chemical Pollution of the Body: All Children Are Endangered by Pesticides," *Townsend Letter for Doctors and Patients*, June 1997.
14. Smith, Bob L. "Organic Foods vs. Supermarket Foods: Element Levels," *Journal of Applied Nutrition*. Vol 45, no. 1, pp. 35-39, 1993.
15. Marwick, Charles. "Genetically Modified Crops Feed Major Controversy," *Journal of the American Medical Association*. Vol 283, pp. 188-190, 2000.
16. Gittleman, Ann Louise, M.S. *Your Body Knows Best*, p.51-52. New York: Pocket Books, 1997.
17. Roberts, HJ. "Aspartame (Nutrasweet®) Addiction," *Townsend Letter for Doctors and Patients*, January 2000.
18. Haas, Elson M. *The Detox Diet*, p. 66. Berkeley, CA: Celestial Arts, 1996.
19. Quan R, et al. "Effects of Microwave Radiation on Anti-Infective Factors in Human Milk," *Pediatrics*. Vol. 89, pp. 667-9, April 1992.
20. "Scientists Link Grilled Meat To Breast Cancer," *Intellihealth Newsletter*, April 6, 2000.
21. Goldberg, Burton. *Alternative Medicine: The Definitive Guide*, p. 816. Puyallup, WA: Future Medicine Publishing, 1994.

Chapter Four

1. Liska, op. cit.
2. Immerman, Alan. "Evidence for Intestinal Toxemia: An Inescapable Clinical Phenomenon," *ACA Journal of Chiropractic*. Vol. 13, pp. 25-36, April 1979.
3. Hoffman, Ronald, M.D. *Seven Weeks to a Settled Stomach*, p. 136. New York: Pocket Books, 1991.
4. Kouchakoff, Paul. "The Influence of Cooking Food on the Blood Formula of Man," *Proceedings: First International Congress of Microbiology*, Paris, 1930.
5. Howell, Edward, M.D. *Enzyme Nutrition: The Food Enzyme Concept*, p. 82. Wayne, NJ: Avery Publishing Group, 1985.
6. Santillo, Humbart. *Food Enzymes: The Missing Link to Radiant Health*, p 14. Prescott, AZ: Hohm Press, 1991.

7. Hurd, Lyle. "An Interview with Dr. Karl Ransberger, The Founder of Enzyme Therapy," *Total Health*. Vol. 19, no. 4. p. 34.
8. Kulvinskas, Victor. *Don't Dine Without Enzymes*, p. 19. Hot Springs, AR: L.O.V.E. Foods Inc. 1994.
9. Ibid., p. 6.
10. Ibid.
11. Cichoke, Anthony J., D.C. *Enzymes & Enzyme Therapy: How to Jump Start your Way to Lifelong Good Health*, p. 134-148. New Canaan, CT: Keats Publishing, 1994.
12. Kulvinskas, p. 20.
13. Lopez, D.A., M.D., R. M. Williams, M.D., Ph.D., and M. Miehlke, M.D. *Enzymes: The Fountain of Life*, p. 246. Charleston, SC: The Neville Press, 1994.
14. Cichoke, op. cit., p. 174.
15. "Plant Enzyme Protease Effective in Reversing Chronic Arterial Obstruction," *Plant Enzyme Therapy: Physicians' Research & Information Series*, April 1991.
16. Lopez, op. cit., p. 14.
17. C. Neuhofer, "Enzymtherapie bei Multipler Sklerose," *Hufeland Journal Biologisch-medizinisches Zentralorgan*, 1986.
18. Pecher, Otto. *Oral Enzymes: Basic Information and Clinical Studies*. Geretsried, Germany: Mucos Pharma, 1992.
19. Howell, op. cit., p. 114.

Chapter Five

1. Hahnemann, Samuel, M.D. *Organon of Medicine, 5th Edition*. New Delhi: B. Jain Publishers, 1993.
2. Percival, Mark. "Nutritional Support for Detoxification," *Clinical Nutrition Insights*. Foundation for the Advancement of Nutritional Education, 1997.
3. " Study: Northeast Power Plants Linked to Sickness, Death," *Intellihealth Newsletter*, May 5, 2000.
4. Percival, op. cit.
5. "Agent Orange Effects Still Being Felt After 25 Years," *Intellihealth Newsletter*, April 24, 2000.
6. "Panel Examines Possible Agent Orange Tie To Diabetes," *Intellihealth Newsletter*, June 12, 2000.
7. Pizzorno, Joseph, N.D. *Total Wellness*, p. 156. Rocklin, CA: Prima Publishing, 1996.

8. Bland, Jeffrey, Ph.D. "A Functional Approach to Mental Illness – A New Paradigm for Managing Brain Biochemical Disturbances," *Journal of Orthomolecular Medicine*. p. 1336, December 1994.

9. Bennett, Peter, N.D., and Stephen Barrie, N.D., with Sara Faye. *7-Day Detox Miracle*, pp. 33, 132, 155. Rocklin, CA: Prima Publishing, 1999.

10. Fincher, Cynthia E., Ph.D. *Healthy Living in a Toxic World*, pp. 40-42. Colorado Springs: Pinon Press, 1996.

11. Stephenson, Joan, Ph.D. "Exposure to Home Pesticides Linked to Parkinson Disease," *Journal of the American Medical Association*. Vol. 283, No. 23, p. 3055, 2000.

12. "Study Cites Chernobyl Health Effects in Poland," *Intellihealth Newsletter*, April 24, 2000.

13. Crinnion, Walter. "Environmental Medicine, Part 1: The Human Burden of Environmental Toxins and Their Common Health Effects," *Alternative Medicine Review*. Vol. 5, no. 1, p. 60.

Chapter Six

1. *Merck Manual, 17th Edition*. West Point, PA: Merck & Co., 1999.

2. Petrakis, NL, King EB. "Cytological Abnormalities in Nipple Aspirates of Breast Fluid of Women With Severe Constipation," *Lancet* 2(8257): 1203-4, 1981.

3. Micozzi MS "Bowel Function and Breast Cancer in US Women," *American Journal of Public Health*, 79(1):73-5, Jan. 1989.

4. Duncan, Lindsey, "Creating A Healthy Colon," *Nutrition Science News*, July 1995.

5. "Natural Prescription," *Natural Medicine Journal*. Vol. 1, no. 10, Dec. 1998.

6. Immerman, op. cit.

7. *Functional Assessment Resource Manual*, p. G7. Asheville, NC: Great Smokies Diagnostic Laboratory, 1999.

Chapter Seven

1. Crimmon, Walter J. "Environmental Medicine, Part 1: The Human Burden of Environmental Toxins and Their Common Health Effects," *Alternative Medicine Review*. Vol. 5, no. 1, pp 52-63, 2000.

2. Ibid.

3. Ibid.

Chapter Eight

1. Shields, JW. "Lymph, Lymph Glands, and Homeostasis," *Lymphology* 25(4); 147-53, Dec. 1992.

2. "Cigarette Smoking Linked to Colorectal Cancer in Major Study," *Intellihealth Newsletter,* December 6, 2000.

Chapter Nine

1. Diamond, op. cit., p. 568.
2. Blonz, Edward R. Ph.D. *The Really Simple No Nonsense Nutrition Guide,* p. 157. Berkeley, CA: Conari Press, 1993.
3. Diamond, op. cit. p. 573.
4. Smith, op. cit.
5. *Family Practice News,* October 15, 1998.
6. Gordon, Sandra. "Could You Drink 597 Cans of Soda?" *Self,* p. 93, Nov. 2000.
7. Fallon, Sally. *Nourishing Traditions,* p. 48. San Diego: ProMotion Publishing, 1995.
8. Whitaker, Julian, M.D. *Health & Healing.* Vol. 9, no. 10, Oct. 1999.
9. "Healthy Beverage Alternatives to Dairy," *Alternative Medicine Digest,* Issue 25, p. 81.
10. Sanchez, Albert, et al. "Role of sugars in human neutrophilic phago-cytosis," *The American Journal of Clinical Nutrition.* Vol 26, no. 11, pp. 1180-1184.
11. Fallon, op. cit., p. 45.

Chapter Ten

1. E. Seifter et al. "Morbidity and Mortality Reduction by Supplemental Vitamin A or Beta-Carotene in Mice Given Total-Body Gamma-Radiation," *Journal of the National Cancer Institute.* Vol. 73, no. 5, 1984, pp. 1167-1177.
2. Null, Gary, Ph.D. *Gary Null's Ultimate Anti-Aging Program,* p. 198. New York: Kensington Books, 1999.
3. Simon, Joel A., M.D., M.P.H. and Esther S. Hudes, Ph.D., M.P.H. "Relationship of Ascorbic Acid to Blood Lead Levels," *Journal of the American Medical Association.* Vol. 281, no. 24, 1999.
4. AI Hecht, K. Mohrmann. "Vitamin E and Low-Dose Irradiation," *The ACA Journal of Chiropractic.* Vol. 14, S89-91, August 1980.
5. Cowen, R. "Soybean Lecithin May Prevent Cirrhosis," *Sci News* 138 (1990): 340.
6. A. Morezek and W. Schmidt, "Effect on the Radiation Syndrome of the Combined Administration of Vitamin B12 and Folic Acid in Whole-Body Radiation in Rats," *Folia Haematol,* no. 90, pp. 401-410.
7. S. Fox, *Journal of Food Science,* vol. 39, no. 2 1974, pp. 321-324.

8. J. Cline, "Effect of Nutrient Potassium on the Uptake of Cesium-13 and Potassium and on Discrimination Factor," *Nature*, 1962, 193: 1302-1303.

9. Reding P, et al. "Oral Zinc Supplementation Improves Hepatic Encephalopathy: Results of a Randomized Control Trial." *Lancet* 1984 Sep;2(8401):493-5.

10. Heerdt, AS, Young WJ, and Borgen, PI. "Calcium Glucarate as a Chemopreventive Agent in Breast Cancer." *Israel Journal of Medical Science*, 1:101-105, 1995.

11. Chen I, et al. "Aryl Hydrocarbon Receptor-Mediated Anti-Estrogenic and Antitumorigenic Activity of Diindolylmethane." *Carcinogenesis* 1998;19(9):1631-9.

12. Michnovicz JJ, Bradlow HL. "Altered Estrogen Metabolism and Excretion in Humans Following Consumption of Indole Carbinol." *Nutr Cancer* 1991;16:59-66.

13. Stoner, GD, Morse MA. "Isothiocynates and Plant Polyphenols as Inhibitors of Lung and Esophageal Cancer." *Cancer Lett* 1997 Mar 19; 114(1-2):113-9.

14. Meister R, et al. "Efficacy and Tolerability of Myrtol Standardized in Long-Term Treatment of Chronic Bronchitis." A double-blind, placebo-controlled study. Study Group Investigators. *Arzneimittelforschung* 1999;49(4):351-8.

15. Gould, Michael N. "Cancer Chemoprevention and Therapy by Monoterpenes," Department of Human Oncology, Madison, Wisconsin. *Environmental Health Perspectives* 105 (Supp 4) 977-979 (1997).

16. Miettin TA et al. "Serum Plant Sterols and Cholesterol Precursors Reflect Cholesterol Absorption and Synthesis in Volunteers of a Randomly Selected Male Population." *Am J Epidemio* 1990 Jan;131(1):20-31.

17. Tabak M, Armon R, Potasman I, Neeman I. "In Vitro Inhibition of *Helicobacter pylori* by Extracts of Thyme." *Journal of Applied Bacteriology* 1996; 80(6):667-72.

18. Offord EA, Mace K, et al. "Mechanisms Involved in the Chemoprotective Effects of Rosemary Extract Studied in Human Liver and Bronchial Cells." *Cancer Lett* 1997;114:275-281.

19. Masterova I, Misikova E, et al. "Royleanones in the Roots of *Salvia officinalis* of Domestic Provenance and Their Antimicrobial Activity." *Ceska Slov Farm* 1996 Sep; 45(5);242-5.

Chapter Eleven

1. Fernandex-Banares F, et al. "Randomized Clinical Trial of *Plantago Ovata* Seeds (Dietary Fiber) as Compared With Mesalamine in Maintaining Remission in Ulcerative Colitis." Spanish Group for the Study of Crohn's Disease and Ulcerative Colitis (GETECCU). *Am J Gastroenterol* 1999;94:427-433.

2. Gonzalez M., Rivas, C, et al. "Effects of Orange and Apple Pectin on Cholesterol Concentration in Serum, Liver and Feces." *J Physiol Biochem* (54) 2: 99-104 1998 Jun.

3. Tazawa K, Okami H, et al. "Anticarcinogenic Action of Apple Pectin on Fecal Enzyme Activities and Mucosal or Portal Prostaglandin E2 Levels in Experimental Rat Colon Carcinogenesis." *J Exp Clin Cancer Res.*, Vol 16, ESS 1, 1997, P33-8.

4. Todd, PA, Benfield P, Goa KL. "Guar Gum, a Review of its Pharmacological Properties, and Use as a Dietary Adjunct in Hypercholesterolemia." *Drugs*, 39(6); 917-28 1990 Jun.

5. Blackburn NA, Redfern JS, et al. "The Mechanism of Guar Gum in Improving Glucose Tolerance in Man." *Clin Sci* 66(3); 329-36 1984 Mar.

6. Weaver GA, Tangel C. "Dietary Guar Gum Alters Colonic Microbial Fermentation in Azoxymethane-treated Rats." *J Nutr.* 126(8),1979-91, 1996 Aug.

7. Fyfe L, Armstrong F, Stewart J. "Inhibition of *listeria monocytogenes* and *salmonella enteriditis* by Combinations of Plant Oils and Derivatives of Benzoic Acid: The Development of Synergistic Antimicrobial Combinations." *Int J Antimicrob Agents* 1997 Jan;9(3): 195-9.

8. Albert-Puleo M. "Fennel and Anise as Estrogenic Agents." *J Ethnopharmacol* 1980 Dec;2(4):337-44.

9. Tinker LF Schneeman BO, et al. "Consumption of Prunes as a Source of Dietary Fiber in Men with Mild Hypercholesterolemia." *Am J Clin Nutr* 53(5); 1259-65 1991 May.

10. Stangroom KE, Smith TK. "Effect of Whole and Fractionated Dietary Alfalfa on Zearalenone Toxicosis and Metabolism in Rats and Swine." *Can J Physiol Pharmacol*, 62(9); 1219-24 1984 Sep.

11. Khorana, M.L., Rajarama Rao, M.R. and Siddiqui, H.H., *Indian Journal of Pharmacy*, 21 (1959), 331.

12. K. Tokura and S. Kagawa, "Anti-Cancer Agents Containing Chebulanin from *Terminalia Chebula*." *Jpn Kokai Tokkyo Koho* JP 07, 138, 165, Sept. 24th, 1995.

13. R. Gulati, S. Agarwal and S.S. Agarwal, "Hepatoprotective Studies on *Phyllanthus Emblica* and Quercetin." *Indian J. Exp. Biol* 33 (4) 261-268, 1995.

14. Abdel-Wahhab, M.A., et al. "Effect of Aluminosilicates and Bentonite on Aflatoxin-Induced Developmental Toxicity in Rat." *J Appl Toxicol* 1999 May-Jun; 19(3) 199-204.

15. Buckley NA, et al. "Activated Charcoal Reduces the Need for N-Acetylcysteine Treatment After Acetaminophen (Paracetamol) Overdose." *J Toxicol Clin Toxicol* 1999;37(6):753-7

16. Masterova I, Misikova E, et al. "Royleanones in the Roots of *Salvia officinalis* of Domestic Provenance and Their Antimicrobial Activity." *Ceska Slov Farm* 1996 Sep; 45(5);242-5

17. Sturdik E, et al. "Mechanism of Antiyeast Activity of Juglone – A Naturally Occurring 1,4-Naphthoquinone." *Biologica (Bratislava),* 38(4): 343-61, 1983.

18. Clark AM, Jurgens TM, Hufford DC. "Antimicrobial Activity of Juglone." *Phytother. Res.,* 4(1):11-13, 1990.

19. Lahiri-Chatterjee M, Katiyar SK, et al. "A Flavonoid Antioxidant, Silymarin, Affords Exceptionally High Protection Against Tumor Promotion in the SENCAR Mouse Skin Tumorigenesis Model." *Cancer Res* 1999 Feb 1;59(3):622-32.

20. "Mechanisms of Anticarcinogenic Properties of Curcumin: the Effect of Curcumin on Glutathione Linked Detoxification Enzymes in Rat Liver." *Int J Biochem Cell Biol* 1998 Apr; 30(4):445-56.

21. Brown Je, Rice-Evans CA. "Luteolin-Rich Artichoke Extract Protects Low Density Lipoprotein From Oxidation *in vitro*." *Free Radic Res* 1998 Sep; 29(3): 247-55.

22. Ko, K.M., et al. "Effect of a Lignan-Enriched *Fructus Schisandra* Extract on Hepatic Glutathione Status in Rats: Protection Against Carbon Tetrachloride Toxicity." *Planta Medica* 1995, 61(2): 134-137.

23. Singletary KW, Rokusek JT. "Tissue-Specific Enhancement of Xenobiotic Detoxification Enzymes in Mice by Dietary Rosemary Extract." *Plant Foods Hum Nutr* 1997; 50(1):47-53.

24. Matsumoto T, Yamada H. "Regulation of Immune Complex Binding of Macrophages by Pectic Polysaccharide from *Bupleurum*." *J Pharm Pharmacol* 1995 Feb; 47(2): 152-6.

25. Lanhers MC, et al. "Hepatoprotective and Anti-inflammatory Effects of a Traditional Medicinal Plant of Chile, *Peumus boldus*." *Planta Med* 57(2): 110-115 1991.

26. Kringstein P, Cedarbaum A1. "Boldine Prevents Human Liver Microsomal Lipid Peroxidation and Inactivation of Cytochrome P4502E1." *Free Radic Biol Med* 1995 Mar;18(3):559-63.

27. Saxena AK, Singh B, Anand KK. "Hepatoprotective Effects of *Eclipta Alba* on Subcellular Levels in Rats." *J Ethnopharmacol* 1993 Dec; 40(3): 155-61.

28. Balzarini J, Neyts J., et al. "The Mannose-specific Plant Lectins from *Cymbidium Hydrid* and *Epipactis Helleborine* and the Plant Lectin from *Urtica Dioica* are Potent and Selective Inhibitors of Human Immunodeficiency Virus and Cytomegalovirus Replication *in vitro.*" *Antiviral Res* 1992 Jun; 18(2): 191-207.

29. Ozaki Y. "Antiinflammatory Effect of Tetramethylpyrazine and Ferulic Acid." *Chem Pharm Bull (Tokyo)* 1992 Apr; 40(4):954-6.

30. Morita K, Kada T, Namiki M. "A Desmutagenic Factor Isolated from Burdock." *Mutat Res* 1984 Oct;129(1):25-31.

31. Duke, James A., Ph.D. *The Green Pharmacy,* p. 545. New York: St. Martin's, 1997.

32. Klayman DL. "Qinghaosu (Artemesinin), An Antimalarial Drug from China." *Science* 228:1049-1055, 1985.

33. Duke, op. cit. p. 553.

34. Guiraud P, Steiman R, Campos-Takaki GM, et al. "Comparison of Antibacterial and Antifungal Activities of Lapachol and Beta-Lapachone." *Planta Med* 1994; 60:373-74.

35. Tomada M, Hirabayashi K, et al. "Characterization of Two Novel Polysaccharides Having Immunological Activities from the Root of *Panax ginseng.*" *Biol Pharm Bull* 1993; 16:1087-90.

36. Lee, BH, et al. "*In vitro* Antigenotoxic Activity of Novel Ginseng Saponin Metabolities Formed by Intestinal Bacteria." *Planta Medica* 1998, 64(6):500-503.

37. Chu DT, Wong WL, Mavligit GM. "Reversal of Cyclophosphamide-induced Immune Suppression by Administration of Fractionated *Astragalus membranaceus* in vivo." *J Clin Lab Immunol* 25(3): 125-9 1988 Mar.

38. Rui T, Yang Y. "Effect of *Astragalus membraneceus* on Electrophysiological Activities of Acute Experimental Coxsackie B-3 Myocarditis in Mice." *Chin Med Sci J*, 8(4): 203-6 1993 Dec.

39. Zhang YD, Shen JP, et al. "Effects of *Astragalus* on Experimental Liver Injury." *Yao Hsueh Hsueh Pao* 27(6); 401-6 1992.

40. Chen J. "An Experimental Study on the Anti-senility Effects of *shou xing bu zhi.*" *Chung His Chieh Ho Tsa Chih;* 9(4); 226-7, 198 1989 Apr.

41. Yuan Y, Hou S, et al. "Studies of *Rehmannia Glutinosa* as a Blood Tonic." *Chung Kuo Chung Yao Tsa Chih* 1992 Jun; 17(6):366-8.
42. Miura T, Kako M, et al. "Antidiabetic Effect of Seishin-kanro-to in KK-Ay Mice." *Planta Med* 1997 Auig;63(4):320-2.
43. Ziauddin M, Phansalker N. "Studies on the Immunomodulatory Effects of *Ashwagandha*." *J Ethnopharmaco;l* 50(2) 69-76 1996 Feb.
44. Praveenkuman V, Kuttan R, Kuttan G. "Chemoprotective Action of *Rasayanas* against Cyclosphamide Toxicity." *Tumori,* Vol 80, ISS 4, 1994 P306-8.

Chapter Twelve

1. "Effects of Acute Physical Exercise on Aryl Hydrocarbon Hydroxylas Activity in Human Peripheral Lymphocytes," *Life Sci* 1990; 47: 427-32.
2. "Exercise May Help Fight Depression," *Intellihealth Newsletter,* September 25, 2000.
3. Anderson, John. "Rebounders: Bounce Your Way to Better Health.," *www.alternativemedicine.com.*
4. Gard, Zane R. "Literature Review and Comparison Studies of Sauna/Hyperthermia in Detoxification," *Townsend Letter for Doctors and Patients,* Aug/Sept 1999, p 76-86.
5. "Oxygen, Life & Health," *Bio/Tech News,* p. 1. Portland, OR: Bio/Tech Publishing, 1999.

Chapter Thirteen

1. Allen, Jane E. "The Down Side of Happy Pills," *Los Angeles Times,* April 10, 2000, p. S2.
2. *Functional Assessment Resource Manual,* p. E16-21. Asheville, NC: Great Smokies Diagnostic Laboratory, 1999.

Chapter Fourteen

1. "Divine Intervention: The Religiously Active Live Longer," *Intellihealth Newsletter,* June 5, 2000.
2. "Study: Optimists Live Longer," *Intellihealth Newsletter,* February 9, 2000.

INDEX

ORDER INFORMATION

Fax orders: (310) 451-4044. Please use this form.

Telephone orders: Call (310) 451-1143.
Have your credit card ready.

E-mail your request to: illuminationprs@aol.com

Postal orders: Illumination Press, P.O. Box 269
Santa Monica, CA 90406

Please send ____ copies of *The Detox Solution* @ $19.95 each, plus shipping and handling.

Please send more FREE information on:

❑ Products ❑ Seminars/Workshops

Name: _____

Address: _____

City: _____ State: _____ Zip: _____

Telephone: _____

E-mail address: _____

Sales tax: Please add 8% for books shipped to California addresses.

Shipping:
US: $4 for the first book and $2 for each additional book.
International: $9 for 1st book: $5 for each additional book (estimate).

Payment: ❑ Check   Credit card: ❑ Visa ❑ Master Card

Card number: _____

Name on Card: _____ Exp. Date ___ /____

Signature: _____